TESTIMONIALS

"This has to be the most exciting prostate book ever written! Dr. Wheeler simplifies a very difficult topic for all to understand."
Charles A. Rogers, M.D. Psychiatrist

"A must read for anyone concerned about the diagnosis and/or treatment of prostate cancer"
David Strong, M.D. (Eminent Urologist and Esteemed Member of the AUA)

"Dr. Wheeler is a visionary! An exciting look at a dreaded disease! The Culture representing the diagnosis and treatment of prostate cancer is about to change! Two Thumbs Up!"
Joseph Cullen, M.D. Neurologist and patient

"This book will help millions of men and all my fans! Every man needs to read this book!"
Randy Owen, Lead singer for the Country Music Group – Alabama and patient

"From a fighter pilot over Vietnam, to a commercial airline pilot around the world, I have always valued my license to fly. Without a valid medical certificate, I would not be able to do so. The diagnosis of prostate cancer triggers an order for immediate grounding. I needed a doctor who had both the medical expertise to treat my prostate cancer as well as the sympathy and understanding necessary to keep me flying. I found both in

Dr. Ronald Wheeler and his clinic in Sarasota, Florida. Not only am I cancer-free but I'm still enjoying my first love; flying."
Pete Carson, Commercial Airline Pilot

"I recently had the privilege of a personal consultation call with Dr. Wheeler. I commend him on his website as having saved my life and certainly the quality of my life, empowering me to intelligently care for myself! I have taken Dr. Wheeler's patented formula, Peenuts® as well as assorted other products he recommends while following his modified Mediterranean Diet. He has put me on the right path! It is working for me! For the first time in a very long time I only got up once last night to empty my bladder. When I woke up and realized it was almost 6:00 am, I couldn't believe it. I feel great and energized! I know I am not done improving but I am so much better than I was! For that, I want to say . . . Thank You!!! I am excited about this book and want to be one of the first to buy it, both in the E-book format and soft bound edition!
Harold Lindsey, Jr.

"The sports world and men in general will be energized and better educated by this fresh look at prostate cancer as presented by Dr. Wheeler! What he states in his book makes 'perfect sense'"!!
Dusty Baker, Major League Baseball Manager

MEN AT RISK

THE DIRTY LITTLE SECRET

PROSTATE BIOPSIES REALLY DO SPREAD

PROSTATE CANCER CELLS

Ronald E. Wheeler, M.D.

authorHOUSE®

AuthorHouse™
1663 Liberty Drive
Bloomington, IN 47403
www.authorhouse.com
Phone: 1-800-839-8640

Published by AuthorHouse   04/05/2012

ISBN: 978-1-4685-4801-3 (sc)
ISBN: 978-1-4685-4802-0 (e)

Library of Congress Control Number: 2012902055

CONTENTS

DEDICATION

This book is dedicated to all men who never knew they had prostate cancer! It is this group of men and their families who have suffered immeasurably through ignorance and the failure to understand that prostate cancer is a disease of healthy men! This group of men never had the chance that men will now have with guidance from my book. Without testing for Prostate Specific Antigen (PSA), men will never know they have a disease (that can be potentially cured) until it is too late. You are the reason I wrote this book!

PREFACE

BEING A MALE with prostate disease has never been more problematic. In the 21st Century, prostate disease and prostate cancer in particular are arguably the most dominant health related risks that men face! The statistics with prostate cancer are particularly troubling. Specifically, 1 in every 5-6 men will contract prostate cancer in their lifetime. It is well known; if men live long enough, virtually all men will contract prostate cancer. Surprisingly to many people, prostate cancer in men is more common than breast cancer in women. According to SEER (Surveillance, Epidemiology and End Results) data within the next 10-15 years, more than 500,000 men will be diagnosed with prostate cancer yearly in the United States. Evidence of an epidemic is noted with 5,000 men turning 60 years of age everyday for the next 20 years! Additionally, data shows that the 7th decade of life (men in their 60s) to be the most prolific decade for the diagnosis of prostate cancer. While experts search for a cure, prevention is likely the best model for success versus this sinister and most unpredictable disease. **At the Diagnostic Center for Disease™, a division of PanAm HIFU™, in Sarasota, Florida, we believe prevention is possible through proper diet, appropriate nutrition, adequate exercise, stress reduction and education!** Evidence is in place that allows men to live with prostate cancer in upwards of 50-60% of patients who contract the disease. Despite this fact, radical prostatectomy remains the most solicited and performed treatment for prostate cancer worldwide! **Let it be known that removal of the prostate is old school.** Any alteration in the frequency of prostate removal must be initiated at the patient level as doctors are biased relevant to what treatment they perform when prostate cancer is diagnosed. Men must understand the issues associated with prostate removal and begin to embrace improved treatment technologies such as High Intensity Focused Ultrasound (HIFU) as well as improved diagnostic testing using 3 Tesla MRI scanning to identify disease before a biopsy, assuming a biopsy remains relevant to an educated population! A generalized lack of academic enthusiasm from Urologists across the United States of America is primarily the single most responsible cause to maintaining the status quo of **conveyor belt medicine**, as I like to call it! Without question, most doctors are withholding validated information and research from patients relevant to Peer Reviewed Journal articles, thereby denying the patient critical data necessary to the decision making process as related to the potential peril of prostate biopsy. Compounding this dilemma; prostate cancer is a disease of healthy men! Typically, men feel little to no pain from prostate cancer until it is too late to make a difference, regardless of treatment. **This book intends to change the way men and women think about the diagnosis and treatment of prostate cancer.** The education gained from reading this book will empower the patient to take charge of his personal health related issues. **This book serves as a "wake up" call to all doctors who share in "The Dirty Little Secret." Patients are encouraged to buy two copies of this book; one as a personal reference and the second for the most arrogant and disparaging of doctors they know!**

Does a biopsy cause prostate cancer to spread?

This is a vexing question for Urologists and sympathetic physicians worldwide. This is an unpopular topic to Urologists primarily as they are used to patients following their advice without question or criticism of the process. Conveyor belt medicine is where patients are expected to do as they are told within a health care model. Not surprisingly, most doctors with whom you will speak will tell you cancer is not spread by a biopsy. They deny that it takes place and state emphatically; there is no credible data or evidence to support its presence. Tell that to the doctors who have authored research articles in various peer-reviewed Journals. Doctors like: **Judd Moul**, Chairman of Urology at Duke University, **Patrick Walsh** from Johns Hopkins Medical Center, **Michael Karin** at the University of California at San Diego, **Katsuto Shinohara** at the University of California at San Francisco, **Haddad** and **Joachim-Ernst Deuster** from Heidelberg, Germany are just a few of the docs to enter the debate with data to support spreading cancer through biopsy! To be sure, prostate biopsy is associated with 'needle tracking', a sinister phenomenon seen when a needle of any size punctures the prostate capsule from any direction. An example that I like to use in the office describes a balloon that contains a highly caustic acid such as sulfuric acid. Assuming the material the balloon is made of will not erode due to the acid, the question is asked if we penetrate the balloon with any needle what happens to the acid. It does not take a rocket scientist to understand that acid will come out of the balloon causing damage to all it comes in contact with. What happens when a needle enters the tip of your finger? Does the injury result in immediate closure of the wound? In a word, no! Do cells come out? Of course, they do! **Patients know this answer because it is intuitive and thereby, makes perfect sense. Doctors on the other hand prefer to ignore the science and common sense while representing needle tracking as a non-issue, hoping patients will respect their knowledge as a practitioner and do as they are told.** If we examine this topic more closely, we will note the needle tracking process was actually prominently described by puncturing a kidney when there was suspicion of renal cancer present based on imaging. Should penetration of the prostate capsule be any different than puncturing the capsule or outer skin of the kidney? I think . . . not! Patrick Walsh from Johns Hopkins stated in 1991 (Journal of Urology article) that doctors would not accept the concept of 'needle tracking' very readily. Can you blame them when upwards of 50% of their income is generated from prostate biopsies? None of this should be about the money but rather about doing what is ethically correct while avoiding risks to the patient, whenever possible! Scientific evidence should define a best practice pattern or standard; not a biased opinion that states, "we would know it by now . . . if there was a problem", quoting Patrick Walsh and others. In November 2002, the **Journal of Urology** read by virtually every Urologist in the world offered proof positive that 'needle tracking' takes place. **The article pointed out a lesion in the rectal wall that treating doctors from the University of California, San Francisco admitted came from a previous transrectal biopsy performed to identify the presence of prostate cancer**. Lost in all of this was the fact that the authors stated that such an event does not occur very often. This was interpreted by Urologists 'en mass' that 'needle tracking' doesn't take place with frequency. Please . . . ! What the authors suggested is that 'needle tracking' is rarely discovered because it is difficult to identify routinely. The truth of the matter notes that 'needle tracking' or seeding of prostate cells beyond the capsule happens 100% of the time with unknown consequences! **No one would argue including yours truly that every biopsy of the prostate results in cells being displaced and growing beyond the prostate capsule.** While there is no doubt 'needle tracking' takes place universally with prostate biopsy, it is doubtful we will ever predict which patients are at greatest risk for seeding cancer beyond the capsule regardless of the biopsy result. To state this more clearly, while I believe there is a chance that cells that escape the prostate will die off in time in many patients; we have no credible evidence that this actually takes place. It would be common sense to assume the greater number of biopsies performed, the greater the chance for an untoward event to take place. Doctors who recommend saturation biopsies are making an egregious misstep. Patients who receive the biopsies have to suffer the consequences of the indiscretion afforded them by less than knowledgeable physicians! Judd Moul, the Director of Urology at Duke Medical Center identified 'needle tracking' with perineal biopsies during his stint at Walter Reed Medical Center in Washington, D.C. The perineum is the space between the anus and the scrotum penetrated during saturation biopsies! **I am humored by doctors who tell their patients . . . once the location of the cancer is identified by biopsy, a treatment plan can be implemented to 'cure' the cancer!** Pretty bold statement without any evidence; is how I interpret this near universal Urology dogma. If 'needle tracking' takes place with any organ biopsy, the prostate is no different and the patient must understand the risk is theirs and not the doctor who performs the procedure. There is a significant concern that 'seeding of tumor cells' beyond the prostate capsule is the reason that 40-60 percent of patients fail to be cured by 7-10 years, referencing the Journal of Urology. **The take home message is to image first and only do a targeted biopsy if you must and then, always try to avoid the consequences of needle tracking through to use of Bicalutamide or similar agent to deprive the cells of much needed Testosterone! I hope you enjoy reading the book as much as I did writing it!**

NOTES:

CHAPTER ONE

Too Many Radicals . . .
Too Many Failures

WHEN YOU HEAR the news that you have prostate cancer, what are you going to do? Rather than panic, you must accept the facts and begin the learning process. Your exit strategy from this dilemma will be to determine how your cancer will be managed. Proven treatment options range from a conservative management program of diet, wellness management, antioxidants and specific nutritional supplements we call chronic disease management (CDM) with no impact on your quality of life to radical surgery with a major impact. Deciding how you will treat your prostate cancer will become the single most important decision you will make for the remainder of your life. Ultimately, your decision must be acceptable to you and your family and be effective while minimizing undue risk, complications and side effects.

Prostate cancer is a disease that does not discriminate, wreaking havoc on all men irrespective of age, ethnicity, education, financial or social status. **When it comes to the topic of prostate cancer, all men are equally ignorant, regardless of education (obviously excepting doctors who should know the topic better than the public at large).** Prostate disease in general and prostate cancer specifically is the most common and dominant disease that men face, while representing a diseased organ that must be understood and dealt with by men of all ages. Often times referred to as a disease of healthy men, prostate cancer has no boundaries, no conscience and will strike most time with no warning other than an elevated prostate specific antigen (PSA) blood test. Your only defense is to become educated on the disease, get motivated and proactive. Your goal is to maintain an optimal PSA of less than 1.0 ng/ml. Many men who fail to heed this warning will pay the ultimate price with their lives. Many more will be spared but asked to endure a life of subtraction, losing many of the qualities from life that make being a man so special.

Statistics on Prostate Cancer

While prostate disease is arguably the number one health risk that men face, prostate cancer is the most prolific organ cancer that men acquire in their lifetime as well as the second leading cause of cancer death, behind lung cancer. One in five to six men will be diagnosed with prostate cancer in their lifetime. Prostate cancer occurs most often in older men. African-American men have a rate of prostate cancer that is twice their Caucasian counterparts. According to the American Cancer Society, an estimated 218,890 men will be diagnosed with prostate cancer this year while in excess of 27,000 men will die from the disease. **This translates into a new case of prostate cancer diagnosed every three minutes while a man dies from the disease every 16 minutes of every day.** With the baby boomer generation aging into their 50s and 60s, at 5,000 men per day; the expectation is for 50,000 men to lose their lives annually from prostate cancer by the year 2020. While men in their 60s or older experience the news that prostate cancer has been detected most frequently, data shows 30 percent of 30-year-old men will acquire the disease only to have their lives spared initially as the cancer incubates for upwards of 15 to 20 years before the impact is realized with a rising PSA blood test. **When you decide to become motivated to learn more about this disease is your decision; what you learn about the disease and how you treat the disease is the heart and soul of this book.**

Radical Prostatectomy—
'Gold Standard' or Educated Guess

Historically, radical prostatectomy (total surgical prostate removal) has been the most common treatment offered and rendered when prostate cancer is diagnosed. The irony of treating the most prolific male cancer most frequently with radical prostatectomy is that the failure rate will be unacceptably high while essentially equal regardless of the approach utilized including the DaVinci Robot technique. While prostate cancer is being detected earlier, there is no convincing data to suggest a significant survival advantage of radical prostatectomy over brachytherapy (radioactive seed implants), as example, with or without external beam radiation, cryosurgery or a treatment strategy called chronic disease management (CDM) (refer to the CDM chapter for a comprehensive review of this concept). **In other words, there is significant data to suggest alternative therapies like CDM may make a better first choice of treatment if overall survival is relatively unaffected by the specific therapy selected. Why should you undergo a major radical surgery with significant complications and side effects if it's not going to make a difference in your survival? You should not!**

If 10 men with prostate cancer are lined up and evaluated, doctors cannot reliably predict who will ultimately be cured and who will fail. In my opinion, this is primarily due to a lack of discrimination regarding where the disease is actually located; principally, the extent of disease. Patients showing more favorable disease characteristics may have better survival rates, but **the fact remains that we cannot predict the final outcome of treatment.** Some patients with "good" cancers will perish of prostate cancer regardless of any treatment we can offer, and some with "bad" or very aggressive cancers may survive even with minimal treatment. **Until we have better tools (or utilize better tools, not currently accepted) that allow us to make truly reliable predictions, the best we can say is that radical prostatectomy can possibly cure 60-70 percent of prostate cancer patients. To state more clearly, we can't accurately predict who will be cured and who won't be cured using our present diagnostic and treatment modalities. To be sure, regardless of our surgical skill level, the outcome and cure rate from major radical prostate surgery is unpredictable. This point is validated by Hendrick Isbarn, M.D. and collaborators at the University Hospital Hamburg-Eppendorf in Hamburg, Germany in their research published in the British Journal of Urology (International Edition) in 2009. Specifically, they found that the biochemical recurrence (BCR) rate for prostate cancer was 40% at 10 years. Unfortunately, this is an unacceptably high rate of prostate cancer recurrence; representative of all radicals performed worldwide, in my opinion.**

So why is radical prostatectomy performed so often? While this is a great question, the answer is very elusive. We hear phrases like, "that's what I was trained to do," "it's the 'Gold Standard' in prostate cancer treatment," "and it's the only way that we can be sure that all of the cancer is gone" or "this procedure gives you the best chance for a cure." **When a patient asks a doctor for his best recommendation and the only procedure he performs is a radical prostatectomy, what do you expect him to say?** Even if the doctor also performs seed implantation therapy and cryosurgery but believes the radical approach is best for most patients; do not expect him to give a glowing endorsement for either of the other two choices. While doctors are supposed to be unbiased in their approach, it is difficult for most physicians to remain completely objective. It's not their fault. They are just expressing what they know based on their training and experience. **The Hippocratic Oath states, "We must first do no harm." This should still be the starting point for any decision related to treatment of prostate cancer.** Finally, remember that treating prostate cancer is also a business. The insurance industry rewards some treatments substantially more than others. Physicians are only human and will tend to be influenced by the very high financial rewards from the insurance industry for surgery or radiation therapy over conservative treatments that aren't reimbursed well. Furthermore, physicians may own shares of radiation therapy centers that are highly reimbursed by Medicare and most insurance companies. **Even given their best intentions, it's hard for many physicians to be totally objective in their recommendations when they can earn $20,000 or more per patient by referring you to their radiation center.**

Physician Practice Patterns

In a survey of more than 500 urologists reported on in the Journal of the American Medical Association (JAMA), the question was asked of urological surgeons; what approach should be taken with a 65-year-old male with a newly diagnosed prostate cancer associated with a Gleason score of 7 and a PSA less than 10 ng/ml? For those unfamiliar with the meaning of Gleason score, refer to the glossary and/or the pathology section of this book for a review. For those more familiar with the term, a Gleason score of 7 represents a moderate to poorly differentiated cell type, commonly encountered in approximately 30-35 percent of all cases of prostate cancer. To the surprise of no one, a traditional urology line of thought or 'party line' was endorsed by 90 percent of the urologists polled, thereby recommending a radical prostatectomy for this patient. While this opinion from a surgeon may come as no surprise, there is minimal documentation to support the strength of such an opinion.

In an effort to establish diversity of opinion, noting that doctors would only recommend what was best for the patient; radiation oncologists were asked their recommendation for the same patient scenario with the same cancer characteristics. The majority of radiation oncologists followed the dictum of their residency-training manual and recommended brachytherapy (radioactive seed implantation) or external beam radiation or a combination of both. **Patients, who seek these professional opinions, must be mindful that it may be difficult to get a totally objective opinion from a physician who is biased based on how he was trained and how he practices. It is often said and bears restating; "If all you have is a hammer, it is amazing how everything begins to look like a nail."**

In this imperfect world, the burden for an improved understanding of the disease and its various treatments, unfortunately, becomes the responsibility for each patient, individually; notwithstanding their lack of adequate education. This doesn't seem quite fair to the vulnerable patient doing little to diminish the anxiety experienced when the diagnosis is made. Based on a likely rush to judgment that is commonly experienced when the diagnosis of prostate cancer is made, patients are encouraged to become increasingly aware of the peril and consequences associated with prostate cancer treatment prior to the diagnosis, not after.

Taking the time to evaluate your options is supported by a research study performed at Johns Hopkins Medical Center. What they demonstrated is that while the diagnosis of prostate cancer must be taken seriously, a delay in treatment of months or even years may not change the course of the disease and the outcome. While this will likely depend on the specific characteristics of disease identified in a given patient, the news is nonetheless heartening as the task to fully understand the disease and the various treatment options is significant. It will take a concerted effort and ample time by all who choose to be well versed.

Better Imaging, Better Decisions, Better Results

This book intends to serve the many worried men with prostate cancer and their families as a fair and objective resource to help in understanding the disease you are now facing and the options available to you. By taking a fresh look at the available scientific information and explaining it in a new and unique way, it's our intention to help you make a truly informed decision about your treatment choices and ultimately about your future.

The true nature of the disease must be completely understood before any meaningful decision is made on how to proceed when the diagnosis of prostate cancer is made. While it is critical to determine the extent of disease in order to select the best treatment strategy, it is equally important to realize the severe limitations of our present diagnostic process based upon our current outdated imaging tools and biopsy techniques. For this reason, we are very excited about Magnetic Resonance Imaging with or without Spectroscopy (MRI or MRIS) discussed in more detail later and throughout this book. MRI performed with a 3.0 Tesla magnet or equivalent alternative may well be the best diagnostic modality for the detection of prostate cancer prior to a biopsy or to establish true organ confinement once the diagnosis of prostate cancer has been confirmed by a biopsy. **Intuitively, imaging must be done before a biopsy (if a biopsy ever makes sense); not after.** The 3 Tesla MRI, diagnostic modality provides the most accurate cancer imaging technology available. The outstanding image quality ensures the best chance for realistic decision-making leading to ultimate success. This scan, which we call the "Ultimate Prostate Scan," provides precision prostate cancer localization allowing us to determine whether the tumor is truly organ-confined prior to any proposed therapy. **If organ confinement is not reliably established, the scientific data does not support radical surgical removal of the prostate.** The MRI Scan provides a true road map of objective imaging excellence to validate cancer localization while spectroscopy, when utilized as an additional sequence, allows us to understand the biochemical components of the tissue in question. Together, these scan sequences are integral to changing the paradigm relevant to the diagnosis and subsequent treatment of prostate cancer.

Chronic Disease Management

Prospective study data associated with our research treatment protocol evaluated the benefit of diet and nutrition versus prostate cancer. The study, entitled, **"Is it necessary to cure prostate cancer when it is possible,"** represented in the Journal, Clinical Interventions in Aging, supports the concept of allowing men the opportunity to live with prostate cancer much like patients would live with diabetes or arthritis rather than undergo surgical organ removal or radiation. If men decide later to attempt to cure the disease with surgery or radiation, their chance of success should not have been significantly diminished by the delay. In other words, **taking our time to evaluate all issues related to the diagnosis and treatment of prostate**

cancer allows us to avoid a rush to judgment. Quite frankly, by delaying the definitive decision making, anxiety is reduced and the advantages and disadvantages of every therapy can be studied in more detail and become better known. **You cannot fully appreciate the consequences of your treatment decision until you completely understand the lifestyle you will have to accept when the choice is made.**

The key to the success of our research treatment protocol relates to the ability to suppress or resolve the signs and symptoms of inflammation (non-bacterial prostatitis) through diet and a prostate-specific patented dietary supplement we developed called *Peenuts®*. This formula represents a unique and synergistic blend of vitamins, minerals, herbs and amino acids. Its special ability to reduce prostatic inflammation has been scientifically validated by improvements in white blood cell counts (a universal sign of inflammation) associated with the prostate secretion or expressed prostatic secretion (EPS) obtained at the time of digital prostate exam, as well as a decrease in PSA levels, given its success with widespread use as a stand-alone treatment for prostatitis. While diet plays an important role, the road to success without surgery or radiation requires optimizing all of our dietary and nutritional resources to fight the cancer. This will become quite apparent once you have reviewed the dietary and nutritional sections of this book.

In our prospective study, mentioned above, 30 patients with known prostate cancer were evaluated over an average time frame of 49 months. During this time, their only treatment was dietary modification and our scientifically designed prostate anti-inflammatory supplement *Peenuts®*. By the end of the study, 28 out of the 30 patients noted a marked improvement or decrease in their PSA levels (the recognized marker of prostate cancer disease activity) averaging 55 percent. This degree of improvement is truly remarkable and has never been reported before in such a large study group without using hormonal therapy, surgery or radiation. While we are certainly pleased with the outcome, we were not really surprised, as we have noted similar significant improvements in thousands of patients over the years while using this supplement. This concept of nutritional optimization and chronic disease management has not been studied adequately as it has never received priority funding. It is our hope that visionary philanthropists who understand and embrace our beliefs, will come together to provide the capital necessary to validate our research as well as promote a prostate cancer prevention trial. The Prospective Study (PROCAP Trial), touched on above, will be described in its entirety in the Appendix.

One of the major advantages of the CDM approach is that you can always change your mind. If the cancer at some point appears to be escalating, notwithstanding a CDM protocol, you can still choose any of the more aggressive treatment options such as radiation therapy, radioactive seed implants, radical prostatectomy surgery, high intensity focused ultrasound (HIFU) or cryotherapy. Meanwhile, you will have enjoyed whatever time the CDM approach provided with minimal side effects or complications.

Clinical Case Study #1

Let's take a look at an actual clinical case that allows us to better understand the present state of prostate cancer treatment and the associated angst that comes with the diagnosis. Jon F., a 54-year-old Caucasian male, was diagnosed with prostate cancer with a Gleason score 6 (3+3) associated with a PSA of 4.2ng/ml. (A Gleason 6 designation comprises the most common prostate cancer cell type identified). It is also recognized to be a cancer type that predicts a reasonably favorable clinical outcome. This is the group of patients that Pat Walsh, M.D. and the team at Johns Hopkins and other major centers of excellence operate on to establish their respective outcome data, thereby validating their treatment choice of radical prostatectomy for prostate cancer. Ironically, this is also the group of cancers that many experts, like Michael Barry from Harvard, believe are over-treated. In other words, it's possible and maybe even likely that many men with this classification of prostate cancer would do equally well with a radical prostatectomy (assuming cure), radiation, radioactive seed implantation, HIFU or with a more conservative approach like Chronic Disease Management (CDM) (reference the Prospective Diet & Nutritional Study). **It is for this reason that word needs to be spread throughout the world that CDM may be a reasonable and viable alternative to radical prostatectomy or radiation when this category of cancer is diagnosed.**

Based on Jon's relative youth and patient fear of impending death from a presumably predictable cancer, the patient agreed to a radical prostatectomy at the urging of his family and surgeon. Six years later, the patient's PSA was rising consistent with a treatment failure. **A progressive rise in PSA following any attempt to cure indicates the failure of the operation (or any definitive therapy) to cure the disease. This is also called biochemical failure or disease relapse.** A rise in PSA despite the complete surgical removal of the prostate tells you that the disease had escaped the prostate prior to or at the time of the surgery. Most often, prostate cancer cells look to find a new source of nourishment in the lymph nodes or bones (or both) when they escape the prostate capsule. It is estimated that the range of disease recurrence following radical prostatectomy or radiation is 30-40 percent and possibly as high as 40-60 percent by 7-10 years. The earlier the rise in PSA following surgery or radiation and/or the failure to lower the PSA to less than 0.5

ng/ml suggests that the disease is more aggressive and was likely systemic at the time of the definitive curative therapy. In other words, when the disease was thought to be localized or confined to the prostate it had already spread microscopically and undetectably to other structures or organs. Unfortunately this information does not help us after the fact except to predict a troubled and probable aggressive clinical course that will likely hasten the patient's demise. The only way to have avoided this outcome is to have avoided the surgery that tried to get rid of the disease in the first place. Confused? Join the millions who, like you, need to learn a new way of thinking about prostate cancer, including how to properly evaluate the various treatments and how to take charge of their care and their futures. **Minimally the failure of Jon F. to be cured calls into question our ability to cure anyone with certainty and should help slow the march of the confused and anxious to the operating room door.**

The medical literature suggests the failure to completely and permanently cure a patient when radical prostatectomy or radiation is performed, bodes poorly for the patient. Specifically, according to Anthony D'Amico of Harvard Medical School and colleagues, when the PSA doubling time (the time it takes for the PSA number to double) is less than three months following radical prostatectomy or radiation, the patient has a 20 times increased risk of dying from prostate cancer within 6-10 years. Our own clinical research concurs, showing the clinical course observed for the patient who isn't cured by radical prostatectomy or radiation will be much more aggressive, giving us less time to fight the battle than the individual who chose a more conservative treatment, such as the strategic CDM protocol. Examples will be provided throughout this book that will make this point very clear.

Returning to the case of Jon F. there were issues other than a rising PSA following the failed attempt at cure with a radical prostatectomy. Ever since the operation, this patient has been a sexual cripple; meaning that he did not achieve adequate erections despite the use of erectile stimulating drugs including but not limited to medications like Viagra (the little blue pill), Cialis, Levitra (PDE-5 inhibitors) or Caverject (an injectable treatment for ED). Jon also complains of urinary leakage, which would have been more tolerable if only the operation was a success. **What is sad is that this patient should have been cured; as his disease characteristics were quite favorable, suggesting that anything short of cure is a significant failure. This case history establishes very clearly why a more conservative approach may have been the better first choice.** Unfortunately, Jon had never been told that he could live a long and prosperous life with the prostate remaining untouched using a more conservative approach like the CDM protocol. Had this happened, Jon would not have been the first patient discussed in this chapter.

This is the reason that patients must become increasingly aware that radical prostatectomy is not always what it is made out to be. **There are no guarantees even when you hear that "the surgery gives you your best chance at cure."** Improved awareness and understanding of the disease is the only defense that will allow the patient to fully comprehend all the options discussed; but more importantly, to walk away and calmly rethink what has been discussed absent the emotion of the moment.

Jon F. made a significant sacrifice for what was ultimately a failed chance at a cure. He would have been willing to live with the quality of life-limiting side effects of impotency and incontinence had the cure been reliably achieved. At this junction in Jon's life, he is now faced with the next set of tough questions that will require intelligent decisions related to how the disease will be managed moving forward. His choice at this point is to consider radiation therapy or CDM (active surveillance). Radiation, replete with its own set of side effects, including but not limited to rectal bleeding, diarrhea, hematuria, urinary urgency, urinary frequency, scarring and radiation cystitis, is likely to worsen his already limited sexual function as well as further decrease his ability to control his bladder. A much more reasonable approach might be the use of a CDM or active surveillance protocol.

At this point, Jon's cancer will respond predictably well to hormone manipulation utilizing an anti-androgen (Flutamide, Casodex or Nilutamide) given intermittently. An anti-androgen prevents the remaining cancer cells from growing by depriving them of the male hormone testosterone, enabling residual cancer cells to die. There will be more about this concept in clinical case study number two. While his PSA was just beginning to rise from the low point of 0.2ng/ml, I would likely defer the use of an anti-androgen until the PSA becomes substantially higher. This would also allow us an opportunity to try other conservative measures to extend the PSA doubling time, as no one knows for sure that the disease cannot be stabilized (when optimal conservative measures are employed), while understanding no two cancers are exactly alike. Furthermore, proactive treatment with an LHRH-analog or anti-androgen (whether alone or in combination) at a lower PSA number may hasten the onset of hormone refractivity (disease resistance), a well-known consequence of hormonal manipulation. Additionally, **we should not discount the potential role of diet and nutrition to assist holding the cancer in check.** In an effort to prevent the PSA from rising to a higher and more definable number, we can use a range of products, supplements, vitamins or formulas associated with various mechanisms of action versus the cancer process in an effort to produce a successful outcome and prolong life. There are no reliable tests or examinations that can tell us with certainty exactly where the cancer is located or that the cancer will not respond to treatment with conservative measures now that the radical prostatectomy has failed to cure the disease. At this point, we will assist Jon regardless of the choice he makes and do all we can to foster his success, including the application of a CDM protocol in the event radiation is chosen and fails. It is not as important why this clinical scenario happened with Jon, but rather, how we can prevent this from happening to the next generation of men diagnosed with prostate cancer.

Clinical Case Study #2

The case history and clinical experience of Carl L. is equally riveting for even the most learned or savvy prostate cancer patient. As a 60-year-old former All-American hockey defenseman at Michigan State University, who now resides in Green Bay, Wisconsin, Carl learned he had prostate cancer when his PSA reached 8.2ng/ml in October 2004. The year prior, his PSA was 3.9 ng/ml. When he asked his Urologist in 2003 if there was anything that could be done to try to lower the PSA, he was told the PSA was still in the normal range and not to be concerned. A 12-core biopsy performed a year later based on the 8.2ng/ml PSA, yielded a Gleason score 4+4=8 cancer in three of six biopsies on the left side and a cancer precursor cell type called High Grade PIN (prostatic intraepithelial neoplasia) on the right side. (See Glossary and Pathology Chapter for an improved understanding of these terms)

His biopsy clinical stage was T2b meaning that significant cancer was located in more than one quadrant on the left side of his prostate. Given the poorly differentiated cancer cell type, Carl went about the process of trying to determine the best way to defeat the disease. Three urologists representing three different urology practices had recommended that a radical prostatectomy was his only or best chance to survive the cancer. **One urologist went so far as to state; if he did not have** the radical surgery, he would be "dead within one year." Concerned for his life and quite frankly scared beyond belief, Carl hastily decided that the radical surgery seemed like the only reasonable option. He had completed his pre-op evaluation and had even received the hospital wristband, identifying him to all hospital personnel as scheduled for surgery. At home, his wife Sandy was feverishly looking for other options as she did not feel comfortable about the choice that the man of her life had made. Several days prior to his early morning arrival at the hospital for the expected surgical procedure, Carl's life changed. Sandy had come across our website, **www.MrisUSA. com** and placed a toll-free call to our clinic. We had a chance to talk to Carl about the disease, his treatment options and what to expect from the surgery.

After a brief factual and straightforward discussion, Carl cut the hospital wristband from his arm and scheduled an appointment at our clinic in Sarasota, Florida. **In our conversation, we said nothing that would diminish his hope for a successful outcome, although we did inform, him that while radical prostatectomy may have provided his greatest statistical chance for cure, as represented by his three urologic consultations, no one informed him that the actual percent chance of a cure was only about 15 percent based on his high Gleason score and the known extent of his disease. In other words, statistically speaking, 85 percent of all prostate cancers represented by Gleason Scores of 8, 9 or 10 will have a disease recurrence within five years after a radical prostatectomy.** Carl was incredibly disappointed that no one had discussed these literature-based facts on the historical surgical outcome associated with this cancer grade, but rather opted for a 'leap of faith' to try to save his life. No one had allowed Carl and Sandy the opportunity to really understand that what they were about to do had very little chance of a cure. Once they were made fully aware of all the facts, they decided that radical prostate surgery made very little sense and was obviously the wrong approach for them.

The Clinical Appointment—A Difference Maker

By making the commitment to see us in the clinic, Carl and Sandy had become a member of our extended family. During the three hour plus clinical evaluation and interview process, we reviewed all the viable alternatives including the option of allowing Carl to live with the disease through a protocol of CDM. Minimally, this option would buy us some time while not burning a bridge; allowing us to be more aggressive later if necessary or if an acceptable option presented itself that made sense when the risk-reward evaluation indicated. We were able to share other patient success stories using the CDM concept with Carl and Sandy. Together we created and accepted a treatment strategy that was intended to at least stabilize the cancer disease process. It was made very clear that we were in this together and we were as close as a telephone call. Based on his heightened disease status and aggressive Gleason Score, we elected to start him on an optimized CDM protocol that included a range of conservative treatments using various mechanisms of action to suppress the disease and make it less aggressive or even dormant.

First, Carl was placed on the Modified Mediterranean diet as well as our nutritional prostatitis supplement, Peenuts® to help resolve prostate inflammation. This was an important step as it has been shown that prostatitis can evolve or transform into prostate cancer. This has been confirmed by many research experts including the American Association of cancer Research (AACR), headed up by Johns Hopkins and independently by Michael Karin, PhD, David Bostwick, M.D., a world-renowned pathologist and collectively, experts on prostate cancer. Carl was also started on Avodart or dutasteride (a 5-alpha reductase inhibitor) at 0.5mg daily to decrease the conversion of Testosterone to Dihydrotestosterone (DHT) as well as promote an anti-angiogenic component (decreases new blood vessel formation) while reducing the size of the prostate. We knew that the PSA could be decreased by some number less than half based on resolution of both benign prostatic hyperplasia and prostate inflammation. We were cognizant of the Prostate Cancer Prevention Trial (PCPT) data where Proscar or finasteride (another 5-alpha reductase inhibitor) was associated with a decreased incidence of prostate cancer by 25 percent when compared to placebo. While we had no data to show any specific benefit versus prostate cancer with this class of drug, we did not want the cancer to be exposed to DHT, the much more active form of the cancer growth promoting male hormone. Vitamin D3 (the active form of Vitamin D) was added for its benefit in decreasing prostate cancer cell proliferation, while Omega 3 fatty acids were added to enhance the heart healthy Omega 3:6 fatty acid ratio while also decreasing prostate cancer proliferation and free radicals.

The final integral piece of the treatment strategy was the use of Casodex (Bicalutamide), a non-steroidal anti-androgen, at 150mg per day. This dosage is much higher than the standard 50mg dose typically used here in the U.S., but is similar to the dose effectively used in Europe. We have had tremendous experience using Casodex at the higher dose as a monotherapy just as it is used in Europe. Notwithstanding the fact that 150 mg represents a higher dose than that typically used in the United States it is quite safe and effective when used intermittently. Specifically, the anti-androgen blocks a prostate cancer cell receptor, thereby inhibiting the growth of cancer. In other words, testosterone remains normal, but is preferentially blocked from its usual action of attaching to the prostate cancer cell receptor at the nucleus, thus, allowing the cell to become disabled, dormant or even die. The concept is similar to what you would expect to see when you put a plastic child-resistant safety cap on an electrical outlet. No matter how hard you try to connect an electrical plug to the source of electricity at that outlet, you can't do it. That's the same way that Casodex blocks the interaction of testosterone with the prostate cancer cell receptor and promotes cell death or dormancy; preferentially over cell growth.

There are a few side effects from the use of Casodex as a monotherapy, including but not limited to a transient elevation in liver enzymes, mild breast tenderness or swelling and the potential for diarrhea. This side effect profile is generally very acceptable for the anticipated short interval of usage. The side effect profile, nonetheless, can be avoided using additional medications or supplements that would minimize and/or eliminate these concerns. Using this approach, we were able to avoid an LHRH-analog (Luteinizing Hormone Releasing Hormone), thereby, by-passing complete chemical castration associated with its host of undesirable side effects including but not limited to: lethargy, increased fasting blood sugars secondary to increased insulin resistance, muscle wasting, hypercholesterolemia, anemia, bone loss, hot flashes, cognitive changes, depression, mood swings and weight gain. When Casodex is used as an intermittent high dose monotherapy, disease specific anti-androgen treatment has a tremendous lifestyle advantage when compared to the more traditional therapy of an LHRH-analog alone or in combination with an anti-androgen (combined androgen blockade), discussed elsewhere in this book.

The decision was made to use the anti-androgen (Casodex) intermittently between PSA action points of 10.0 ng/ml and 1.0 ng/ml. This meant that at a PSA number of 10 ng/ml or higher would mark the point where Casodex would begin and 1ng/ml or lower would indicate the point where the Casodex would be discontinued. Carl remained on the treatment protocol for 17 months total. During this timeframe, the Casodex was used for the first two months only, dropping the PSA (the marker of disease activity) from 13.0 ng/ml to 0.3 ng/ml. In effect, Carl had been off of Casodex for 15 months, while his PSA had remained stable at 1.7 ng/ml. This response represents a truly remarkable positive response for a very aggressive cancer. In his yearly follow-up appointment at our clinic, Carl's expressed prostatic secretion (EPS) white blood cell count (the number of WBC's associated with the expressed prostatic secretions) had gone from TNTC (too numerous to count) down to only 45 white blood cells when examined microscopically. This decrease in inflammatory cells is consistent with the use of the Peenuts® formula at 3 capsules daily as described in the Appendix. In effect, this represented a 91percent decrease in the inflammatory response (a process that we believe promotes prostate cancer evolution). The reduction in white blood cells in the expressed prostatic secretions can only be attributed to the dietary therapy and unique nutritional supplements used. Carl's urinary symptoms had also improved from a score of 10.5 (moderate symptoms on the International Prostate Symptom Score Index [IPSS-Index] to 1.5 (mild symptoms) in the same time frame, representing an improvement in symptoms of 86 percent. (Refer to the Appendix for the complete IPSS-Index.)

In his follow-up, rather than discussing his impending demise as predicted by one of his urologists, we celebrated a measure of victory versus an unpredictable and potentially deadly disease. We had demonstrated the success of CDM in a very difficult and potentially dangerous clinical scenario. While we believe this case represents one of the more spectacular responses of prostate cancer to CDM, highlighting Casodex as a monotherapy, this should not diminish the impact of key nutrients and medications as outlined previously. While this case sounds "too good to be true," we always welcome calls from patients, critics and colleagues to discuss our approach or for an update on how Carl and Sandy are doing. Carl and Sandy would be happy to share their joyous experience with those who care to contact them as well! **Maybe someday, Carl and Sandy will be able to tell their story on a bigger stage, thereby bringing more than just hope to the hundreds of thousands of men who face the same uncertainty of prostate cancer every day.** Now, with the disease suppressed, Carl and Sandy decided to take yet, another step. They decided to take a calculated risk to get rid of the disease once and for all, by undergoing high-intensity focused ultrasound (HIFU) at a site outside of the U.S. under our supervision. HIFU is still under FDA review (at the time of book publication) and therefore not currently offered, in the United States of America as of March 2009. Carl's progress will be monitored by an MRI analysis of his prostate, using 3.0 Tesla Magnet MRI or equivalent to determine the extent or absence of disease **without the need for confirmation by additional biopsies.** Refer to the section on Magnetic Resonance Imaging (MRI or MRIS) for a better understanding of this technique as well as an explanation for the possible elimination of prostate biopsies as the procedure of choice to confirm treatment success or failure. **As of March, 2011, Carl's PSA number was less than 0.05 ng/ml or statistically the same as zero!** Not bad for a patient who was supposed to be dead within a year without a radical prostatectomy performed.

What will you do when Prostate Cancer is diagnosed?

So when the diagnosis of prostate cancer is made in your case, what will you do? Will you try to live with the disease or will you want to remove the cancer at any cost? Is your goal a cure and if so, is this realistic and worth the price of side effects and potential complications? **While we never want to deprive you of hope; false hope and unrealistic expectations are unfair to you, the patient, who so desperately wants to succeed.** If a cure is possible, what are the true chances of success? Is it worth the risk when your chance of success is less than 50 percent? If a cure is impossible, what is the best strategy to ensure the best outcome? This is not as simple as just applying a radical prostatectomy or radiation therapy to a cancer but rather lies in **a multi-factorial approach** that may include a radical prostatectomy, HIFU or radiation but only if the odds of success are overwhelmingly in your favor and you are willing to take the risk. Our inability to reliably predict success or cure versus prostate cancer suggests that we should take our time and consider all of our options very carefully before the commitment is made to proceed with any definitive treatment. Get a second and even a third opinion. **If you act on impulse and make the wrong choice, you will have a lifetime to lament the error in judgment.**

An Icon in Urology Speaks Out

William Fair, M.D., former Chairman of the Departments of Urology and Surgery at the esteemed Memorial Sloan-Kettering Cancer Center was so frustrated with his inability to predict a successful outcome with radical prostatectomy or radiation for prostate cancer patients that he stated in a now famous speech from 2000; **"Based on everything we know about prostate cancer, I am not sure that it should not be treated as a chronic disease."** While we are not saying that radical prostatectomy is obsolete, we are saying that if we continue to apply the same therapy to every patient without a realistic understanding and appreciation for the risks involved and our limited ability to predict treatment success, we should limit the procedure to only those who best qualify for the procedure, thereby supporting the greatest chance for success. **The future of radical prostatectomy may ultimately be doomed based on the public's increasing perception suggesting lack of physician understanding of the disease, greed and/or inappropriate dogma tied to a disease we know too little about.** What Dr. Fair may truly have been seeking was a moratorium on radical prostatectomy and radiation therapy until he and other research experts could figure out the natural history of the disease, thereby selecting patients for a treatment based on a sound strategy as opposed to a **"one size fits all"** mentality. **There is rarely a doctor among us who will share Dr. Fair's commentary with his newly diagnosed prostate cancer patients, much less investigate and embrace valid conservative options as appropriate care.** These conservative yet effective options will be addressed in later chapters that discuss minimally invasive treatment like high-intensity focused ultrasound (HIFU).

Will You Be Proactive or Reactive?

For men with PSA levels of greater than 1.0 ng/ml, it is not too premature to begin to think about the educational process in front of you. As you will learn later in this book, 20-30 percent of all prostate cancers are present in the PSA range of 1-4.0 ng/ml. **If you choose to wait, as you believe yourself to be too healthy, you could face the same tough decisions that Jon F. faced! In Jon's case, he never knew he had another option until it was too late.** On the other hand, you can think ahead and begin planning your strategy as if you had the disease while possibly avoiding the disease altogether. Will you be a willing participant when a biopsy is recommended when your PSA exceeds 4.0 ng/ml (20-30 percent or more of biopsies are positive when the PSA exceeds 4.0 ng/ml) or will you reach out first to an improved technology like that available at the Diagnostic Center for Disease™ in Sarasota for a confirmational MRI scan? Random biopsies should be discouraged based on the sampling bias as well as the relatively low risk of prostate cancer on any given prostate biopsy procedure; not to mention the possible risk of spreading cancer cells (if present) beyond the prostate. Will what you have read thus far stimulate you to be proactive and try to avoid an inevitable disease by controlling prostatitis with dietary modifications and appropriate nutritional supplements? Or are you content to be reactive and take your chances that the disease won't come your way? Whatever your personality, whatever your choice, we are dedicated to making a difference with you when the time comes. **If cancer is inevitable, we want your case to be predictably successful giving you the opportunity to continue to take from life all that is yours.** The remaining chapters in this book are instructional and will make you think. What makes this book different from other prostate books is that we have brought together unique ideas and concepts, as well as international experts who are prepared to stand by the facts in a fair and balanced manner as well as respond to tough questions where they may not have the answer. For these and many other reasons, we encourage you to use this book as a learning tool, as a reference and as a guide to keep you health conscious while protecting your prostate and your heart. It has taken us years to do the research and additional years to write this book, so please take your time. Read it carefully and absorb it so that you are equipped to face the battle, should the disease ever present itself to you or a loved one.

NOTES:

CHAPTER TWO

Everything You Ever Wanted to Know About Chronic Prostatitis

"A CRITICAL UPDATE ON PROSTATITIS AS A CAUSE OF PROSTATE CANCER"

INTRODUCTION:

CHRONIC **PROSTATITIS** (INFLAMMATION or infection of the prostate) is common to virtually all adult men. Not surprisingly, **Prostatitis is associated with virtually all cases of prostate cancer and present in nearly every prostate biopsy, regardless of other findings.** According to Drs. Krieger and Berger, Urologists at the University of Washington, in Seattle, "All men either have *prostatitis* or will get *prostatitis* in their lifetime." Prostatitis has received some unexpected, but welcomed, publicity with the movie, **"The Green Mile"**, starring Tom Hanks as the Prison Warden as well as the revelation that the now deceased former leader from Iraq, Saddam Hussein had an attack of prostatitis while incarcerated. Interestingly, and notwithstanding the above comments, *prostatitis* **has been termed the "trucker's disease",** based on the fact that truck drivers sit on their backsides, (better stated, prostates), all day long, while driving a truck. While I can't change the historical reference, truckers manifest the signs and symptoms of ***prostatitis*** by virtue of sitting all day, driving mile after mile. The sitting position does not create the disease, but rather allows the disease to be readily identified clinically. **Just for the record, all men are equally likely to contract *prostatitis* regardless of job description.**

Chronic ***prostatitis*** may not cause significant symptoms in many men, but in others it can be a devastating disease that severely affects the quality of life of those afflicted. For many Professionals, ***prostatitis*** is difficult to diagnose and even more difficult to treat. A wide variety of therapies are available but few actually work in more than a small percentage of men. While none of the standard treatments available is able to improve the health and wellness of the prostate long-term, a proven approach, with a patented formula, may be your best first step. We'll review the current knowledge about *chronic* ***prostatitis***, your treatment options, and the science linking an inflammatory disease to prostate cancer.

THE PROSTATE:

All men are born with a prostate that grows and enlarges throughout life based on various forms of stimuli. The prostate gland (in health) is a spongy, walnut sized, mucus-producing organ that lies just below the urinary bladder and superior to the rectal wall. The prostate surrounds the urethra, a channel through the prostate, which carries urine from the bladder to the outside. The most significant growth of the prostate, associated with an increase in the number of cells (hyperplasia), begins in the early to mid 40s and is believed to be related to Dihydrotestosterone production. **Inflammation or growth of the prostate commonly causes difficulties in urination that should be addressed at the earliest sign.** The only known function of the prostate is to produce a secretion that nourishes and protects sperm during reproduction. It has no other known proven purpose.

THE DEFINITION:

Prostatitis is defined as inflammation or infection of the prostate. **Simplistically, *prostatitis* can be divided into two groups; bacterial and non-bacterial.** Bacterial may be divided into acute and chronic while non-bacterial *prostatitis* is generally recognized as chronic. The National Institute of Health developed and accepted the latest definition of *prostatitis* primarily guided by the presence of chronic pelvic pain associated with the more traditional acute and chronic clinical presentation. While I refer you to the formal paradigm presented by the NIH for a complete understanding, the most common presentation is Type IIIA or non-bacterial, inflammatory *prostatitis*. While *prostatitis* may be acute, (associated with systemic findings of fever, chills and rigors (shakes), most cases of *prostatitis* are chronic and tend to be incurable, with relatively frequent recurrences despite optimal, yet ineffective traditional treatment. Unfortunately, traditional therapy involves the use of antibiotics, which are effective in less than 5% of cases, as a remedy for non-bacterial *prostatitis*, although, antibiotics may improve symptoms temporarily secondary to an anti-inflammatory mechanism.

NIH Classification of Prostatitis

- I. Acute bacterial prostatitis: acute infection of the prostate
- II. Chronic bacterial prostatitis; recurrent infection
- III. Chronic nonbacterial prostatitis; chronic pelvic pain syndrome (CPPS)—no demonstrable infection
- IIIA. Inflammatory CPPS: WBCs in semen/EPS [voided bladder urine (VB3)]
- IIIB. Non-inflammatory CPPS: No WBCs in semen (EPS or VB3)
- IV. Asymptomatic inflammatory prostatitis: no subjective symptoms; detected either by prostate biopsy or presence of WBCs in prostatic secretions (EPS) during evaluation for other disorders

---

THE CLINICAL PRESENTATION:

Symptoms of **prostatitis** (also common to [EP, enlarged prostate] or [BPH, benign prostatic hyperplasia]) are the number one reason that men seek the advice of their primary care physician or Urologist. The most significant symptom of *chronic* **prostatitis** is pelvic pain, followed by various voiding symptoms, impotence and/or infertility. Referred pain from **prostatitis** is commonly located in the groin, testicles, lower back, penis, an area circumferentially around the rectum, the perineum and/or in the suprapubic area above the bladder. Additionally, pain is not uncommonly associated with ejaculation. Typical urinary symptoms produced by **prostatitis** include getting up at night to void (Nocturia), frequency of urination, urgency of urination, incomplete voiding, decreased force of the urinary stream, intermittency of the stream and a need to push or strain to void.

POSSIBLE CLINICAL SCENARIOS TO
CHRONIC PROSTATITIS PRESENTATION

POSITIVE EPS ------------------------	NO SIGNIFICANT VOIDING SYMPTOMS/PSA < 1
POSITIVE EPS ------------------------	SIGNIFICANT VOIDING SYMPTOMS/PSA < 1
POSITIVE EPS ------------------------	**NO SIGNIFICANT VOIDING SYMPTOMS/** PSA ≥ 1
POSITIVE EPS ------------------------	SIGNIFICANT VOIDING SYMPTOMS/**PSA ≥ 1**

NOTES:

SIGNS & SYMPTOMS ASSOCIATED
WITH CHRONIC PROSTATITIS:

Perineal Discomfort/ Pain	Inguinal Discomfort/Pain	Lethargy
Penile Discomfort/Pain	Ejaculatory Discomfort/ Pain	Epididymal/Testicular Swelling
Burning on Urination	Hematuria (Microscopic)	Scrotal Discomfort/Pain (Including testicular)
Blood in the ejaculate	Voiding Symptoms	Dysuria (Pain/Stinging on Urination)
PSA ≥ 1	Irritability	Decreased Sexual Performance/Impotency
Depression	Hematuria (Gross)	

Prostatitis is a troubling disease that remains a health risk to most of the adult male population for far longer than is necessary. Frequently, men don't realize they have *prostatitis*, requiring a Prostate Specific Antigen (PSA) blood test to be performed to prove it. **A PSA of ≥ 1 ng/ml indicates *prostatitis*,** based on research presented at the NIH in 2000. Historically, men under 50 years old, with voiding symptoms or pelvic pain, had *prostatitis* until proven otherwise. Men over 50 years old, with the same symptoms, were assumed to have had an enlarged prostate (EP) or BPH. A study presented at the NIH in 1999 has shown that most men with voiding symptoms, regardless of age, actually had *prostatitis* when properly tested. In a trial of 235 consecutive men who exhibited even mild voiding symptoms, greater than 80% were found to have *chronic prostatitis,* regardless of their age based on an evaluation of the expressed prostatic secretion (EPS).

THE DIAGNOSIS:

Prostatitis has been termed **"the waste basket of clinical ignorance"** by prominent Stanford University Urologist-Emeritus Dr. Thomas Stamey because of the difficulty it presents in diagnosis and treatment. *Prostatitis* is usually identified or suggested by the symptoms it produces and the findings of a sore or tender prostate when a digital rectal examination is performed. Prostate Specific Antigen (PSA), a blood test designed to identify patients at risk for prostate cancer, will also be increased in most cases of *prostatitis.* The presence of a specific urinary tract infection, together with pelvic pain, fever, chills, rigors, voiding symptoms and a sore or tender prostate on rectal examination, will identify the 5% of patients with *acute bacterial prostatitis,* a true infection. Chronic bacterial *prostatitis* is also quite uncommon, but devoid of the acute symptoms including fever. While it would not be surprising to identify men with chronic *prostatitis* who have no symptoms at all, the PSA provides a virtual 100% sensitivity to predict the diagnosis when the PSA number is ≥ 1.0 ng/ml.

While obtaining an EPS requires some knowledge and skill on the part of the Care provider, the ability to perform this procedure is critical to the ability to obtain representative outcome data as well as judge the benefit of a treatment plan. To be sure, one should not expect a Urologist or Primary Care Physician to perform this test with any degree of accuracy or skill if they rarely perform it. **If you have concerns about prostatitis, you must go to a physician who is understands the importance of the EPS and understands how to get the specimen to be evaluated.** Unfortunately, most Urologists do not understand the disease or the diagnostic principles with significant clarity to assist you. When patients ask me how to find a doctor who performs the EPS procedure, I suggest they call the office and ask if the doctor(s) perform the test. If the receptionist hesitates with the response, they likely do not.

The prostatic secretion (fluid) is commonly obtained by gentle to moderate massage of the prostate during the digital rectal examination (DRE). The secretion is obtained from the tip of the urethra. When the secretion is examined under the microscope, a finding of ≥ 10 white blood cells per microscopic field (400X) is considered definitive proof of non-bacterial inflammation or *prostatitis*. Additionally, a histological examination of a prostate biopsy (a tissue sample) can also show definitive signs of inflammation and diagnose *prostatitis*. Unfortunately, inflammation tends to be under diagnosed when prostate biopsy specimens are reviewed by the Pathologist, based on its presence in virtually every tissue sample. Ultrasonographically, the presence of enhanced blood flow (seen commonly with color flow, power Doppler) in combination with calcium deposits herald the diagnosis of *prostatitis* as well. **Despite the fact that examination of the prostatic fluid or EPS makes the definitive diagnosis, the rare family physician and fewer than 10% of all Urologists perform it** because of difficulty in obtaining a proper sample, lack of interest, test complexity, lack of time, inadequate testing equipment, uncertainty of treatment or a lack of knowledge. In the busy world of a medical practice, uncertainty of treatment and a lack of time are likely the two most common reasons physicians prefer not to deal with this disease.

Based on challenges inherent with obtaining an accurate EPS, many physicians (including Urologists) have resorted to an evaluation of the post massage urine (VB-3) for the diagnosis of **prostatitis**. This concept has been popularized by Curtis Nickel, M.D. (Member of the **NIH Prostatitis Collaborative**) and others as an acceptable diagnostic alternative to the EPS. In an effort to validate the post massage urine as a surrogate diagnostic marker, a direct comparison of EPS and VB-3 was performed on 49 men believed to have **prostatitis** based on any degree of urinary symptoms and PSA (Reference the **EPS/ VB-3 Comparative Study** in the Appendix section of this book). In this study comparison, all 49 men had **prostatitis** based on a diagnostic EPS with a median white blood cell count of 145 WBCs/HPF (High Power Field) or (400X). The post massage urine (VB-3) performed immediately following the collection of the EPS noted a non-diagnostic median white blood cell count of 5-6 white blood cells/HPF. **Using ≥ 10 WBCs, as diagnostic for prostatitis, the VB-3 (post massage urine) missed 61% of patients with prostatitis.** In other words, a test that was heralded as an acceptable alternative for the EPS missed almost two thirds of patients with the disease that it was intending to diagnose.

For this reason, patients and physicians should be discouraged from using the VB-3 (post massage urine) as a definitive screening test for **prostatitis**. To restate, there are too many false negatives to suggest that this test has any redeeming diagnostic clinical value. On the other hand, if the pre-massage urine (a typical urinalysis) is compared to the post massage urine quantitatively for white blood cells, there is value to the test technique from a relative point of view. **In my opinion, any increase in the number of white blood cells per high power field from one specimen to another will identify prostatitis patients definitively when the PSA is ≥ 1.0 ng/ml.** Unfortunately, the mere diagnosis does not provide an adequate and dependable marker for follow up based on variability of massage technique from one office visit to another. Acceptance and clinical application of flawed test procedures by physicians merely underscores the ignorance and confusion that trickles down to the suffering patient. With a clear understanding of the above, patients empowered with this knowledge will be able to take a more active role in treatment decisions with their physician while ultimately improving their outcome. While nearly everyone recognizes that medicine is an inexact science, physicians are obligated to separate fact from fiction. In other words, **if a test fails significantly to identify the disease it is intended to find and cannot be reliably repeated, we should not use the test. Failure to understand this principle from a professional point of view merely widens the chasm of ignorance between the educated and the under-educated masses allowing confusion to remain rampant.**

In *prostatitis,* any combination of pelvic and urinary symptoms are possible, individually or concomitantly as well as the common presentation of an individual (with a PSA blood test result of ≥ 1.0 ng/ml), who is without pain, discomfort or urinary problems, yet still has *prostatitis,* based on an abnormal assessment of the prostatic fluid or EPS. **In other words, it is not unusual to have *prostatitis* without signs and symptoms common to the disease.** Our data shows conclusively that the PSA blood test is the most convenient marker to identify the presence of *prostatitis.* Furthermore, our research demonstrates the Sensitivity and Specificity of PSA as a diagnostic tool to be 100% when the PSA is ≥ 1.0 ng/ml.

THE ETIOLOGY (CAUSE) OF PROSTATITIS:	
—Viruses	—Idiopathic (Unknown) Factors
—Bacteria, Nanobacterium, Mycoplasma, Chlamydia	—Stress and Psychological Factors
—Yeast	—Immune System Related Disease (Including AutoImmune Diseases)
—Dietary Factors	—Social, Genetic or Environmental factors
—Crystal Deposition and Biofilms	—Any Combination of the Above

TREATMENT OPTIONS:

Treatment of **prostatitis** has been anything but a sure proposition. According to noted **prostatitis** expert Dr. Curtis Nickel of Kingston, Ontario and the NIH, **"there is widespread frustration, discomfort, and lack of knowledge in both primary care physicians and urologists' ability to manage prostatitis".**

Those patients who truly have an identifiable bacterial infection of the prostate (culture proven) will certainly benefit from antibiotics. Antibiotics may need to be continued for 2-6 weeks; while in rare cases, long-term or indefinite antibiotic suppression therapy may be necessary. We don't have any data that looks at recurrent disease over many years, but, it is believed by this author that **bacterial prostatitis may transition to non-bacterial prostatitis.**

Campbell's Urology, the Urologist's most authoritative reference text, identifies only about 5% of all patients with **prostatitis** as having a *bacterial component*, which can be "cured", at least in the short term, by antibiotics. In other words, 95% of men with **prostatitis** have little hope for a cure with antibiotics alone since they don't actually have any identifiable bacterial infection. As a male, it is wise to request a culture & sensitivity (proving bacterial **prostatitis**) of either the urine or EPS, before consenting to the use of antibiotics. While antibiotics are over used, if your doctor insists on an initial trial of antibiotics, despite your concerns, it may be most prudent to follow his instruction as he likely has your best interests in mind. Repeated trials of antibiotics are discouraged based on concern for suppression of the immune system and the possibility that a super-resistant organism may result, not to mention the needless expense.

In the treatment of **prostatitis**, physicians have traditionally recommended everything from doing nothing to multiple and extended courses of antibiotics, synthetic drugs and lifestyle changes. **It is not unusual to hear a doctor tell his/her patient that he needs to learn to live with it; referencing prostatitis.** Among the various treatment options; alpha blockers (Hytrin®, Rapaflo, Cardura®, Flomax® and Uroxatrol®) are designed to relax the muscle tension at the junction of the prostate and bladder neck region (like a hammock) to improve urinary flow. This class of drug does tend to improve voiding difficulties by relaxing tension at the bladder neck region (space between the prostate and the bladder); but are expensive, need to be taken indefinitely, may have significant side effects and don't cure the underlying problem or prevent prostate growth.

Finasteride (Proscar®) or Dutasteride (Avodart®), synthetic drugs that block the conversion of Testosterone to Dihydrotestosterone, can shrink prostate tissue but there is no proof it helps in the treatment of **prostatitis** as defined by decreasing white blood cells found in the prostate secretion. Allopurinol, a drug that reduces uric acid levels in the body, has been used to treat **prostatitis,** based on the theory that uric acid crystals may form in the prostate secondary to refluxing urine and cause inflammation. Most clinicians, who have tried Allopurinol for **prostatitis,** report disappointing results from this therapy. Anti-inflammatory agents (Motrin®, Alleve or Advil®) and hot sitz baths have been helpful in treating the discomfort caused by **prostatitis** in many patients, but neither of these treatments actually cures the disease and the benefits wear off rapidly. Irritative voiding symptoms may be relieved by a myriad of bladder relaxing agents such as oxybutynin (Ditropan®) or solifenacin succinate (Vesicare®), while anti-depressants such as amitriptyline (Elavil®) have been helpful in various chronic pain conditions such as *prostatitis* associated with depression. Nanobacterium (one hundredth the size of an E. Coli bacterium) has been postulated as a cause of prostate stone formation. Unfortunately, there is no definitive data to suggest that this microbe is problematic, much less a concern for prostatitis evolution. Biofeedback, behavioral therapy, referral to a pain clinic, and/or psychological treatment has been recommended for patients with *prostatitis* and occasionally offers some relief to selected individuals. For the most part, current treatment methods for *prostatitis* are generally rather disappointing.

Prostatic massage plus antibiotics deserves further review. Proponents of prostate massage (championed in the Philippines) have little reproducible data to support their enthusiasm. My personal experience with prostate massage demonstrates only temporary results with transient prostate size reduction and relief from congestion. Unfortunately, long-term benefit for the resolution of *prostatitis* based on prostate massage (as measured by EPS), over time, is unrealistic and is not likely to occur. Other drawbacks include intense discomfort/pain at the time of massage, the need for accurate cultures of the prostatic fluid and a dependence on antibiotics to ultimately affect the cure.

Dr. John Krieger, noted Urologist at the University of Washington and member of the Prostatitis Collaborative at the NIH, appropriately **points out the following multiple factors preclude accuracy of the culture technique involving urine, semen or prostatic secretion for diagnosing or treating** *prostatitis:*

1. **The presence of inhibitory substances**
2. **The unknown effects of many previous courses of antibiotics**

3. The fact that most bacteria from the prostate do not readily grow on conventional culture media
4. The high number of uncharacterized bacteria that infect human prostate tissue
5. There is inherent difficulty in obtaining a pure specimen from the prostate, which has not been contaminated by possible infectious organisms of the urethra or urinary passage
6. The fact that most cases of *prostatitis* are not infections in the first place

NOTES:

CHRONIC NON-BACTERIAL PROSTATITIS OPTIONS:					
PRODUCT OR PROCEDURE	**Effects on LUTS** (lower urinary tract symptoms) **Voiding Symptoms**	**EFFECTS ON PSA**	**EFFECTS ON EPS**	**ABILITY TO CURE**	**IMPROVED SEXUAL PERFORMANCE**
Antibiotics	Possible	Yes	No	No	No
Avodart/Proscar	Yes	Yes	No	No	No
Alpha—Blockade (Hytrin, Rapaflo, Cardura, Flomax and Uroxatral)	Yes	No	No	No	No; also causes retrograde ejaculation commonly
Peenuts® (all natural Patented formula)	Yes	Yes	Yes	Yes	Yes; secondary to prostatitis resolution
Surgery	Yes	Yes	Possible	Possible	No
Chronic Prostatitis is non-bacterial in ≥ 95% of all cases					

PROSTATE SPECIFIC ANTIGEN (PSA) AND PROSTATITIS:

Prostate Specific Antigen (PSA), referenced earlier, was originally designed as a blood test for prostate cancer surveillance. Historically, PSA blood levels of 0-4 were designated as "normal", but this range was arbitrarily selected and never meant to become gospel for normalcy; therefore, does not necessarily indicate a healthy prostate. ***Prostatitis* represents the number one reason that PSA elevates.** Additionally, we know that up to 30% of all prostate cancers occur in patients with PSA levels less than 4.0 ng/ml. Since prostate cancer obviously cannot be considered normal, this suggests that the original "normal" PSA range of 0-4 ng/ml is much too high. It's been suggested that any PSA level greater than or equal to 1.0 ng/ml indicates an unhealthy prostate, with active ***prostatitis,*** as confirmed by an NIH presentation in 2000 (R. Wheeler). Data from a Johns Hopkins white paper from 2002 corroborates the importance of PSA to prostate cancer. **Based in part on the Baltimore Longitudinal Data, Ballentine Carter and colleagues confirmed a 3-4 fold** increased incidence of prostate cancer development in men aged 40-60, when the PSA level was in excess of 0.6-0.7 ng/ml. Peter Gann and colleagues have shown through their research that a PSA between 2.0-4.0 ng/ml is associated with a 5-9 times increased incidence of an aggressive cancer within the subsequent 10 years. This is sobering data that predicts disease and must be understood; even though many men choose to be unknowing and/or ignorant regarding prostate disease markers rather than choosing a proactive or preventative course of action.

As noted earlier, it's well known that ***prostatitis*** increases the PSA level. In fact, it is much more likely that any unexplained increase in PSA level is due to ***prostatitis*** than to BPH or prostate cancer. A few Urologists commonly treat their patients with high PSA levels with 4-6 weeks of antibiotics and repeat the PSA level before recommending a biopsy when the DRE (digital rectal exam) findings are non-diagnostic. In this scenario, only if the second PSA level remains elevated will a biopsy be ordered. **My approach to this clinical scenario would be to recommend imaging for all patients, thereby replacing biopsy. Moreover, instead of antibiotics (unless a bacterial infection is isolated); I would recommend the patented *prostatitis* formula, Peenuts®.** A minimum of 6-12 months on this nutritional formula would be required to adequately make an impact on a disease that may be worsening at the time the patient is first evaluated.

I believe that a significant percentage of any elevation in PSA level in the blood (associated with a normal digital prostate examination) should be considered ***prostatitis*** until proven otherwise. This is based on the fact that 70-80% of all biopsies are negative when an elevated PSA is encountered. While prostate cancer is certainly a concern and should be considered carefully and appropriately, ***prostatitis*** is much more likely from a statistical point of view. PSA can serve as a very useful marker or indicator of the degree of prostatic inflammation present and help determine the effectiveness of *prostatitis* therapy through comparative testing.

THE LINK BETWEEN CHRONIC PROSTATITIS AND PROSTATE CANCER:

Virtually all men will develop *prostatitis* at some point in their adult lifetime. This has been shown in several studies including one done in 1979 by Drs. Kohnen and Drach who found 98.1% of 162 prostates removed surgically (for prostate cancer) had evidence of inflammation (*prostatitis*). Dr. Timothy Moon, Urologist at the University of Wisconsin, and many others, report that virtually 100% of the biopsy and surgical prostate specimens they examine show evidence of *prostatitis*.

Compounding the issues, virtually all men eventually get prostate cancer if they live long enough. In 2004, according to the American Cancer Society (ACS), 32,000 men died from prostate cancer; while over 232,000 new cases were diagnosed. Prostate cancer is the most common malignancy to affect men and the second leading cause of cancer death in men (lung cancer is first). In the United States, one in four men who undergo prostate biopsy will be found to have prostate cancer, but all of them will have *prostatitis*. These findings have led Dr. Timothy Moon and others to suggest that prostate cancer is always associated with *prostatitis*.

Young men in their thirties typically are quite prone to *prostatitis* and are not generally thought to be at risk for prostate cancer. But a study from Memorial Sloan-Kettering Cancer Center, in New York, found that 30% of 525 American men aged 30-39 actually had microscopic prostate cancer. Is it postulated then that *chronic* **prostatitis** may increase the risk for and/or promote the growth of prostate cancer? There is evidence that suggests this may be so. The importance of this data is confirmed by the Detroit Autopsy Study, headed up by Weil Sakr, which corroborated that 30% of 30-year-old men had *prostatitis* and prostate cancer.

It is well known that chronic inflammation of several other organs is associated with various cancers. Examples include but are not limited to: the inflammation of the lower esophagus (Barrett's Esophagitis), which leads to esophageal cancer, hepatitis that may lead eventually to hepatic cancer and ulcerative colitis, which often develops into colon cancer. Since chronic inflammation causes cancer in other organs, it is not unreasonable to suggest that chronic prostate inflammation *(prostatitis)*, if left unattended, may ultimately lead to prostate cancer. This concept has been demonstrated more clearly by the American Association of Cancer Research (AACR) and corroborated independently by David Bostwick, M.D., world-renowned Pathologist. Specifically, the AACR has shown that *prostatitis* (an inflammatory disease) represents cellular oxidative stress resulting in cellular dysplasia, proliferative inflammatory atrophy, subsequent cellular mutation associated with changes in DNA (Deoxyribonucleic Acid), prostatic intraepithelial neoplasia (PIN), and ultimately prostate cancer.

Prostate cancer is always found together with *prostatitis* while all men will probably get both diseases if they live long enough. Both prostate cancer and *prostatitis* raise Prostate Specific Antigen (PSA) levels and occur most often in men in their 60s. Both conditions are currently at epidemic, if not pandemic levels. While prostate cancer and *chronic prostatitis* are clearly associated, further research and epidemiologic studies are required to add additional clarity to the exact nature of the relationship.

Based upon the now well-recognized association between Prostatitis and Prostate Cancer, *prostatitis* resolution is a key component to Chronic Disease Management (CDM). CDM is a competing option to more traditional therapies that allows men to live with their cancer, while preventing Impotency, Incontinence and the stigma of failure to cure. **Living with prostate cancer is realistic and is analogous to living with Arthritis or Diabetes.** Living with prostate cancer becomes more attractive when it is realized that successful intervention for cure (replete with the negative side effects) adds only 3 years to the life expectancy of a man in his 50s, 1.5 years to a man in his 60s and 0.4 years to a man in his 70s. This data comes from the elegant work of Michael Barry and colleagues at Harvard. For many prostate cancer patients, the risk of treatment failure is often too big of a gamble to take. Thus, as the male becomes better informed through prediction nomograms (statistical clinical models) and up-to-date treatment outcome data, an attempt at formal therapy may lose some of its luster, as quality of life takes center stage and becomes the dominant issue for our remaining years.

THE LINK BETWEEN PROSTATITIS AND INFERTILITY:

The inflammatory process of ***prostatitis*** has been shown to affect sperm quality primarily by decreasing the motility of sperm. Couples who are trying to conceive a child should look at the very real possibility of prostatitis treatment as the most cost effective and best "first step" to improving sperm quality. While the identification of ≥ 10 white blood cells in the prostate secretion is sine qua non for the diagnosis of ***prostatitis***, the presence of any white blood cells in a sperm sample (ejaculate) would also herald the presence of concurrent disease in most cases. Additionally, my clinical acumen suggests that a PSA blood test result of ≥ 0.5 ng/ml may also be associated commonly with ***prostatitis*** and decreased fertility. (Please review data regarding my patented natural remedy Peenuts® for resolution of signs and symptoms consistent with prostatitis).

CONTEMPORARY RESEARCH:

Present research dollars in **prostatitis** are so few, that at our present pace generations will come and go with countless innocent men suffering and possibly dying needlessly (related to prostate cancer developing from inflammation) before the true answers are known. A reflection of the paucity of academic support to **prostatitis** research is noted with the 1998 National Convention of the American Urological Association, (attended by American and International Urology experts). Specifically, 51% of all the papers and studies presented involved prostate cancer, while only 3% addressed **prostatitis**. The trend has not changed since then. While a few studies relevant to antibiotics as a treatment for bacterial **prostatitis** are underway (funded largely by a pharmaceutical industry that manufactures antibiotics), there is virtually no other significant research currently being done in the United States on this disease. Clearly, there is no disease topic more worthy of research and research dollars than the number one health risk that men face. Whether we are speaking about **prostatitis,** enlarged prostate (EP) or prostate cancer; these diseases are individually and collectively epidemic while individually and collectively equally germane to male health and wellness.

To state further, practically every man alive has **prostatitis,** making it one of the world's most common diseases, if not the most common. Diagnosis is difficult and current treatments are frequently inadequate. The association between **prostatitis** and prostate cancer is irrefutable. With all this in mind, it is particularly disturbing that **prostatitis** research has been so significantly under-funded for years. Leroy Nyberg, M.D., associated with Urology Research for the National Institutes of Health (NIH) has stated: **"It's amazing to me that we can't reliably treat the majority of men with *prostatitis".*** The NIH has organized a research arm that expects to bring a fresh look to *chronic **prostatitis,*** but the results of this research are not expected for many years, if ever. **Today, *chronic prostatitis* for many represents an enigma, but clearly qualifies as the single most under diagnosed, misunderstood and inappropriately treated medical disease in the world.**

In an effort to demonstrate the impact of ***prostatitis*** resolution to the evolution of prostate cancer, **I have proposed the "ProCap" (Prostate Cancer Prevention) Trial.** This is a randomized, double blind, placebo controlled, age matched study that is intended to prove the patented Peenuts® ***prostatitis*** formula can prevent prostate cancer by resolving ***prostatitis.*** **This study, intended to underscore the importance of inflammation resolution to an avoidance of prostate cancer, is the most ambitious effort to date to establish validation for prostate nutrition in men's health.** As noted earlier in this article, the American Association of Cancer Research, Pathologist, David Bostwick, M.D. and others have shown that ***prostatitis*** evolves into prostate cancer. While this study seeks funding, the concept grew out of clinically significant results from a Prospective Prostate Cancer Study that showed benefit of diet and nutrition on men with moderately well differentiated prostate cancer (Gleason 5/6). **Specifically, 90% of men enrolled in the study (n=23), noted suppression of their PSA (the marker of disease activity) over a surveillance period in excess of 40 months.** The remaining 10% noted stable disease. While the study findings suggest that 50-60% of all prostate cancer cases (consistent with a Gleason scores of 5 or 6) are being over treated with traditional treatments, the Prospective Study was a designed effort to prove that ***prostatitis*** resolution (partial or complete) with the Peenuts® formula would have an impact on prostate cancer. In this study, the improvement in the white blood cell count associated with the EPS (the most significant biological representation for **prostatitis** resolution) was noted to be 73% which mirrors the 66% reduction in white cells (based on previous clinical research) presented to the US Patent & Trademark Office regarding the patent application which was granted in 2001.

THE PROSTATE BIOPSY REVOLVING DOOR:

The inability to maintain a normal PSA (less than 4.0 ng/ml for most labs) will put you (the patient) in a unique group of men asked to consider a biopsy of the prostate. **Men unique to this group who fail to stabilize the PSA (less than 4.0 ng/ml) will become the hunted.** Once the biopsy scheduling (merry-go-round) begins, it is difficult to prevent subsequent biopsies! It is PSA anxiety that drives repeat biopsies in the absence of a cancerous result. As doctors, it is important to find disease, seemingly at any cost, in men who will benefit the most from our therapies. If your PSA is high ($\geq$ 4.0 ng/ml), your prostate will become the target of a biopsy needle with virtually any Urologist you meet, except me. **Therefore, your only defense is to be proactive and know your PSA number! If your doctor says it is fine . . . ask what the number is and take a copy of the PSA with you for your records. To be healthy, your PSA must be minimally less than 1.0, while preferably less than 0.5 ng/ml; like mine! For the record, my PSA has been flat-lined for more than 10 years at 0.3 ng/ml, consistent with a healthy prostate (0.2 ng/ml is the same as 0.00 statistically speaking)!**
While my thought process might be an exception to the traditional urologist, there are basic principles that need to be

applied when a clinical scenario presents itself as concerning for prostate cancer. In my clinical practice, men with a non-cancerous digital prostate examination can defer the biopsy and definitive imaging when prostatitis is identified and the PSA value is less than 5.0 ng/ml. Conservative management is the preferred and recommended treatment course, when added to proper diet, appropriate nutrition, adequate exercise, stress reduction and education. Obviously, the Peenuts® prostate nutritional formula is an integral and proven part of the program. The inability to resolve the disease as determined by a normalized or stable PSA will put us back at square one where the biopsy becomes the diagnostic choice of most urologists! **For me, a 3 T MRI scan is the best objective marker to a diagnosis of prostate cancer.**

A classic example of a patient's experience in the traditional doctor's office involves a 65-year-old man from Lubbock, Texas who had noted a PSA of 18 ng/ml. His 'traditional' Urologist appropriately offered and performed an ultrasound examination and prostate biopsy. The biopsy result noted *chronic **prostatitis*** with no evidence of cancer. Antibiotics were ordered despite the lack of a positive culture and sensitivity, with no other therapy considered. **Remember that less than 5% of cases of *prostatitis* are actually caused by bacteria; potentially curable with antibiotics.** His PSA was repeated after 6 months and found to be unchanged. The patient underwent a second prostate biopsy, at the doctor's insistence, which again showed only *chronic **prostatitis.*** When the patient asked his doctor what he could do, the urologist offered to repeat the PSA in another 6 months and consider an additional biopsy at that time. This is a clinical scenario that is all too common across the United States every day, whereby, men are given no alternative in an attempt to avoid a future biopsy. Clearly, this patient would have benefited with an MRI scan using a 3.0 Tesla magnet. I believe, as physicians, we must become better educated regarding relevant scientific concepts that may radically change the diagnostic or treatment course of any patient. Far too many men are asked to return to the biopsy arena over and over, without a well thought out, patient-friendly strategy or "master plan". In this case, the patient was aware enough to research *prostatitis* on the Internet. Eventually, he discovered a nutritional product that improved his urinary symptoms substantially and reduced his PSA by almost half in only 3 months. This was accomplished by merely using Peenuts®, the advanced nutritional therapy for the prostate, which he was able to purchase without a prescription! While this patient's response was outstanding, not all patients respond identically. **The use of the Peenuts® formula is not intended to replace the advice of your doctor but your thoughts (as a patient) will play a role in the physician's decision.**

Another equally riveting case involved a 75 year old male who had experienced five previous biopsies (all negative) associated with a PSA of 22.6 ng/ml. Using only Avodart® (Dutasteride) and the Peenuts® prostate nutritional formula, his PSA dropped to 7.88 ng/ml by the end of 11 months and 5.1 ng/ml at 24 months. Without the presence of prostate cancer, Avodart® would have been expected to cut the PSA in half (11.3 ng/ml). The improvement to 5.1 ng/ml is exceptional and validates further the benefit of the Peenuts® nutritional formula related to the resolution of *prostatitis*. Furthermore, his EPS decreased from 400 WBCs to 130 WBCs in only 9 months. While this approach likely shows the benefit of Avodart® and Peenuts® in combination, the need for additional biopsies is now gone as the patient's prostate health status has improved markedly. While further studies with this treatment protocol are encouraged, the expectation remains high that similar results will be forthcoming.

CLOSING THOUGHTS:

To declare your prostate healthy, your PSA must be less than 1.0 ng/ml with a complete absence of urinary symptoms; To Check your PSA (as a screening test only) in the comfort of your home, call today for your **PSA "Diagnostic Home Kit"**—Toll Free: 1-866-PSA-CHEK (772-2435).

A PSA of ≥ 1 indicates an unhealthy prostate. It is obvious that the lower the PSA, the lower the risk of prostate cancer. Anything you can do to lower your PSA level will likely reduce your risk of eventually getting prostate cancer.

Keep track of your PSA level for your own records. The risk is too high if you do not! Never accept the words from a doctor that your PSA is normal or nothing to worry about unless it is truly less than 1.0 and stable. If your PSA is 1.0 or higher, your brain must not accept what you have just heard, because most doctors do not know the real facts and do not keep up. **You must know the number!!!** If your PSA is between 1.0-4 ng/ml, there is a 20-30% chance prostate cancer exists. Likewise, if your PSA is between 4.1-10.0 ng/ml, there is a 20-30% chance that prostate cancer is present. Given this data, the healthiest number for you is a PSA of less than one; remembering that prostate cancer has been reported with a PSA of less than one, as well, but the odds of not having cancer with such a low number are in your favor.

Have your PSA and digital rectal examination performed regularly, usually at least every year for men aged 30 or older. Get the PSA on your birthday so you can remember! **You must know that 30% of 30 year old men have prostate cancer.** This is referenced in the research from Memorial Sloan-Kettering and Weil Sakr's work with the Detroit Autopsy Study! Men at greater than average risk for prostate cancer, such as men of African-American descent and men with a positive family history of prostate cancer should be checked yearly starting at age 30 with a PSA blood test minimally. Men with known elevations in their PSA levels and those with inconclusive or "suspicious" previous biopsies may need to be checked more often.

Don't be afraid to ask questions of your physician or get a second opinion about your prostate health. A true professional will take the time to answer your questions and be open to suggestions about alternative therapies as well as be willing to follow you clinically.

Research from the American Association of Cancer Research (AACR) and others indicate **the link between *prostatitis* and prostate cancer is real!** Practically all men with *prostatitis* will eventually get prostate cancer (if we live long enough) as the diseases are commonly found together. **Remember, understanding *prostatitis* is your best first step to helping yourself.**

Learn all you can about *prostatitis* and treat it as aggressively and effectively as possible. Peenuts® may be your best and least expensive initial opportunity to establish and/or maintain prostate health and may delay or even prevent the development of prostate cancer. Validation will be identified by any combination of biologic disease marker improvement, as determined by a decrease in PSA, a decrease in EPS and/or a decrease in Urinary Symptoms.

Be aware that your physician may not be an expert on the treatment of *prostatitis*. Ask him about the various validated diagnostic tests and therapies available and which ones are appropriate for you.

For more information on Peenuts® and other nutritional products for the prostate, call **SunVita™ at 1-888-733-6887** or log onto the Peenuts® website at **www.Peenuts.com**. Also, check out the National Institutes of Health (NIH) Website (**www.nih.**

gov) for more general information on *prostatitis* and prostate cancer research.

EDITORIAL COMMENT:

By Stephen W. Leslie, MD FACS (Urologist and Chairman of the Department of Urology at Creighton Medical School)

The widespread incidence of prostatitis is well known to urologists and other doctors, but its association with prostate cancer has previously been considered incidental. In this chapter, Dr. Wheeler has suggested that prostatitis may actually cause prostate cancer based on evidence supportive of inflammation leading to cancer consistent with a number of other organ cancers, the research of the American Association of Cancer Research, David Bostwick, Michael Karin, PhD and others. While the association alone between these two conditions may fall short of being considered definitive, it is certainly plausible and deserves more study. **Even a limited causative link between prostatitis and prostate cancer would cause a dramatic change in our attitude and approach to prostatitis.**

Currently, prostatitis therapy consists primarily of antibiotics, alpha blockers and other drugs. This chapter correctly points out that these remedies are often inadequate. Dr. Wheeler recommends considering nutritional agents in the absence of successful definitive therapy. **Although nutritional therapy has been widely used and studied in Europe, it is not routinely recommended by many U.S. physicians for a number of reasons.** Nutritional therapy is not taught in most U.S. medical schools and many American physicians are unfamiliar with the available scientific research on the subject. Published studies on nutritional therapy are criticized for using different preparations and dosages, having too small a sample size with limited numbers of participants, being of inadequate duration, and bias in the selection of patients to be tested. Commercially available nutritional therapies are usually not manufactured to a pharmaceutical grade standard, which means each bottle, even from the same company, may have different biological effects. There is no universally accepted dosing schedule for many of these natural remedies and their mechanism of action is often unknown. Further, no specific combination nutritional product for either prostatitis or symptoms of prostate enlargement has ever been properly tested in a well-designed, scientific study.

Dr. Wheeler describes a study he performed at the Diagnostic Center for Disease™ on a unique combination nutritional therapy called Peenuts®. He reports outstanding objective and clinical results, but the scientific details of his research need to be carefully reviewed and his findings duplicated by other medical experts. **If further research indicates he has indeed found a safe and highly effective therapy for the signs and symptoms of prostatitis and prostate enlargement, this would be a major contribution to the health and wellbeing of American men while saving the health care system tens of millions of dollars. Further elaboration of the prostatitis to prostate cancer model would qualify as a major medical breakthrough. Minimally, Dr. Wheeler's research offers a unique patented formula with little downside with a potentially tremendous upside for motivated men.**

CHAPTER THREE

Chronic Disease Management

~Defining the Role of Integrative Medicine in
Prostate Cancer Prevention and Treatment~

PROSTATE CANCER TREATMENT means different things to different people. While all traditional therapies are judged on patient survival statistics, there is very little difference among the various therapies relevant to this point. Based on the fact that men will generally live 15 plus years regardless of the treatment rendered when prostate cancer is diagnosed, it may be more appropriate to be speaking about quality of life while living with a disease using a chronic disease management (CDM) strategy whenever possible. Surely, we want to live long productive lives but who among us wants to live life at any cost? It is one thing to make a concession to have our sexual abilities compromised and yet another to tolerate wet undergarments or pants from a stress-provoking procedure like lifting a daughter, a grandson, a granddaughter or suitcase. But it is, nonetheless, a completely different story when we are told the disease saga continues as witnessed by a rising PSA (prostate specific antigen), despite a definitive therapy. This is a sacrifice we did not bargain for; this was not the way we were told it would be. Depression, despair, anxiety, anger, frustration, fear and devastation are a few of the emotions and conditions that you must live with. Whom can you turn to with this high degree of despair and frustration? The truth is there are very few salvage concepts (treatments with hope) that can effectively give you a new "lease on life." The uncertainty of survival and cure heightens as the Gleason score rises. In other words, a Gleason score of 7 (3+4 or 4+3), 8 (4+4), 9 (4+5 or 5+4) and 10 (5+5) are associated with immense uncertainty and a lack of predictability with definitive treatment procedures. To state more clearly, these disease states are predictably unpredictable. It is this dilemma that suggests a treatment concept like chronic disease management (CDM) that integrates complementary and traditional medical disciplines.

Chronic disease management (most closely aligned with active surveillance) is defined by a unique, highly successful integration and application of various treatment modalities representing multiple mechanisms of action versus prostate cancer. Patients with a Gleason score of 6 (3+3) represent the ideal candidate to live with the disease, much like people living with rheumatoid arthritis or diabetes. This concept has been validated by the peer-reviewed research article entitled, **"Is it necessary to cure prostate cancer when it is possible?"** This article is referenced in this book. The protocol speaks to proper diet, appropriate nutrition, adequate exercise, stress management and continuing education as the keys to health and/or management of a disease. The diet of choice is a modified Mediterranean cuisine where the primary objective is to decrease Arachidonic Acid (AA) from the diet. Arachidonic Acid is problematic as it is pro-inflammatory, thereby favoring cellular oxidation and free radical formation. It also increases cancer cell proliferation and aggressiveness when present.

Controversial Ingredients that should be avoided

Inflammation as example, such as joint aches and pain commonly referred to as arthritis is nurtured by dietary indiscretion primarily associated with fatty acid consumption and/or abuse. To reduce AA most markedly, I principally recommend an avoidance of fats associated with red meat (beef, pork and lamb) and dairy (milk, cheese, ice cream and egg yolks). Similarly, it is necessary to reduce carbohydrates and simple sugars; food stuffs cancer preferentially feed on. Nutritionally, I try to limit consumption of nutrients of marginal value while avoiding controversial ingredients/supplements including Flax, Chondroitin, Beta-Carotene, Lycopene and Co-enzyme Q10. It is my belief, nutrient distributors have taken advantage of the purported benefit associated with many nutritionals and have applied a less than credible sales promotional program for almost everything on their shelves. Personal belief or folklore commonly replaces facts. Unfortunately, this dilutes the veracity of nutrient products or formulas while building an army of skeptics. Far too many consumers are gullible when they think nutritional supplements alone can turn around years of toxicity, disease and aging by wiping the "proverbial slate" clean. Selective nutritionals provide a valued component to systemic health for various disease signs and symptoms, however, are often times overmatched when facing a full blown disease like prostate cancer. Therefore, it is for this reason that I think nutritionals generally contribute far more in disease prevention models as well as an adjunct to traditional medicine. Therefore, be realistic and don't ask too much of your nutritionals. While it is never too late to make an impact with your health, the contribution of nutritionals should be well defined in dose and purpose while toxic doses are to be avoided. If you think a little bit of something does well by you, don't fall into the abyss of ignorance thinking that more is better.

I have witnessed a rejuvenation of hundreds, if not thousands, of patients realizing that what is done for one organ affects all other organ systems as well. To state further, a diseased organ is generally the result of systemic mismanagement related to diet, nutrition, exercise and stress. It is important to remember, while we treat the diseased organ, we must not treat that organ at the expense of another. While we are all familiar with side effects associated with traditional medications, the same concept can occur with nutritionals. In effect, because we do not treat disease in a vacuum, we must be mindful of the advantages and disadvantages of everything we consume including nutritionals. You will learn later in this book why the controversial ingredients mentioned above should be limited, if not eliminated from your diet.

To state further, chronic disease management (CDM) embraces the integration of complementary medicine (for example, nutritional supplements) and traditional medicine through multi-modality, multi-mechanistic approaches that begin with the resolution of inflammation and ends with the elimination of disease. As you will see, these same principles, when applied to prostate cancer, can change the course of the disease dramatically. Controlling inflammation is not as easy as turning a light switch off. There are a series of events, whereby inflammation is associated with a veritable control panel of switches that must be managed internally. In effect for every action, there is a reaction or response changing the dynamics or pathway of inflammation. Controlling for Arachidonic Acid may be the single most important concept or best first step. Therefore, I cannot overstate the importance of reducing inflammation to the overall health of a patient. Any successful health program must include a mechanism to reduce, if not eliminate inflammatory processes. **While no one seems surprised by the revelation that prostatitis (prostate inflammation) evolves to prostate cancer, it is equally important to avoid inflammatory promoting food groups associated with saturated fats and Omega 6 fatty acids.** Suffice it to say, it is important to consume a diet rich in nutrients that potentiate cell vitality while blocking enzymes that enhance cellular oxidation or destruction. This would include Cyclo-oxygenase (COX) and Lipoxygenase (LOX) as catalysts to inflammation through oxidation mechanisms. The expected end result is to decrease the production of Eicosandoids called Prostaglandin E-2 and Leukotrienes principally. Individuals interested in learning more about the topic of inflammation with its biochemical algorithms are urged to consult references that speak to these concepts.

Also, encouraged in a CDM protocol is tea, primarily green tea but also black. Tea is replete with powerful antioxidants that discourage prostate cancer cells from growing while preserving the integrity of the cell. Tea is believed to be a natural alternative to Celebrex, a popular anti-arthritic prescription medication. Specifically, tea is a beverage rich in Polyphenols including Epigallocatechin Gallate (EGCG) representing an anti-oxidative mechanism that blocks the COX II enzyme when consumed in sufficient quantity as a beverage or when taken as an extract. If individuals enjoy tea, I generally recommend 2-3 cups of warm tea daily served with a wedge of lemon squeezed into the tea to stabilize the active compounds. Celebrex, on the other hand, provides a predictable pharmaceutical dose, with predictable results, in altering cellular oxidative reactions. In many patients who are experiencing signs and symptoms of arthritis, I often encourage the use of a non-controversial dose of Celebrex at 200 mg/day. To state further, Celebrex is patented to block the COX II enzyme, thereby predictably blocking one pathway to joint pain and/or cancer growth. Similarly, reducing the inflammatory process of prostatitis is also critical to the success of my CDM protocol based on the viable pathway of prostatitis evolution to prostate cancer. Prostatitis arguably represents the most common and significant site of inflammation in all men. Even for men who have had their prostates removed, the *Peenuts®* formula makes sense based on its various mechanisms of action (anti-inflammatory, anti-oxidant and immune boosting). **My preference, however, for men who have had a prostatectomy or radiation is to consider UroStar™, a sister product to Peenuts® but more comprehensive systemically and less organ specific.** Research data is available in the appendix to show the benefit of the *Peenuts®* formula versus biological markers (PSA, EPS and voiding symptoms) associated with prostatitis.

Bill Nelson, M.D., noted cancer research specialist at Johns Hopkins, has described in his research how carcinogenic stimuli (for example, heterocyclic cancer causing compounds like charred meat off the grill) require a site of inflammation to begin a genetic and bio-molecular transformation into cancer. Not surprisingly in men, the prostate gland provides the most prolific and widespread example of an inflammatory process that virtually all men experience throughout their lifetimes. For this reason, one should not be surprised that prostate cancer is also the most prolific cancer that men get.

Vitamin D is recommended in the form of Vitamin D3. Unfortunately, experts in Vitamin D biochemistry do not agree or uniformly understand with validated confidence (based on research data) how much Vitamin D3 is required in the diet or nutritionally available through supplements to achieve an absolute recommended dose requirement. These concerns, notwithstanding, I generally recommend a minimum of 5,000-10,000 units of Vitamin D3 taken daily. Vitamin D, in its active form, has been shown to decrease prostate cancer cellular proliferation. Obviously, support for this mechanism of action does not require further explanation when I am speaking to a man with prostate cancer.

When men experience voiding symptoms that are not allayed by the *Peenuts®* formula alone at either 2 or 3 capsules per day, I would recommend Uroxatral (an alpha 1a inhibitor) at 10 mg/day. The benefit of this recommendation is based on the relative frequency of bladder neck hypertrophy in middle aged to older men. In this scenario, the bladder neck cannot relax, thereby slowing the passage of urine. The reason I favor Uroxatral over Flomax is based on studies that have shown this formulation to cause cellular apoptosis (cell death) in prostate tissue. This can only be a favorable process when either prostate cancer or an enlarged prostate (EP) is suspected. While a common side effect can be mild lethargy for the first week or so and retrograde ejaculation, most men tolerate this drug quite well.

Omega 3 fatty acids are discussed in the diet section but it bears repeating that Omega 3 fatty acids are essential for both males and females as we balance our Omega 6 (dietary component) to Omega 3 ratio systematically; closer to a 1 to 1 ratio. Noting the typical American diet produces a ratio of Omega 6 to Omega 3 closer to 20 to 1, any improvement in the consumption of Omega 3s will have a positive impact. It is important to remember that Omega 3 fatty acids are pro-health while Omega 6 fatty acids are pro-inflammatory. Research has been reported that suggests that Omega 3 fatty acids inhibit the proliferation or growth of prostate cancer cells in addition to decreasing the inflammatory process. Associated with the cardiovascular system is a decrease in plaque formation associated with a decrease in the oxidation of cholesterol. For these reasons, Omega 3 fatty acids, not found in a normal diet, must remain a part of your daily routine.

It is not uncommon for men with prostate cancer to have difficulty controlling their cholesterol. Frankly, many men with prostate cancer are overweight. This is based primarily on poor dietary and exercise habits. If men cannot improve the LDL and HDL components as well as decrease cholesterol and triglycerides, I commonly recommend an anti-cholesterolemic medication while monitoring the lipid panel using the Vertical Auto Profile (VAP), a comprehensive lipid analysis. As a side benefit, many medications that decrease cholesterol also provide a mechanism of anti-angiogenesis (decrease new blood vessel formation). Clearly, this type of medication, if indicated for cholesterol, adds another mechanism of action versus prostate cancer proliferation, as cancer requires blood flow to expand its base of operation.

Why Should I Use Avodart?

Based on the findings of the Prostate Cancer Prevention Trial (PCPT), I recommend Avodart daily at .5 mg. Avodart is the obvious choice to me as it inhibits type 1, type 2 and even type 3 isoenzymes of 5-alpha Reductase. This is the enzyme that predominantly enables the conversion of testosterone to Dihydrotestosterone (DHT), remembering that prostate cancer prefers DHT for maximal growth potential. In effect, when the enzyme is blocked, the cancer can only access the least potent form of testosterone. By virtue of this action, it is believed that the aggressiveness of the cancerous process is diminished. Furthermore, this class of drug is pro-apoptotic (enables cell death) while decreasing the size of the prostate by 20-30 percent. **In our Prospective Diet and Nutritional Prostate Cancer Study, it is my belief this class of drug creates an additive effect relative to prostate cancer suppression complementing the prostate nutritional formula *Peenuts*®.** Research continues in an effort to establish statistical benefit with this concept. This class of drug also makes sense in men with voiding symptoms and a prostate gland volume of greater than 30 grams.

When to Use an Antiandrogen

Beyond these various mechanisms, it is my preference to reserve an anti-androgen for those patients who don't respond to a conservative dietary and nutritional regimen. Rather than begin an anti-androgen or an LHRH-analog at the first sign of disease or disease recurrence (example—a rising PSA) following a failed treatment, I support the various mechanisms of action described previously to benefit the patient with a preference to never allow the PSA to go above 10.0 ng/ml. As you will see throughout this book and in my Prospective Diet and Nutritional Prostate Cancer Study, this may be all that is needed. **While patients familiar with my protocol will have the option to validate their success using the 3 Tesla MRI scan (with its various sequences) while avoiding repeat biopsies, those who cannot contain the disease as witnessed by a rising PSA approximating 10 ng/ml, will begin a short trail of an anti-androgen using either Casodex (bicalutamide) or Flutamide.** The anti-androgen will generally continue for 4-6 weeks allowing the PSA to drop commonly to 1 ng/ml or lower at which point the anti-androgen singularly, will be discontinued. This pattern can continue intermittently and indefinitely until a decision is made to perform a more definitive procedure, thereby rolling the dice for a chance at cure. Notwithstanding, the success of the CDM approach, it is not uncommon for the educated patient to take a run at the disease with a definitive form of therapy at some point in time. Notwithstanding the consideration of traditional therapies like prostatectomy and radiation, newer and less traditional treatment concepts like high-intensity focused ultrasound (**HIFU**) may be poised as a technology to dominate the treatment landscape as an effective, yet conservative, patient friendly, treatment for prostate cancer. While not yet approved by the FDA in the United States as of this writing, the early trials on HIFU from Europe, Mexico and Canada demonstrate results that provide evidence of a complete kill of cancer cells in the prostate while preserving sexual, urinary and bowel function. Likewise, this has commonly been my experience with the HIFU technique in treating patients for many years. Beyond this therapy, other patients have commonly chosen brachytherapy or cryotherapy as reasonable less morbid procedures than radical prostatectomy.

Patient Case Presentation with CDM

An example of the benefit achieved with the Chronic Disease Management protocol can be witnessed through the clinical disease course of Bryce Zender, a 68-year-old male from Central Florida. In this compelling case for CDM therapy, prostate cancer was suggested less conclusively by using color flow "Power Doppler" ultrasound at our clinic when only 6 short months prior a biopsy performed by his local urologist, failed to show any evidence of cancer. An MRI scan was not available to me at the time of this patient's evaluation. In this particular case, the color flow "Power Doppler" highlighted suspicious areas of blood flow to the prostate that ultimately served as vascular targets for the biopsy needle. The rationale for this concept is based on the fact that prostate cancer requires blood flow to proliferate. While I personally feel that Color Flow Doppler ultrasound adds a measure of validation as to where prostate cancer cells live, data in the literature does not overwhelmingly support this referencing Pelzer's research. Once I diagnosed prostate cancer with a Gleason score of 6, his urologist recommended a radical prostatectomy while I recommended chronic disease management.

Bryce chose CDM, the path that predicted the best quality of life possible and was placed on Flutamide, an anti-androgen, as a monotherapy for slightly more than two months. During this time, his PSA had dropped like a rock from 10.7 ng/ml to .5 ng/ml, an improvement not unexpected with this medication. Bryce continued with the diet, nutrient supplements and medications recommended without any compromising side effects. What he did not anticipate was what followed ... unbelievably and to the surprise of everyone; his PSA had favorably remained in the range of 4.2 ng/ml to 4.4 ng/ml (± 1.2 ng/ml) for more than four years. The single use of the anti-androgen (Flutamide) in combination with the basic components of the CDM protocol had allowed the PSA to remain stable at 4.4 ng/ml for 51 months and counting. To my knowledge, this type of incredible result has never been experienced or discussed extensively in the literature. In effect, his level of clinical success validated the decision made by Bryce and his wife MaryAnn to remain conservative and reject a radical prostatectomy. In an effort to objectively prove that his PSA was truly reflective of stable disease, my Monday morning quarterback physician critics have requested saturation biopsies. Rather than succumb to the pressure to perform a procedure biased by sampling error and replete with "needle tracking," Bryce was objectively evaluated using a 3 Tesla MRI scan; currently available to our practice patients. The scan results showed the cancer to be organ-confined within the capsule showing no sign of tumor extension or breach. This result was outstanding and consistent with my prior belief that his disease would be organ-confined as suggested, albeit, not confirmed by allied testing. **Once we had established stability of disease by PSA, imaging of the prostate had appropriately replaced biopsy as a point of validation for organ confinement. For men monitoring their cancers with relatively low PSA readings, 3 Tesla MRI scanning or the equivalent has made**

biopsy obsolete. To read Bryce's story in his words, I invite you to access his case report presented in the appendix.

The Risk of "Definitive" Prostate Cancer Treatment Failure is high

Recently, I was asked to consult with a 60-year-old male who only 10 days prior had received the 'shocking news' that he had been diagnosed with prostate cancer. A successful businessman in the prime of his life, this man was told to have his answer regarding prostate cancer treatment in two weeks. The recommendation was made by his urologist for Radical Prostatectomy based on his age and inability to predict cancer aggressiveness. His PSA was 11.0 ng/ml while his digital exam was non-diagnostic for cancer. The pathology showed a Gleason pattern 4+3/7 and a stage T2b (cancer limited to one side). A ploidy (DNA analysis) was not requested as the surgeon's plan was to remove the prostate. This patient needs to have a 3.0 Tesla MRI as well as a prescription for an anti-androgen to clean up the spill of cancer cells spread beyond the capsule. Once the staging is complete with the MRI scan, a decision can be made regarding what form of definitive therapy makes most sense based on quality of life issues and predicted outcome data! This individual would have a HIFU procedure performed by me if his prostate size allows for the treatment and the patient is seeking the most patient friendly treatment for the most common male malignancy. In my opinion, radical prostatectomy and radiation offer too little for this active male based on the significant side effects associated.

While it is tragic for any man to hear the four words, "you have prostate cancer," the far greater tragedy is the evolution of a group of men who represent the next wave or epidemic of treatment failures. This scenario plays out every day across the U.S. Ever present is a group of stoic and dogmatic physicians who fail to identify any group of patients who fail to qualify for a "definitive procedure" while ignoring the fact that the literature has shown 30-56 percent of men are over treated when prostate cancer is diagnosed. Allan Partin's data from Johns Hopkins provides the statistical edge for prediction of clinical failure in the decision-making process. Essentially, if the total PSA value is greater than 10 ng/ml; with a diagnosis of prostate cancer, you have a legitimate 50 percent risk the disease process is already outside the prostate capsule (extra-capsular). While this can be validated with a 3 T MRI scan, why remove a diseased organ when there is high likelihood the disease is no longer confined to the prostate? **If the odds do not favor success, you should look carefully at all other options; including a vaccine currently being studied outside the USA, through my research efforts (www.czbiomed.com).** To be sure, our ability as physicians is to predict with accuracy exactly where the cancer process lives amounts to nothing more than an educated guess. Any combination of diagnostic tests, such as Prostascint Scan, AMAS test, PSA, Gleason score, CAT scan, PET scan, Ploidy, Prostatic Acid Phosphatase, NMP-48, Kallikrein assay or any other diagnostic test, excepting a 3 T MRI (with or without spectroscopy), fails to adequately improve the sensitivity and/or specificity to make the case for organ-confinement.

Prostate Cancer May Be Systemic at the Time of Diagnosis

Validation that prostate disease cannot be accurately and dependably staged is noted through a study presented by Robert Vessella, Ph.D., in Toronto. Forty-nine study patients scheduled for Radical Prostatectomy, presumably based on the ability to cure, underwent a bone marrow cellular aspirate to look for prostate cancer cells prior to the initial incision. After adequate tissue nourishment of the specimen obtained, 87 percent of patients were found to have prostate cancer cells metastatic to the bone marrow at the time of surgery. **While there should always be an attempt at a scientific explanation for this type of phenomenon, the best interpretation is that all patients are at risk for local spread beyond the capsule at the time of diagnosis regardless of the best surgical opinion offered and/or rendered. This ideology is not as much about the selection of treatment as it may be about the lack of understanding for the natural history of the disease.** Patients are reminded that while the mere presence of prostate cancer in the bone marrow does not guarantee a site of metastasis; it is also safe to say, there is no guarantee that it will not develop into one either. Adding more fuel to the fire of controversy, a study from Northwestern demonstrated the presence of free-floating prostate cancer cells in the ambient blood suctioned from the surgical site in 92 percent of men undergoing radical prostatectomy, substantiating the spread of prostate cancer cells with operative intervention. Therefore, **it is my opinion that patients are at far graver risk of quality of life reduction, if not life itself, with a failure of radical Prostatectomy to cure than living with the disease with the benefit of other successful disease stabilizing modalities including Intermittent Hormone Blockade (IHB) or selecting a less morbid procedure in an attempt at cure. Less morbid definitive treatment options include cryosurgery or high-intensity focused ultrasound (HIFU).** None of this should suggest that Radical Prostatectomy is obsolete although changes in patient selection and the treatment paradigm must be made. While many physicians endorse this thought, I nonetheless, do not condemn using radical Prostatectomy in a select group of well-informed patients who qualify by age, low total PSA and a Gleason score of 6 or less. Those **individuals must also know, there is a risk of over treatment inherent in the decision made to remove the prostate.** Notwithstanding this comment, Jon Freda's inability to be cured at age 62 with a Gleason score of 6 and a PSA of less than 5 ng/ml would argue against the recommendation to remove the prostate. That stated . . . other treatments mentioned would qualify equally well for this same group of patients.

Additional Patient Case Reports

Prostate cancer attacks real people every day, often times changing their lives forever. I am reminded of a case that supports the need for a less dogmatic approach to prostate cancer treatment. I received a desperate call from a 51-year-old male from New York who was told by his urologist that radical prostatectomy was his only option for cure with a total PSA of 35 ng/ml and a Gleason score of 8. This opinion came from a very prominent urologist at a major New York University Hospital teaching center. **In my opinion, this case represents a blatant mismatch of surgical skill versus the unknown biology of prostate cancer. Given this clinical scenario, the patient had a greater chance for failure than success from a radical prostatectomy suggesting the argument to remove the prostate represents questionable judgment that cannot be overlooked.** Even cases that should be slam dunk for cure; fail. So why put a patient with poor predictive markers through a meaningless, traumatic exercise at the cost of significant emotional stress when a better plan can be created? **A desperate patient looking for any suggestion of hope is not of the mindset to make a decision of this magnitude much less discuss a topic he knows too little about. I can't state it any more clearly; a radical prostatectomy gives this patient, only false hope. To suggest otherwise is a gross misrepresentation that serves little more than filling a hospital bed and an ego.**

In another representative case, I received a call from a 55-year-old male from Virginia who was diagnosed with a

Gleason 8 prostate cancer in association with a total PSA of 6.5 ng/ml. Seeking the advice of a highly skilled referral urologist in the Washington D.C. area, the patient became convinced by his doctor that the only real option remaining for him was a Radical Prostatectomy. Despite my best efforts to alter history, the patient felt compelled to follow through with the operation as his surgeon was highly regarded in the community and nationally known. Following the surgery, the patient was given the "thumbs up" sign by his urologist, indicating that all cancer had been removed. In other words, the prostate capsular margins were clear of disease. **Within three months of his operation, the PSA had elevated to 1.5 ng/ml; consistent with the failure to be cured.** People often ask me, how can this be? Either cancer cells were inadvertently left behind at the time of surgery or the cancer was already extracapsular at the time of surgery and we just didn't know it. **The issue here is generally not our skill level in removal of the prostate gland, but rather our misjudgment for the extent of the disease process at the time of clinical presentation as well as the natural history of a Gleason 8 cancer.**

This type of scenario is all too common with Radical Prostatectomy recipients whom in my mind are by and large undereducated and not prepared for the devastation they are asked to experience. In other words, the system we use to qualify men for this procedure is inadequate, flawed and/or obsolete. These cases bring to light the uncertainty that goes along with the gamble for cure. **As long as surgeons see the opportunity to seize success in the face of predicted failure, the group of prostate treatment failures will continue to rise.** Why take the risk? I frequently tell patients that if a curative procedure looks good today, it will likely still look as good in 6 months. **If no urologist can guarantee success with radical prostatectomy (and we do not) with 20 plus years of training and experience, how can you (the patient) make your most important health**

RONALD E. WHEELER, M.D.

decision of your life in four weeks or less, absent adequate education. Truth is, you cannot and should not.

Currently, there are excellent educational resources available that will allow you to get up to speed on prostate cancer disease decision-making, including: **PCRI (www.pcri.com)**, The Prostate Forum, our websites at: **www.safebiopsy.com, www.Peenuts.com, www.MRISUSA.com, www.PanAmHIFU. com, www.ProstateCancerPreventionFoundation.org (www. PCPFUSA.org),** and others will provide the essential data and/ or information that will serve as a platform from which your decision will ultimately come. Patients are reminded that prostate cancer support groups located throughout this great country of ours provide an additional educational resource. The patient survivors in these groups often speak quite candidly in the form of a testimonial on all issues of life after treatment failure. The fact that these groups are growing should create national concern and suggest that there has to be a better approach associated for the topic of prostate cancer cure. While I am not trying to come between a patient and his physician, the inability of a physician to speak effectively to all viable options and/or delay a treatment option of choice in deference to a patient's educational needs, will ultimately result in a loss of confidence by the patient.

Treat Prostate Cancer as a Chronic Disease

While the population across the U.S. is littered with our prostate surgical and radiation therapy failures, I continue to remind patients that if we can't get it right with Arnold Palmer at one of this country's most prestigious institutions, what makes you think that you'll succeed at the institution you select? The alternative to treatment failure is to avoid definitive treatment altogether. **The late William Fair, M.D., noted urologist from**

Memorial Sloan-Kettering may have said it best when he suggested, "Based on everything we know about prostate cancer (in the year 2000), I am not certain that it (the disease) shouldn't be treated as a chronic disease." We should all learn from one so noble and honored in the field of urology.

Our Prostate Disease Protocol

At the Diagnostic Center for Disease™, all of our prostate cancer patients are offered all viable treatment options. Following a lengthy dialogue including a comprehensive question and answer session, patients most frequently select CDM complemented by Intermittent Hormone Manipulation or blockade. The reason for this is simple; it gives patients an opportunity to explore all options through extensive research in the absence of impending doom. The addition of intermittent hormonal manipulation to the therapeutic approach represents the least invasive, least traumatic, yet equally effective format of disease suppression, assuming the failure of a conservative diet and nutritional protocol to succeed. Using the PSA as a guide, action points are selected, whereby patients understand the parameters of when to begin therapy and when to discontinue. Generally, an anti-androgen is selected as the initial best first step for therapeutic response once side effects have been addressed thoroughly. This protocol generally allows for all quality of life issues to continue unchanged. Sexual activity is not uncommon while a patient is using an anti-androgen without an LHRH-Analogue. Examples of an anti-androgen used as a first line of therapy include Casodex (Bicalutamide), Flutamide, Ketoconazole (an antifungal) or Nilandron (Nilutamide).

Regardless of the form of therapy selected, an intermittent application of this monotherapy is the standard of care implemented when the PSA reaches approximately 10 ng/ml or higher. Critics argue that intermittent therapy has not shown to be a benefit in overall survival. While this may be true, we don't have compelling validated data to suggest it does not. Furthermore, the more important message is that continuous therapy (anti-androgen alone, or in combination with an LHRH-analogue) will fail to respond at some defined, yet unknown time. The literature supports refractivity at 2.5 years (on average) with continuous usage. Therefore, continuous therapy predicts disease refractivity or lack of responsiveness to the therapy and generally should be avoided whenever possible. Avoiding refractivity should be a goal of all treating physicians. Even while therapy has proven to be successful, we should not be unwilling to give the patient a holiday from the therapy causing osteoporosis, muscle wasting and lethargy. With intermittent therapy, it is not infrequent for a patient to be on a therapeutic agent for a month to 3 months and then remain off of therapy for many months or years at a time regardless of Gleason score as noted with Bryce Zender, Jim Walker, Carl Lackey, Jim Fouche, Jude Deplaizes, Larry Yohe, and others. Critical to this approach is the patient's responsibility to make lifestyle changes. **Prostate cancer is not felt to be a stand-alone disease but rather reflective of a series of unintentional (less than favorable) habits throughout life.**

Defeating Prostate Cancer is More Complex than Radical Prostatectomy Alone

In an effort to make a difference, I believe that the multi-faceted approach associated with the CDM protocol must be initiated as early as possible and include: proper diet, appropriate nutrition, adequate exercise, stress reduction and continued education. Beyond this, a plan or strategy is crafted that is patient specific and consistent with the most precious of quality of life issues. We expect our patients, as an example, to remain sexually active throughout their treatment course and never be incontinent of urine.

While our prostate cancer management program is successful, I am never quite satisfied. The only way to decrease the incidence of treatment failures is through education and prevention of the disease. Prostate cancer survivors, therefore, are urged to step forward and promote their message as a living legacy to all men who cross their path. **All men who have lived to see another day while fighting prostate cancer have the responsibility to preach to their sons about being proactive versus prostatitis while being vigilant of their PSA value from age 30.** Without this proactive approach we cannot make headway versus the ignorance that currently dominates the traditional treatment arena.

As I have previously stated, when prostate cancer is diagnosed, I recommend an intermittent application of hormonal manipulation or intermittent hormone blockade (IHB), assuming the PSA is approximating 10.0 ng/ml. This allows for a cooling off period so that the patient does not feel undue pressure from family, physician or friends to make a decision he is not prepared to make. This is also a time to develop the infrastructure for the decision that will be made later. This decision requires the knowledge of the positives and negatives associated with all options considered. Patients are reminded that all viable treatment options should theoretically be considered at this point. It is only through the comprehensive evaluation and understanding of all treatment risks and benefits that quality of life issues can be preserved while in many cases must be preserved for the sanity of the patient. This period of consideration and/or education should last no less than six months. Obviously, patients who have more extensive disease at the time of diagnosis do not fit this model and should respond immediately with intermittent hormonal blockade using PSA action points to guide their future course. In my opinion, patients do not need to die from prostate cancer any longer. With an improved awareness program, prostate disease will be diagnosed earlier giving all men many more viable options for future care. Medically, any good coaching staff has the tools with which to suppress the disease activity for an as yet undefined period of time. With that said, quality of life issues, important to all of us become the focus of attention as we live with the disease. Using this methodology, patients may find that their disease is non-aggressive and may not need to be treated at all as witnessed by many of the patients participating in the prospective diet and nutritional study or CDM protocol independent of any study.

Patient Case Report

I am reminded of a 70-year-old male from New Hampshire who had prostate cancer diagnosed in associated with a PSA of 6.4 ng/ml and a Gleason score of 7 (4+3). A recommendation was made by his urologist to have a radical prostatectomy. The urologist made this recommendation as the patient was in fairly good health without evidence of life limiting disease such as heart disease, hypertension or diabetes. Given the fact the patient was ready to leave on his yearly winter trek to Florida; the gracious urologist suggested a second opinion with a Florida urologist would be in order given the time constraints. It was good karma; the patient came to see me. After an intensely comprehensive visit at my office, I suggested that we consider diet alone with our patented prostatitis formula *Peenuts*® as plan A. In the event this very conservative approach failed, as witnessed by a progressive rise in PSA, plan B would incorporate the addition of an anti-androgen as a monotherapy. His PSA action points were arbitrarily set at 8 and 1, suggesting the point where the anti-androgen treatment would begin and the point where the anti-androgen would discontinue respectively. I recommended the patient get his PSA at monthly intervals to establish disease volatility, suppression or stabilization. If the PSA remained quiescent, we would go to a 2-3-month PSA schedule. In approximately one year, the patient returned for follow-up. In follow up, the expressed prostatic secretion (EPS) (the diagnostic test for prostatitis) showed significant improvement from his initial visit, while his PSA had lowered to 4.2 ng/ml; without the need for the anti-androgen. Realizing that this patient controlled his prostate cancer using basic lifestyle change, highlighted by dietary adjustments and a prostate nutritional product (Peenuts®), I asked the patient what his urologist back home thought of the success of his conservative measures. His urologist concurred with his patient's noted success by stating, **"I guess you no longer need the radical prostatectomy."** In effect, a victory had been achieved for all who cared for this patient because of his desire to remain conservative. Thus, the patient avoided the threat of incontinence, impotency and possibility of disease recurrence; all possible with a radical prostatectomy. He was in effect, living with his disease in a suppressed or non-advancing biologic state. Additionally, he was not threatened by bone loss, muscle wasting, hot flashes, impotency, weight gain and lethargy from taking LHRH-Analogue drugs that would have been more than the disease required at this time. This patient now counts his success versus prostate cancer at 2-3 month intervals with the PSA blood test. Our coaching process allowed for the patient to understand the risks and benefits of all pertinent therapies realizing that the best therapy for him was associated with no definitive therapy at all.

Awareness Fails When Professionals Do Not Understand the Significance of PSA

The battle versus prostate disease does not always turn out so well. I recently heard from a 65-year-old gentleman from Nebraska who had understood and appreciated the benefit of yearly PSA screenings. For the previous 5-6 years, his PSA had held stable in the dangerous and unpredictable range of 3.5 ng/ml. His digital exam was non-diagnostic according to his physician. The medical consensus opinion, explained to him suggested that his PSA was within normal limits and that a yearly PSA should continue, although was not absolutely necessary. A year following this encouraging news and a month after he retired, his PSA was recorded at 29 ng/ml. The biopsy of the prostate revealed the obvious. He had prostate cancer. Not only did he have prostate cancer but also he had cancer that had aggressively invaded his bones. Despite an orchiectomy (removal of the testicles) to wipe out virtually all of the testosterone that fed this cancer, he died within two months of the diagnosis. Fortunately, this clinical presentation is not routinely seen. Nonetheless, this sad case shows the vulnerability of a healthcare system that had failed to prevent the demise of a patient who understood the words: "proactive and awareness." He was misinformed on what a normal PSA level really was while never told of any proactive preventative concepts. He merely followed the directions of his health care provider and paid the ultimate price because he thought his doctor knew best. **Regardless of what the healthcare system says, patients are advised to get the PSA, know the number, be proactive and keep reading and learning. Patients must become aware that the best number for PSA is less than 1.0 ng/ml and to do whatever they can to get it there and keep it there. This patient's life may have been spared if this information, were known by his health care providers.**

Prevention Makes Sense

The only paradigm to adequately complement patient survival from prostate cancer treatment and management of treatment failures is to implement an aggressive attempt at prostate cancer prevention through awareness. The interpretation of the PSA, "the barometer of prostate health," must be enhanced significantly to identify disease in a more timely fashion. Historically, the 0-4 ng/ml range has been associated with 20-30 percent of all prostate cancer cases. Despite this, we have been telling patients since 1986 that 0-4 ng/ml is normal. Most notable to this group, of so-called "normal" patients is the former Gulf War General, Norman Schwarzkopf. He was diagnosed with prostate cancer with a PSA of only 1.8 ng/ml. Once he understood his options, he responded by having his prostate removed. While I trust the General continues to do well, he remains active as a proponent of PSA testing and improved awareness through education. As a medical profession, we must stop representing as normal something that is far from normal. Patients are losing options and time to treat as PSA rises consistent with a greater aggressiveness of disease (prostatitis and/or prostate cancer). Despite the criticism that PSA has received relevant to prostate cancer detection, the PSA blood test has excellent sensitivity and specificity for detection of prostatitis, a precursor disease of prostate cancer.

The Application of PSA to Chronic Disease Management

In data I reported on at the NIH in 2000, I demonstrated that a PSA of 1.0 ng/ml or greater indicated prostatitis in 100 percent of patients (n=177). This was validated with the EPS (expressed prostatic secretion), the diagnostic test for prostatitis. **This exercise proved PSA is a surrogate marker for prostatitis.**

This sentinel research was corroborated by Ballentine Carter at Johns Hopkins in March 2002 and touched on throughout this book. Suffice it to say, we have only seen the tip of the iceberg on a devastating disease associated with this organ. The real epidemic is the new generation of prostate cancer patients disguised today as prostatitis patients. **Unfortunately, if we don't recognize the disease earlier and/or offer proactive options to the unwitting public, we will pass the baton of disease ignorance from one generation to another. Without an improved algorithm on prostate health, future generations of men will stand in front of a new generation of physicians with the same level of dogmatism and arrogance, while failure to cure will be perpetuated over and over, ad infinitum.**

Chronic Disease Management Begins
With Prostatitis Resolution

While there are many theories for the evolution of prostate cancer, there is no one factor that can be isolated as the etiology of the disease process. While the component parts are multi-factorial, the most glaring and least understood element to me is the oxidative damage/destructive process of prostatitis or inflammation. Furthermore, an improved understanding for the role of glutathione may hold the key to unlocking the pathogenesis of prostatitis to prostate cancer. This is currently being investigated at Johns Hopkins. While much work needs to be done as we continue to validate the cause and effect of the inflammation to the cancer, no one will dismiss that inflammatory disease leads to other cancers and that prostatitis and prostate cancer coexist at the time of prostate cancer diagnosis. While my thoughts on the role of prostatitis to prostate cancer are more clearly outlined in the chapter on prostatitis, there is no doubt in my mind that the inflammation associated with prostatitis is causative to prostate cancer. This opinion is corroborated by an elite group of research specialists including doctors: Bostwick, Lieberman, Issacs, Nelson, Moon and others. These experts recognize prostatitis as a disruptive cell pathway that leads to prostate cancer. In this scenario, prostate cells become atypical and then dysfunctional through a process affected by chronic inflammation associated with proliferative inflammatory atrophy. Subsequent cellular change or mutation creates PIN (prostatic intraepithelial neoplasia) or ASAP (atypical small acinar proliferation) that ultimately evolve into a prostate cancer cell.

Closing Thoughts

Clearly, the evolution of prostate cancer and response to therapy varies from patient to patient and is based on many as yet unrecognized factors. Every patient should recognize that the fear of what cancer will do must play no role in the treatment decision process. Time is generally on your side! Therefore, patients are encouraged to get educated with a physician coach who will guide them using an unbiased approach, even if the best approach doesn't include surgery, radiation, cryosurgery or HIFU. As physicians, we must not abandon our patients if they choose a less than definitive approach. Through our efforts, we will empower the patient with education, experience and professional knowledge to know what is best. The lack of data to prove adequate and predicted success with definitive treatment options speaks loudly and clearly for change. What we know at this point with prostate cancer is an inexact science where physician judgment and surgical operative skill are divergent and minimally related. **The only way to blend judgment and skill is to realize that we have limitations to cure.**

Specifically, we must let go of the belief that everyone can be cured with something. We must give up the "one size fits all" mentality as well as focus our treatment only for the most qualified candidates using improved realistic guidelines for all options with their inherent success. Only in this manner, can the medical profession restore a modicum of integrity to the treatment paradigm. The influence from this thought pattern will push awareness toward earlier evaluation and diagnosis and therefore, hopefully yield greater success in a smaller group of qualified participants for longer periods of time.

It is often said, sometimes, 'the more we learn, the less we know'. It is only through vision and acceptance of our outcome data that we will realize that maybe the late William Fair, M.D. was right when he recognized that prostate cancer was far too complex of a disease to subject to any single procedure or process. **There can be no "Gold Standard" treatment when failure to cure is so common. Clearly, there are disease treatments that are performed commonly, but commonly performed procedures (standard of care treatments) do not fit the definition of a "Gold Standard." None of what I have said should diminish the strides that have been made, but make no mistake about it; the disease course for most men remains an enigma. It is our collective inability to cure prostate cancer predictably that prompted the late William Fair, M.D. to stand for the patient while suggesting we should treat prostate cancer as a chronic disease.** Why hasn't anyone altered his or her treatment pattern based on Dr. Fair's epiphany? Not even in his untimely death from colon cancer, have we gained inspiration to emulate an icon in urology. **If we haven't learned anything more from Dr. Fair, it is clear that the choice in prostate cancer treatment is anything but definitive and the patients need to know it.** For this reason, a program based on diet and nutrition may not be so far-fetched after all as we begin to understand that living with the disease through chronic disease management (CDM) may be the best option of all. Maybe we have reached the cross roads and it is finally time to treat all prostate cancer as a chronic disease. **The predictable predicament is what should drive research and prevention models.** This is not some new revelation but a disease pattern that has been ongoing for decades. Our lack of understanding for the pathway of disease should clear the way for meaningful open discussion between all interested parties. We should all be humbled by a disease that takes our loved ones from us at such an alarming rate. Likewise, we should all be humbled by a disease that presents itself every three minutes of every single day across America. If you have ever seen a man die from prostate cancer, you wouldn't have to see it again to remember the loss of weight, the loss of appetite, the loss of energy and muscle mass, the loss of mobility, the ashen look, the bone pain or the loss for the will to live. It is this image (emblazoned in my mind's eye) that drives my will to explore more closely what we know and what we do not know about this epidemic disease.

NOTES:

CHAPTER FOUR

Definitive Treatment for Prostate Cancer Targets All Men with the Disease . . . Inappropriately

THE "ONE SIZE fits all" . . . "get the cancer out at any cost" philosophy is often times more than the disease requires. Noting that men live 15-20 years regardless of the treatment modality offered, men are encouraged to be cautious in their decision making process when the diagnosis of prostate cancer is established. Studies (from Johns Hopkins principally) show that delaying a treatment for six months or longer has no impact on the ultimate outcome in men with favorable histology (Gleason score (GS) ≤ 6) and 'low volume disease'. The term 'low volume disease' is difficult to get my arms around as the extent of disease should never be based on biopsy (due to sampling error or bias), but rather on imaging with a 3 Tesla MRI scan. That said, delaying your decision makes most sense as it gives you ample time to improve your understanding of all your options as well as to realize, in most cases, **the treatment offered may be associated with side effects that may be worse than the disease itself.** After all, there is no reason to suffer from impotency, incontinence or rectal injury unnecessarily.

While no guarantee of outcome will ever be offered with surgery, radiation, cryosurgery or any other credible treatment including HIFU, patients should become educated relevant to a minimally publicized study that speaks to an effective management plan, primarily through diet and nutrition. The study findings associated with a Gleason 6 prostate cancer suggests this treatment approach called Chronic Disease Management (CDM) may make sense for the majority of men with prostate cancer; noting that 50-60 percent of all prostate cancer cases are a Gleason 6. While this prospective study had been presented to the Society of International Urology (SIU) in Bariloche, Argentina and to the Prostate Cancer Symposium sponsored by the American Society of Clinical Oncology (ASCO) and published, it is, nonetheless, not part of the mainstream commentary regarding prostate cancer treatment options. With additional publicity, more men will become better informed, improving their decision-making ability. Furthermore, the reason that men must take a lead role in their personal health and disease status is based on studies that show doctors generally recommend the treatment option consistent with their training as opposed to an objective assessment of all options. **When physicians get paid for performing the treatment concept of their choosing, what incentive do they have to refer the patient to competitors or treat the patient conservatively?**

In the prospective study **'Is it necessary to cure prostate cancer when it is possible'** relevant to the benefit of diet and nutrition versus prostate cancer, men have achieved significant success in the excess of seven years while the average surveillance period in excess of 36 months. Validation that this protocol works is confirmed by Prostate Specific Antigen (PSA) suppression; a reduction in disease activity in excess of 58 percent. This user-friendly treatment strategy, while effective, is arguably the best first choice for men with a GS of 6 (3+3) or less. Equally important, these patients suffer no decrement in lifestyle issues and no side effects. Specifically, the threat of impotency and incontinence is avoided as men treat their disease chronically through the program called, Chronic Disease Management (CDM). While this approach is discussed in greater detail in the chapter on CDM, what makes this data even more compelling is that every patient encountered with a GS of 6 and a PSA value of less than 15ng/ml was enrolled. Thus, there was no selection bias to enhance the outcome.

When our study group was compared to a treatment group, with similar cancer characteristics, representing the academic talents and surgical skill of expert physicians from across the country, the findings were even more spectacular, favoring CDM. **What I found was a group of men who experiences a much different (poorer) outcome when the decision was made to attempt to cure rather than live with the disease. While there may be many theories on why these men failed to be cured, the most intriguing thought relates to the possibility that the treatment itself was related to the failure.** While it is easy to be critical in hindsight for the decision to try to cure these patients, it could be that the operative procedure or radiation in some manner accelerated the cancer growth process. While it is commonly recognized that disrupting the primary cancer focus can spread cancer cells locally, no one has ever studied a group of failures and/or compared them to an alternative non-surgical, non-radiation treatment concept. To be sure, the treatment attempt exposes the possibility that the biology of the disease has not been well understood, while the patient was exposed to unnecessary risk. The decision to try to cure patients may have underestimated the complexity of the disease or failed to understand the true risk as measured by readily available nomograms that predict outcome data. To state further,

Gleason 6 prostate cancers are not supposed to fail definitive therapy and in fact, represent the majority of patient treatment success at major institutions like Memorial Sloan-Kettering, MD Anderson and Johns Hopkins. Based on some patient examples that will follow, I would encourage a randomized study with a major treatment facility to further validate the strengths and weaknesses of immediate therapy versus delayed therapy and/or the benefit of CDM.

NOTES:

Prostate Cancer—Gleason Score 6 Comparisons
Treatment versus Non-treatment

Disease Characteristics	Treatment Group (National Experts)	Non-treatment Group (The Diagnostic Center)
Number of Patients	N=20	N=23
Median Age	64 years	64 years
PSA @ Diagnosis	12.7 ng/ml (mean)	6.8 ng/ml (mean)
Clinical Stage	T1c, T2a, T2b, T2c, T3, T4	T1a, T1c, T2a, T2b, T2c
Treatment Rendered	Radical, Radiation, Cryosurgery, Hyperthermia	Chronic Disease Management (CDM)
% Success or % Failure	100 % Failure	100% Successful
Time to Failure	37.7 months (mean)	Non-applicable (N/A)
Surveillance Period	N/A	38.5 months (mean)

Patient Examples

While every attempt has been made herein to present the following cases in an educational manner that stimulates academic discussion without prejudice or malice, we cannot hide from the fact that these are real cases involving real men who made the wrong choice with their doctor. These cases point out quite clearly, the current level of ignorance as well as why both physicians and patients must continue to learn. Failure to cure a patient in association with a definitive disease treatment can only be avoided through improved preparation of the patient primarily with heightened awareness and education allowing for the best decision making while minimizing quality of life altering risks. Reflecting back to the year 2000, Dr. William Fair, former Chairman of the Departments of Surgery and Urology at Memorial Sloan-Kettering may have stated it best when he said in a now famous quote, "**Based on everything we**

know about prostate cancer, I am not sure that it should not be treated as a chronic disease." While poignant, his words speak to the frustration regarding the inability to predictably select the most appropriate group of men for cure; reducing the odds of success with any treatment process to little more than a process of chance or a "crap shoot." Minimally, CDM allows us the time to make better choices in disease management while realizing that CDM may be the best choice available.

NOTES:

Case Comparison #1

61	**Age**	56
9.1 ng/ml	**PSA @ Diagnosis**	9.1 ng/ml
T2a	**Clinical Stage**	T1c
58%	**% Chance of Organ Confinement**	75%
6	**Gleason Score**	6
Radical Prostatectomy	**Treatment Selection**	Chronic Disease Management (Diet & Nutrition based)
Immediate; Margin Positive at Surgery	**Time to Failure (if applicable)**	N/A
Treatment Failure despite adjuvant radiation therapy	**Outcome of Treatment**	40% Decrease in PSA @ 58 months
Fair-Poor	**Quality of Life**	Excellent

Case Comparison #2

64	**Age**	56
7 ng/ml	**PSA @ Diagnosis**	4.4 ng/ml
T2a	**Clinical Stage**	T2c
58%	**% Chance of Organ Confinement**	32%
6	**Gleason Score**	6/7
Radical Prostatectomy	**Treatment Selection**	Chronic Disease Management (Diet & Nutrition based)
84 months	**Time to Failure (if applicable)**	N/A
Treatment Failure despite adjuvant radiation therapy	**Outcome of Treatment**	61% Decrease in PSA @ 39 months
Fair-Poor	**Quality of Life**	Excellent

Case Comparison #3

57	Age	64
13 ng/ml	PSA @ Diagnosis	14.4 ng/ml
T2a	Clinical Stage	T1c
42%	% Chance of Organ Confinement	62%
6	Gleason Score	6
Radical Prostatectomy	Treatment Selection	Chronic Disease Management (Diet & Nutrition based)
12 months	Time to Failure (if applicable)	N/A
Treatment Failure despite adjuvant radiation therapy	Outcome of Treatment	90% Reduction in PSA @ 29 months
Fair-Poor	Quality of Life	Excellent

Case Comparison #4

59	Age	56
8.3 ng/ml	PSA @ Diagnosis	9.1 ng/ml
T1c	Clinical Stage	T1c
75%	% Chance of Organ Confinement	75%
6	Gleason Score	6
Radiation	Treatment Selection	Chronic Disease Management (Diet & Nutrition based)
72 months	Time to Failure (if applicable)	N/A
Failure	Outcome of Treatment	40% Reduction in PSA @ 58 months
Good-Fair	Quality of Life	Excellent

Case Comparison #5

58	Age	56
7.5 ng/ml	PSA @ Diagnosis	4.4 ng/ml
T2c	Clinical Stage	T2c
46%	% Chance of Organ Confinement	31-55%
6	Gleason Score	6/7
Radiation	Treatment Selection	Chronic Disease Management (Diet & Nutrition based)
29 months	Time to Failure (if applicable)	N/A
Failure	Outcome of Treatment	61% Reduction in PSA @ 39 months
Fair	Quality of Life	Excellent

Case Comparison #6

59	Age	71
8.1 ng/ml	PSA @ Diagnosis	8.6 ng/ml
T2b	Clinical Stage	T1c
49%	% Chance of Organ Confinement	43%
6	Gleason Score	7 (4+3)
Radiation	Treatment Selection	Chronic Disease Management (Diet & Nutrition based)
36 months	Time to Failure (if applicable)	N/A
Failure	Outcome of Treatment	66% Reduction in PSA @ 17 months
Fair-Poor	Quality of Life	Excellent

Case Comparison #7

73	Age	43
5.3 ng/ml	**PSA @ Diagnosis**	5.4 ng/ml
T1c	**Clinical Stage**	T1c
80%	**% Chance of Organ Confinement**	80%
6	**Gleason Score**	6
Radiation	**Treatment Selection**	Chronic Disease Management (Diet & Nutrition based)
24 months	**Time to Failure (if applicable)**	N/A
Failure	**Outcome of Treatment**	61% Reduction in PSA @ 41 months
Poor	**Quality of Life**	Excellent

Case Comparison #8

60	Age	71
17 ng/ml	**PSA @ Diagnosis**	8.6 ng/ml
T2c	**Clinical Stage**	T1c
30%	**% Chance of Organ Confinement**	43%
6	**Gleason Score**	7 (4+3)
Radiation	**Treatment Selection**	Chronic Disease Management (Diet & Nutrition based)
36 months	**Time to Failure (if applicable)**	N/A
Failure	**Outcome of Treatment**	66% Reduction in PSA @ 17 months
Good-Fair	**Quality of Life**	Excellent

Case Comparison #9

64	Age	56
4.27 ng/ml	**PSA @ Diagnosis**	7.3 ng/ml
T2a	**Clinical Stage**	T2a
66%	**% Chance of Organ Confinement**	58%
5	**Gleason Score**	5/6
Radiation	**Treatment Selection**	Chronic Disease Management (Diet & Nutrition based)
12 months	**Time to Failure (if applicable)**	N/A
Failure	**Outcome of Treatment**	38% Reduction in PSA @ 40 months
Good-Fair	**Quality of Life**	Excellent

Case Comparison #10

64	Age	64
4.56 ng/ml	**PSA @ Diagnosis**	4.7 ng/ml
T1c	**Clinical Stage**	T1c
80%	**% Chance of Organ Confinement**	80%
6	**Gleason Score**	6
Cryosurgery	**Treatment Selection**	Chronic Disease Management (Diet & Nutrition based)
60 months	**Time to Failure (if applicable)**	N/A
Failure	**Outcome of Treatment**	64% Reduction in PSA @ 72 months
Fair-Poor	**Quality of Life**	Excellent

Case Comparison #11

58	**Age**	56
5 ng/ml	**PSA @ Diagnosis**	4.4 ng/ml
T2c	**Clinical Stage**	T2c
55%	**% Chance of Organ Confinement**	31-55%
6	**Gleason Score**	6/7
Hyperthermia Germany	**Treatment Selection**	Chronic Disease Management (Diet & Nutrition based)
36 months	**Time to Failure (if applicable)**	N/A
Failure	**Outcome of Treatment**	61% Reduction in PSA @ 39 months
Fair	**Quality of Life**	Excellent

While I am always pleased to hear about the successes **(recognized only at 10 years post-therapy)**, I am equally concerned regarding why men fail. Could it be that the definitive treatment with surgery or radiation represented more than the disease required? Even more concerning; do definitive treatments impart undue risk to a selected group of patients? Could it be that my group represented the more favorable group for cure and that the group representing doctors from around the country, who failed to be cured; represented the better group for CDM therapy? While that may be true, I am certain that my patients would not want to trade places and try to push the envelope when success was already in hand. My point in all of this; based on my success rate and a lack of physician consensus for best treatment, it would appear that conservative management may be the best first option for all men with a GS of 6 or less. In my opinion, men need to take additional time to truly understand the risks they are taking by making a quick decision related to a disease that is unpredictable at best. Furthermore, **a recent study from Johns Hopkins noted that men who delayed surgery for several years had the same chance of success or failure as men who opted for immediate care. This is a mandate for all men to put the brakes on a definitive action plan when the diagnosis of prostate cancer is established.** In this scenario, men may actually realize that living with the disease is an advantage when the comparison is made to treatment with failure as witnessed with these case histories. Failure is defined as incontinence, impotency, and worse yet, the return of the disease associated with a rising PSA blood test result post-therapy.

The men with prostate cancer, who have already been treated and failed their therapy based on a rising PSA, have lost the opportunity to experience CDM first hand as a primary treatment modality. While I will always encourage further studies, **it is truly the men who failed to understand the concept for early detection or prevention of prostate cancer, which get a second chance with Chronic Disease Management when they receive the diagnosis of prostate cancer.**

NOTES:

CHAPTER FIVE

You Are What You Eat

THE BEST DIET is one that is nutritious and uses sound dietary principles! To be successful, a dietary protocol must be easy to follow, easy to access and be affordable. The basic principle of any diet relies on the intake of calories (from your dietary choices), as energy resources, as well as the requisite expenditure of energy (calories lost) associated with daily activities. Any imbalance in the exchange of calories over a 24-hour period will tip the scales to enhancing weight gain or conversely weight loss. Beyond a diet that supports a healthy lifestyle, questions surround the source of calories that complement the basic food groups.

My belief is the Mediterranean Diet embodies most of the principles of healthy eating, and with some modification, can become an even better diet, which does not support the growth of cancer. The Modified Mediterranean Diet has become known, to my patients, as the "Wheeler Diet" or "Prostate Diet." This diet is built on sound nutritional doctrines and avoids controversial foods or nutrients, including animal fat, dairy fat, Co-enzyme Q10, Lycopene, Chondroitin, Flax and Beta carotene that may hasten the growth of prostate cancer cells. The principles of the modified Mediterranean diet with appropriate nutrition, adequate exercise, stress reduction and education, enable prostate cancer patients to thrive with the disease, while avoiding lifestyle altering treatments, such as radiation or surgery (refer to Prospective Diet and Nutritional Study). In effect, many patients with known cancers are living a better life with cancer than prostate cancer patients who have received definitive treatment. Additionally, a nutritionally validated diet supports systemic health enhancing maximum output from the various organ systems. In other words, the "Wheeler Diet" specifically promotes a healthy heart, a healthy prostate in men, a healthy colon, a healthy brain and so forth. **Interestingly, the 'South Beach Diet' while favorable to the heart is not entirely favorable to the prostate!**

Dedication to any dietary plan must come from within. Without question, commitment comes with some level of sacrifice and requires a measure of dedication. After all, most people do not "tune in" to dietary needs until they are in their forties and by then the junk food, fast food, muffin munching, cola guzzling and sugar-swallowing habits have made a mess of their bodies both internally and externally. Frequently, weight gain is the only indication of real problems that lie within. Years of dietary abuse leave indelible marks such as diabetes, hypertension, weight gain, heart disease, stroke and an increased risk for prostate cancer proliferation, when present.

While many of us see the physical display of dietary recklessness with a quick daily glance in the bathroom mirror, it takes meaningful blood tests to gauge the destruction and/ or compromise that have occurred within. For most men, an evaluation of lipids and prostate specific antigen (PSA) is all that is required to improve your understanding of risk with the two most prominent diseases men face. Specific to the lipid panel; a comprehensive lipid panel is recommended to evaluate the sub-types of Low Density Lipoprotein (LDL or bad cholesterol), Triglycerides, High Density Lipoproteins (HDL or good cholesterol) as well as meaningful ratios of one fat component to another. By making these assessments, a lifestyle-altering plan can be implemented while meaningful change can be accurately documented. Once the various components of the lipid panel are understood, effective change can be validated by monitoring these levels on a 6-12 month basis. Beyond the LDL/HDL ratio and triglyceride/cholesterol ratio, there is the Arachidonic acid/ EPA (Eicosapentaenoic Acid) ratio, as well as the EPA/DHA (Docosahexanaenoic Acid) ratio, that evaluates systemic Omega 3 fatty acids. These ratios have been shown to be predictive for heart disease, if unfavorable, while predictive for heart health when they become normalized.

Rather than waste money on a basic lipid panel, associated with a 10-12 hour fast and less than accurate calculations, which may give us a false sense of health and well-being, my patients are encouraged to take advantage of the Vertical Auto Profile (VAP) test, **a real time accurate assessment of the lipid metabolism within your body without fasting**. This is a comprehensive microanalysis of your systemic fat composition. Based upon the fact that minimally 50 percent of patients with normal lipid panels (using the basic lipid profile) persist with heart disease, the Vertical Auto Profile test is essential to providing the best methodology for understanding heart disease risk. We cannot allow a genetic history of high cholesterol; for example, to be an excuse or barrier for not exercising or trying to change dietary habits. Fortunately for those who are genetically predisposed to hypercholesterolemia (high cholesterol), there are medications that can control, if not correct, the problem, once identified. Unfortunately, in many cases, a sentinel event must take place; to serve as a "wake-up call" that mandates change. Former President Bill Clinton needed chest pain and a diagnosis of heart disease to cause him to alter his dietary milieu. In other words, it literally took a life-threatening event to knock some health sense into him. With heart bypass surgery behind him, chances are he will not be passing through the "arches" of his favorite fast food eatery anytime soon. Like many others, he now bears the scar of a surgical procedure that will forever remind him why proper diet and exercise is as important as life itself.

Just like the former President and his "awakening," many patients I see have had the same type of life changing experience with the diagnosis of prostate cancer. Fortunately for my patients, my interests lie not just with the prostate but systemically as well. I realize and understand the responsibility of treating the total patient. I believe, in my heart, that most diseases and cancers are a culmination of a series of interrelated systemic events or battles lost and are not organ-specific. In many cases, prostate cancer is systemic when we had every reason to believe it was organ-confined. For this reason, all patients should be coached and treated as if their disease process is beyond the capsule of the prostate at the time of diagnosis and hope that it is not! In this manner, patients will become more aware; the worst case scenario does not necessarily mean loss of quality of life or life itself! **Specific to my clinical practice, I coach patients regarding dietary principles! While our goal is prostate disease resolution, a healthy prostate means little without a healthy heart.** Health of one organ system should never be encouraged at the expense of another. In this regard, we do not treat disease in a vacuum, but most understand what is good for one disease or organ, may cause conflict with another. From my position of understanding, this translates into a controversy and controversy must be avoided.

We have all heard; **"you are, what you eat".** While this sounds trite or simplistic, what you eat determines disease and aging of the organ systems. Type II Diabetes, for example, results primarily from pancreatic burnout associated with years of dietary abuse. To be sure, the simpler the sugars, and the less complex the carbohydrates in your diet, the more frequent will be the call to the pancreas for insulin production.

Over time, the incessant demand for insulin results in organ failure or adult onset diabetes; whereby the pancreas cannot keep up with what you are eating and gives up. Diabetes is commonly associated with visual disturbances, weight gain (obesity), peripheral neuropathy (tingling and numbness of the hands and feet), inadequate circulation of blood, loss of bladder control, loss of erectile abilities and much more. It is estimated that there are minimally 11 million adult-onset diabetics in the U.S., while millions more are doing their level best to join the ranks through poor eating habits and a lack of exercise. What is more revealing is that a better diet could have prevented the body from breaking down. Unfortunately, the under-educated are most prone to this disease process, but we will all succumb if we are unwilling to push back from the table and/or change 'what's for dinner'. There is no excuse for this disease in a large percentage of adults. More importantly, no specific assortment of vitamins and minerals will have an impact without a basic dietary understanding of the Glycemic Index (a measure of how quickly your blood glucose level from carbohydrates will rise) and a commitment by the individual to consume an improved diet. The Glycemic Index (GI) is, therefore, related to the complexity of the carbohydrates we eat (refer to a GI chart of carbohydrates for specific details). Specifically, the GI correlates to the relative insulin required to offset or balance the sugar entering the blood stream. To state further, food selections with higher GI numbers will raise blood glucose levels more easily and thereby trigger the pancreas to enhance its production of insulin while lower numbered food groups accommodate a slower insulin release, thereby, decreasing the demand on the pancreas. **To summarize this; the more complex the carbohydrates we eat, the less is the demand on the pancreas (a good thing), making more complex carbohydrates better for you.**

Before we can fix a problem, we must first recognize that there is a problem. Let's look at an example of a diet concept that has figuratively gone south. It is amazing to me the number of people who hang out at eateries that serve chicken wings. This is one commodity that you must do without! Wings are loaded with saturated fat and very little protein with a modicum of nutritional value; not to mention, the fat that they were fried in; is artery clogging. It amazes me how people pick up a chicken wing and pick it clean to the bone without any sense of remorse for the dietary misadventure that just occurred. The only meritorious comment is that your stomach is now full, albeit, you are filled with grease and chicken skin mixed in with a disproportionately small morsel or two of legitimate protein. Wash it all down with a couple of beers and you are good to go; lunch, supper or snack was fat, more fat and microscopic protein and carbohydrates. WOW! This is nothing to feel good about. You would have been better served with a grilled chicken breast (without the skin, of course) with a piece of lettuce, tomato, a slice or two of onion (a source of natural Quercetin, a bioflavonoid) and a couple of pickles on a whole wheat Kaiser bun. **Do I need to remind you to use a condiment other than mayonnaise?**

While I personally and professionally discourage red meat consumption, it is obvious that various steak cuts including: chuck, rib eye, New York strip, prime rib, London broil and sirloin, have significantly more fat than a filet mignon (without the bacon, of course). Men at risk of prostate cancer (approximately 50 percent of 55-60-year-old men) or men, who are currently battling the disease, are encouraged to avoid red meat as it has been shown to enhance the growth of cancer. A fatty acid called, Arachidonic Acid, common to red meat, has been shown to promote aggressive growth of prostate cancer when present. For this reason, men at risk of the disease based on age alone are cautioned about the risks of red meat consumption.

While I probably don't need to talk about hamburgers, I will, as over 150 million have been sold over some specified time frame by fast food outlets with no letup in sight. If the threat of mad cow disease or E. coli (Escherichia Coli or the animal's bowel bacteria) wrapped within your "burger" at no extra charge does not discourage you to avoid this dietary indiscretion, think in terms of hormones injected into the meat, the saturated fat, the fat on the griddle, as well as a meal full of fatty acids that promote cancer growth, precocious puberty and heart disease. Did I hear anyone ask for seconds or double on the all-beef patty? In this case, when you are hungry while wanting to avoid the temptation of eating less nutritiously, try a garden fresh salad with a skinless chicken breast added. Extra virgin olive oil with red wine vinegar (vinaigrette) will top this selection nicely.

Typically hot dogs, sausage, scrapple, spam and kielbasa are made from scraps of meat, representing the poorest quality of meat that can't be used elsewhere. Commonly, chemicals are added to kill bacteria and add color to the final product. If this is your selection for the grill or for eating out, it really doesn't matter if your selection was blessed by a Rabbi or not, as the selection represents anything but what you should eat. If anything, you should receive a blessing from the Rabbi for eating it. Come on people, let's get our priorities straight; are you living to eat or are you eating to live? Few knowledgeable people believe that eating hot dogs is living large. The proverbial silver lining in an otherwise dark cloud; what you are eating will keep someone in a job. Congratulations! Now you may take a bow and be proud of what you have been doing, even if it is unhealthy! You are doing your best to support the economy!

While some of what I have described previously may be part of American culture, what I have described is associated with a premature exit from life associated with heart disease and prostate cancer growth (when present) and therefore, must only be consumed as a rare event, if ever. The risk to living a fruitful quality of life with a measure of longevity will be seriously challenged by a lifetime of hot dogs and hamburgers. Free-range chicken and turkey (white meat) is the best selection when given the choice. Unfortunately, we are not always in the most convenient location when hunger strikes. In those instances, I urge you to consider a grilled chicken sandwich on a whole wheat bun **appropriately undressed of mayonnaise** or a salad with sliced grilled chicken on top with a non-creamy dressing!

Whether it is hormones injected to fatten the meat we eat, poor preparation that contaminates the meat we eat or the pollutants in our stream, oceans and waterways; we need to avoid toxins whenever and wherever possible. The public, for example, may want to consider a boycott of farm-raised salmon unless the grocer can assure us that the pond where the salmon were raised is devoid of pollutants like PCBs (poly-chloro-Benzene, a cancer causing chemical), animal waste and heavy metals that are commonly downstream from landfills or Industrial Manufacturing plants. To make matters worse, the fish are often fed a diet of fishmeal (ground up fish), a common source of additional mercury as well as Omega 6 fatty acids (corn meal) to fatten them up, thereby depleting the anticipated Omega 3 fatty acid benefit. The net effect of this activity results in a less than stellar dinner choice that could be more toxic than nutritional. Unfortunately, if you are not armed with information that gives you the assurances you need, I suggest that you should not eat the fish that was farm raised.

The best fish to consume are cold-water varieties that are high in Omega 3 fatty acids. The reason for this is that the standard American diet (SAD) offers far more Omega 6 fatty acids than Omega 3s. Omega 6 fatty acids are precursors to cellular oxidation and pro-inflammatory processes leading to a variety of diseases including arthritis, asthma, psoriasis and who knows what else. While most Americans have an Omega 6: Omega 3 ratio in the neighborhood of 20:1, **the ideal is 1:1**. Fish that qualify as being full of the favorable Omega 3 fatty acids include: wild Salmon, Halibut, Tuna, Mackerel and Sardines. Other fish types like Grouper, Ono, Redfish, Snapper and Trout are examples of fish that serve as wonderful protein sources but do not have the Omega 3 fatty acid content that you may have thought you were getting. This is the reason that I personally supplement with Omega 3 fatty acids as part of my daily routine. I generally recommend a 2:1 ratio of Omega 3s; consisting of 1400-1600mg of EPA daily with approximately 700-800mg of DHA daily.

Without question, arguably, the most studied and proficient diet to enhance systemic health and longevity of life is the Mediterranean Diet. No other diet is as comprehensive and beneficial to the prevention of disease. Other diets when studied carefully are flawed, while subsequently counterproductive to health. All experts are in agreement that the diet you consume should provide the core nutrients to enable a healthy lifestyle. The modified Mediterranean Diet is a step up from the traditional core Mediterranean Diet, in that, it recognizes the sacrifices that Americans must make if they want to undo the years of dietary abuse. The core ingredients of this dietary plan are protein, carbohydrates, fruits, vegetables, fats and non-toxic water. Specifically, the protein sources allow you to enjoy fish, white meat chicken, white meat turkey, peanut butter, egg whites and beans prepared in many delightful combinations. The vegetables recommended are always fresh (when available) and should highlight the cruciferous or Brassica classification of garden delights including but not limited to: broccoli, broccolini, Brussels sprouts, collard greens, mustard greens, kale, cauliflower and cabbage. This class of vegetables contains cancer-fighting plant nutrients called phytonutrients including

DIM (di-indoyl methane), fiber and I-C3 (Indole 3-Carbinol). More importantly, the sources of these core nutritional ingredients are integral to the image you will portray, while being mindful that a caloric intake in excess of your daily metabolic needs will result in weight gain. Complementing your caloric intake with an adequate exercise program should allow you to maintain your weight while exercising more often and decreasing the calories consumed will result in predicted weight loss. We should all be mindful that a marked decrease in daily caloric intake could result in unnecessary hunger and decreased productivity at home or in the work place. Starvation or food deprivation "fad diets" are discouraged as they are doomed to fail as the ability to comply with such a regimen decreases daily. The inability to comply with any diet ultimately results in a rebound weight gain with no lessons learned except the diet did not work.

Let's begin to understand some of the essentials of the diet I recommend. As the diet develops, you will readily see the difference from what you currently eat and a diet concept that you need to embrace. For more information on what's for dinner, please consult the "Wheeler or Prostate Diet".

The Prostate ("Modified Mediterranean") Diet

In summary, the most nutritionally replete diet for all men and women is a Modified Mediterranean cuisine. The benefit of this type of diet includes heart health, prostate health and serves as a mechanism to slow the aging process. Heart disease is prevalent in all ages but most commonly in men aged 40-70. Similarly, prostate disease is prevalent in all ages beginning as early as our teen years and extending throughout our adult lives. **The Wheeler or Prostate Diet is ideally intended for all men who want to prevent heart disease and prostate disease as they age.** For men who already have heart or prostate disease, it is never too late to start with a proper diet. **You can expect to lose weight on this diet**. Beyond the dietary commentary, I encourage prostate nutritional support with the patented *Peenuts*® formula, regular daily exercise, stress reduction and continued education. Remember, don't stop reading, don't stop learning and enjoy the change in menu as you now; eat to live.

Fresh Fruits

A great source of antioxidants, fresh fruit provides very important vitamins and minerals. The only down side is the sugar content. For this reason, fruits make a great snack or addition to any meal. Consumption should be moderate while not excessive. Examples include but are not limited to: oranges, tangerines, bananas, cherries, grapefruit, watermelon, pineapple, cantaloupe, guava, kiwi, strawberries, blueberries, raspberries, blackberries, cranberries, papaya, grapes, apples, pomegranate, plums, etc. **Minimal to moderate intake of fruit juice is recommended.**

Fresh Vegetables

Eat fresh, never canned, with the exception of tomato paste and stewed tomatoes! Vegetables supply a much needed source of vitamins, minerals and health-related properties including but not limited to: Quercetin, Indole-3-Carbinol, sulforaphane, di-indoyl methane (DIM), capsaicin and roughage. Examples include but are not limited to: cruciferous vegetables belonging to the Brassica classification including: broccoli, broccolini, Brussels sprouts, kohlrabi, kale, collard greens, bok choy, mustard greens, cabbage and cauliflower. Non-Brassica vegetables include but are not limited to: tomatoes and tomato related products including the aforementioned tomato paste, stewed tomatoes, tomato soup or juice, V-8 juice, ketchup (moderate intake secondary to the sugar content) and tomato sauce; peppers including chili pepper, bell pepper, habanera pepper, etc. Also, onions, peas, carrots, spinach, beets, string beans, mushrooms (shitake, portabella, morel, maitake, oyster, porcini, etc.); steamed, sautéed or wok-prepared vegetables are most nutritious. **Minimize corn and corn related products (corn syrup) in recipes and also try to avoid fried onion rings**.

Cooking Oils

Olive oil is best; canola oil is an alternative where olive oil can't be used. **Avoid palm oil, coconut oil, corn oil and vegetable oil**.

Garnish

Garnish and/or accentuate any dish with garlic, cucumbers, lettuce, greens, celery, curcumin, cilantro, pepper, oregano, ginger, rosemary, thyme, parsley, sage, mustard, pickles, olives and pimento.

Protein Sources

Cold water fish including but not limited to: fresh or canned tuna (best in water or olive oil), wild salmon, halibut, sardines and mackerel. Other protein sources include: turkey and chicken (white meat only, without skin) turkey bacon, turkey sausage, beans (all types), egg whites and peanut butter; scallops, shrimp, crab, lobster and calamari are OK depending on the preparation. **Avoid red meat including: hamburgers, hot dogs, sausage, kielbasa, chili with ground beef, barbecued beef, steaks, prime rib, pork or lamb,** wild game, chicken wings, sloppy Joes, bacon, pork roll, prosciutto, pepperoni, salami, bologna, Lebanon bologna, head cheese, organ meats, spam, ham and smoked meats. Fish to avoid include: tile fish (tilapia), swordfish and farm-raised salmon (when the origin of the fish pond or fish feed is not known). Additionally, you should not need to be to be told to avoid the 'cheesy bacon bowl' at one of our fast food eateries!

Dairy

Non-fat yogurt, egg whites or eggbeaters, skim milk, non-fat cheese and non-fat cottage cheese are good choices. **Avoid fat associated with dairy including: cheese, whole milk, half & half, cream, ice cream, egg yolks, mayonnaise, miracle whip and cream sauces including but not limited to hollandaise, béarnaise and giblet gravy.**

Pasta and/or Carbohydrates

Complex pasta made with spinach, whole wheat or rice is best, and whole grain breads are encouraged. Moderate consumption of pizza is permitted (absent the cheese is best), while whole wheat crust is best when served with pizza sauce or marinara. Sweet potatoes are preferred over white baking potatoes although the skins of both are nutritious. **Limit simple pasta like spaghetti and noodles while avoiding bread sticks, white bread, white rice and simple sugars such as refined white sugar and honey. Also, avoid: French-fried potatoes unless they are fried in olive oil.** Sugar substitutes include: Stevia and Xylitol while Splenda could be used for cooking.

Salads

Fresh garden greens with cucumbers, tomatoes, avocado, raisins, radishes, onions, peppers, olives, carrots (occasionally), nuts and fresh vegetables to suit. Minimally eat one salad daily; the best dressing is extra virgin olive oil and balsamic vinegar. **Examples of salad dressings to avoid include but not limited to: thousand island, creamy Italian, creamy garlic, French, blue cheese and ranch. Avoid croutons as well (unless homemade).**

Whole Grains

Granola (homemade), oatmeal, grape nuts, rye, wheat and sesame are great choices. **Avoid flax whenever possible.**

Crackers

Whole wheat (Example: Low Sodium/Low fat Triscuits) is best. **Avoid crackers made with partially hydrogenated oils including but not limited to cottonseed oil and soybean oil, which represent trans-fats.**

Soups

Tomato soup with vegetables, tomato soup without vegetables, chicken with rice or chicken noodle are great appetizers or may be a meal by itself. Based on the need to avoid dairy whenever possible, avoid cream-based soups.

Desserts

Seasonal berries or a piece of dark chocolate (if you must) are great. Dark chocolate is a source of stearic acid; favorable to prostate health in moderation. **Avoid pastries, doughnuts, cheesecake, cookies, ice cream and pies.**

Soy

Minimal intake of soy including Genistein and Diadzein subtypes. Additionally, soy that may be consumed but is not necessarily recommended includes: soymilk, soy cheese, soy nuts, soybeans, miso, tofu and tempeh. **Avoid soy sauce because of its high salt content.**

Snack Foods (in moderation)

Non-fat pretzels, peanuts, hazelnuts, pistachios, brazil nuts, almonds, walnuts, pecans, filberts, grapes, dark chocolate, trail mix (homemade), Triscuits with peanut butter, dried fruits, air-popped popcorn, matzos, a piece of fresh fruit. **Avoid soft drinks (promotes osteoporosis), potato chips, corn chips, candy, milk chocolate, pork rinds, microwave popcorn, cookies, goldfish, cheese twists or products made with partially hydrogenated cottonseed oil or soybean oil.**

Beverages

Reverse-osmosis water is best (3-4, 6-8 oz. glasses per day); green and red teas are best (source of polyphenols) with a wedge of lemon squeezed into the tea prior to consumption; Concord grape juice, red wine as an evening beverage (one to two 6 oz. glasses is recommended for men while one 6 oz. glass for women) daily. Moderate the intake of any alcoholic beverage including vodka, whiskey, tequila, gin, scotch, rum, beer, assorted after dinner drinks and wine. **Avoid: milk shakes, soft drinks, cream liquors and schnapps.**

Nutrition

Any validated prostate formula (example: the patented *Peenuts® formula*) that has been proven to be beneficial versus prostatitis by lowering the white blood cell count associated with the Expressed Prostatic Secretion (EPS) would be best. Nutrition should never be a substitute for a proper diet! Omega 3 Fatty Acids including 1400-1600mg of Eicosapentaenoic Acid (EPA) and 700-800mg of Docosahexaenoic Acid (DHA) daily in an effort to decrease prostate cancer cell proliferation and balance lipids including LDL/HDL, total cholesterol/HDL, and EPA/Arachidonic Acid ratios are beneficial! Quercetin found in apples and onions may assist chronic pelvic pain syndrome. **Avoid: flax, beta carotene supplement, co-enzyme Q10 supplement, Chondroitin supplement and Lycopene supplement, alpha lipoic acid and methyl sulfanyl methane (MSM).**

General Dietary Considerations

- **Avoid fried foods whenever possible in favor of broiled or baked.**
- **If dieting, precede every meal with a 6-8 oz. glass of water.**
- **Heart health and prostate health is directly related to a proper diet (see modified Mediterranean diet), appropriate nutrition, adequate exercise, stress reduction and education.**
- **Always eat food fresh and/or fresh frozen; canned goods generally should be avoided due to preservatives and sodium. An exception would be tomato-based products including tomato sauce or tomato paste.**

- If you grill your dinner, do not overcook or burn what is to be consumed, as this is associated with the production of pre-cancerous heterocyclic compounds.
- Avoid the use of butter or margarine remembering, "If it is solid at room temperature, you probably shouldn't use it."
- Fifteen percent of your daily calories should come from acceptable fats. Olive oil is best!
- An interesting APP for the many phones that help you count calories is called: Lose It! (This is a free download; as of this writing)

NOTES:

CHAPTER SIX

The 'Dirty Little Secret' Doctors Won't Tell You . . . 'Prostate Biopsies Really Do Spread Prostate Cancer cells'

ARGUABLY, MORE THAN a million men per year receive the news that a biopsy must be performed; as the risk of cancer is significant when the Prostate Specific Antigen (PSA) rises above 4.0 ng/ml. According to historical data from the American Cancer Society and others, 20-30 percent of men biopsied will be found to have prostate cancer when the PSA is associated with 4 or higher but less than 10.0 ng/ml. Unfortunately, when a biopsy is performed, many men suffer immeasurably from the trauma inflicted when intrusive needles have been punched through the rectal wall repeatedly varying in numbers from 12 to 24 cores (most commonly), and upwards of 86 biopsy cores when a mapping procedure is performed transperineally. Interestingly, the highest number of biopsies I have ever noted was 86; a dubious record when saturation or a mapping biopsy was performed by a physician in Central Florida. While the majority of men experience 12 biopsy needle punches, virtually all men experience something negative or untoward related to lifestyle issues with the procedure. To be certain, virtually all men experience passage of blood in their urine, bowel and ejaculate while still others experience unremitting pain, incontinence and assorted sexual dysfunctional challenges including impotency.

Still others may follow the path of a Neurosurgeon concerned about his rising PSA who went to a major Medical Institution on the East coast. While it is unclear whether this physician ever had prostate cancer, he never made it out of the hospital; dying from septic shock in 2010. Biopsied men are hospitalized upwards of 5% of the time due to high fever, chills and non-stop shaking called rigors. It is my opinion, the contamination of bowel bacteria, (principally E. Coli) into the blood stream is far more common than reported. **While death rarely occurs (less than one percent of the time), it is 100 percent for the man who dies.**

Competing with a biopsy is a 3 Tesla magnetic resonance imaging scan described by Peter Scardino, M.D., Chairman of the Departments of Urology and Surgery at Memorial Sloan Kettering (MSK) as the **"next greatest diagnostic test"** in improving our understanding of prostate cancer. **Men have a choice of biopsies or imaging to find a cancer at the Diagnostic Center for Disease™.** The decision for biopsy is associated with significant false negatives while imaging can be associated with false positives. When the skill set in imaging can be correlated to biopsy in a blinded manner, evidence will show that only the most skilled in prostate MR interpretation will have the fewest false positives, while the false negative rate with random 12 core biopsies can only be enhanced by a needless, expensive and life threatening saturation biopsy. When you compare a 20-30 percent yield from biopsy to a greater than 90 percent positive yield of cancer from imaging, there is little debate that random biopsies, common place in medical practices across the country, must be replaced by imaging or minimally preceded by imaging allowing for a targeted biopsy assuming a biopsy is ever done.

Let's put this into perspective. Doctors will generally wait until your PSA reaches 4.0 ng/ml or higher before a prostate biopsy is recommended. They will tell you (the patient) it is "the standard of care" which actually means virtually nothing. What I am asking for from any "expert" is a clarification for the quality associated with the so-called "standard of care." Is it a Gold Standard, a Silver Standard, a Bronze Standard or a Tin Standard? **From where I sit, a Tin Standard fits as a 20-30 percent yield for prostate cancer fails to win Gold, Silver or Bronze in any competition. In fact, the last time I looked, a student who scores a 20-30 percent on any test, fails that test.** Who among us would establish a standard of care and allow it to be enduring for decades with a paltry yield of 20-30 percent? In four words: "no one," except urologists. Why would well-educated men and women in urology practice support this diagnostic exercise if they know of the risk for tracking cells beyond the prostate (needle tracking) as evidenced in the literature? **In three words, they should not.** Why aren't doctors as concerned with a rising PSA under 4 as over 4 when prostatitis is the number one reason PSA rises? Among others: David Bostwick, M.D., Michael Karin, Ph.D. and the American Association of Cancer Research (AACR) have been saying for years that inflammation of the prostate leads to prostate cancer. **Why aren't more resources put into prevention than cure? Why don't doctors at least admit the chance of needle tracking, knowing that references exist in their respective journals that support the spread of prostate cancer cells with a biopsy?** In two words, **they should.** How is it that imaging rules diagnostically with virtually every other visceral (organ) disease yet with prostate cancer, we refuse to accept imaging or advance the cause for understanding imaging better? How is it in the twenty-first century that a leader in urology like Peter Scardino, M.D. is allowed to protect the "diagnostic turf" in favor of biopsies simplistically by stating, "At our institution (MSK), we diagnose prostate cancer through random biopsies."! I can only assume that if university leaders stand in unity for random biopsies, they would also support fishing in the Dead Sea or duck hunting in the parking lot of any supermarket by firing random rounds of buck shot into the air expecting a duck or goose to land in their basket. If all I have stated seems preposterous, how about playing darts without a dart board. Who among us would take a drive of any distance in an unknown city without a map or GPS with high confidence of returning to the original starting location? The chance of being successful in any of these scenarios is virtually non-existent. There is only one reason doctors would eschew imaging in lieu of random biopsies. **Follow the money.** It has to be about the economics of medicine that dictate trying to hold onto a practice pattern that is not supported by the best science. Maybe this is a defined plan of obsolescence or futility in a $2.5 billion dollar a year business, called: Prostate Biopsy.

Despite the fact that biopsies spread prostate cancer cells, treating physicians who have a vested interest in the biopsy business as it relates to the application of high-intensity focused ultrasound (HIFU) have convinced the Minister of Health in the Canadian Government, **'all men treated for prostate cancer in Canada must have a documented malignancy or no treatment can be rendered'. How can any governmental entity support a process that represents risk to its patient population without an independent review of all options by an unbiased panel of experts?** My Canadian colleagues have stated I have an unfair advantage by scanning prostates with a 3 Tesla MRI scanner, despite the fact I have correlated scans and biopsies in more than 200 patients proving the value of imaging to be far superior to random biopsies. This validated data was presented at New York University (NYU) in the summer of 2010 and supported by the research of Jurgen Futterer, M.D. from Nijmegen, the Netherlands.

In a case presentation at the NYU Meeting on Focal Treatment of prostate cancer, a well-known but traditional urologist was asked how he would manage a 62-year-old male with a 12 core biopsy proven GS 6 prostate cancer on the patient's right side (in 2/6 cores) and a stable PSA value of 4.5ng/ml over the past two years. The patient was interested in focal therapy as a means to eliminate the anxiety associated with living with a cancer that is less than predictable and without a question; less than a certainty of remaining indolent. The left side of the prostate noted no evidence of cancer associated with the previously performed biopsy. This particular doctor, who trained at Memorial Sloan-Kettering, stated he would now do a saturation biopsy to confirm the cancer previously diagnosed was in fact on the right side and that no cancer was noted on the left side prior to treating him for cure. I had trouble stomaching this absolute insanity of thought. Once the biopsies had confirmed that cancer is only present on the right side, focal treatment for cure would ensue using the HIFU technology.

Dr. Wheeler's response:

First of all, the notion that patients who undergo saturation biopsy can be cured is a stretch at best. The data would suggest that this just couldn't happen. Furthermore, why would any doctor want to impose on a patient intense pain and high risk for sepsis, not to mention bleeding from every conceivable pelvic orifice, when a 3 T MRI scan could be performed to validate the previous cancer diagnosis? In my model, I do not encourage random or saturation biopsies, however, I would not discourage a targeted biopsy under very controlled conditions assuming the scan does show specific suspicious regions of interest on the left side and the patient accepts the risk of needle tracking. Therefore, without evidence of cancer on the left side, based on imaging, the patient would be scheduled for a partial HIFU procedure while protecting all structures on the left side including the neurovascular bundle (enables erections) as well as the urethra. **Compelling research data from the Diagnostic Center for Disease™ and others establishes that the 3 T MRI scan must dictate the next best steps for a patient previously diagnosed with prostate cancer, not repeated biopsies.** When given the choice of additional biopsies with their inherent risks versus imaging with a 3 T MRI, the patient will walk quickly away from the MSK trained physician's opinion supporting additional biopsies.

In my opinion, doctors will not change their practice patterns so the burden to change medicine must lie with outraged patients who must demand a scan from their insurance carriers in lieu of a biopsy as the best first step when a PSA value predicts the need for a biopsy or further evaluation.

Unless doctors begin to proactively advise patients of all risks associated with biopsies including "needle tracking," my prediction is some patient advocacy organization will support an investigation into legal proceedings for doctors who fail to offer adequate informed consent. For this reason, **I urge all doctors to tell their patients that the risk of the prostate biopsy for spreading Prostate Cancer cells is real with every prostate biopsy performed.** While individual doctors may believe the risk is minimal or non-existent, the literature does not corroborate this thought process. The best advice is to be "fair and balanced" in your presentation and allow patients to consider all options carefully before they commit to a biopsy. After all, **it is well documented through the work of Michael Barry, M.D., and others that 30-56 percent of all cases of prostate cancer are over treated while arguably 50-60 percent of prostate cancers are associated with a GS of 6 (3+3). This is a cancer that can be managed conservatively in most cases, so . . . what's the rush?**

Patrick Walsh, M.D. from Johns Hopkins Medical Center with fellow colleagues; Sheldon Bastacky, M.D. and Jonathan Epstein, M.D. (noted pathologist), are quoted in a Journal of Urology article (May 1991) stating, **"Our data suggest that subclinical seeding is a more prevalent process than was formerly believed. In particular, tumor seeding within the needle track can occur following transrectal biopsy, a phenomenon that had never been previously recognized. Furthermore, our study also demonstrates the novel finding of seeding following the thin needle biopsy gun technique. . . . This information seems not to be common knowledge among many physicians."**

In another area of intriguing thought, Mark Schoenberg, M.D., the Medical Director of International HIFU, the manufacturer and distributor of Sonablate 500 HIFU technology has recently gone out on a limb academically and declared that he and the Medical Advisory Committee at the Charlotte, N.C. based company have categorically dismissed the diagnostic skill set of the treating doctor and research of Jurgen Futterer, M.D., Claire Allen, M.D. and myself (MRI experts) as it relates to the 3 T MRI scanner, effective May 1, 2011. In a time when strength of conviction and doctors (not manufacturers) are deciding what is best for their patients, Dr. Schoenberg may be responsible for making a most egregious error in medical judgment, while flexing his academic muscles. His medical judgment or lack thereof could be the "kiss of death" for a fledgling business like International HIFU. Dr. Schoenberg's lack of leadership is evident as he has cowered to the pressure from traditionalists and walked away from the future of prostate cancer diagnostics while cementing his legacy to the past. Dr. Schoenberg has taken what I believe is an ill-advised step in declaring a procedure already approved in the U.S. for treatment of benign disease in females (Uterine Fibroids) and also indicated for BPH (benign prostatic hyperplasia) in men and changed the rules preemptively exceptionalizing prostate cancer. He has declared that "old school" prevails; while assuring male patients who are treated with the Sonablate 500, high-intensity focused ultrasound technology, are also going to have to endure "needle tracking," to qualify for that technology. Dr. Schoenberg's best diagnostic model no longer supports the benefit of MRI imaging (at the very least), as an equivalent to a very poorly performing needle biopsy procedure. As stated earlier, **imaging has proven to be superior to the biopsy concept for all reasons.** Dr. Schoenberg has also eschewed the commentary of Sonablate 500 user, Joachim Deuster, M.D., from Heidelberg, Germany, who is concerned about biopsies causing "needle tracking," and has stated so in an article referenced in the appendix of this book. Finally, Dr. Schoenberg also puts Mark Emberton, M.D., a treating and research urologist in London, in a precarious position as Dr. Emberton is conducting MRI research sponsored in part by International HIFU and part of a much larger consortium of European urologists favoring 3 T MRI for its diagnostic capabilities in men suspected of prostate cancer. Patients are advised that MR Imaging is an acceptable and outstanding diagnostic tool for competing high-intensity focused ultrasound technology used primarily in Europe. Patients are also advised that additional information is available on the PanAm website (www.PanAmHIFU.com) or by calling the Diagnostic Center for Disease™ in Sarasota, Florida at (877) 766-8400.

In closing:

1. Doctors cannot and should not have the privilege to insist that patients get a biopsy when the number one reason PSA rises is prostatitis. Historically, very few MDs understand prostatitis!

2. Most doctors do not have the knowledge base or an adequate understanding of what the literature really says regarding "needle tracking" and therefore, do not have the right to categorically deny that "needle tracking" takes place with any patient at any time. To do otherwise is admitting ignorance and puts patients at undue risk!

3. Doctors must stop telling patients that "needle tracking" no longer is an issue since we have gone to smaller needles. The question here is whether the cell is smaller than a needle opening! There cannot be any doubt about this one! A cell is always smaller than the diameter of a needle!! I am surprised very qualified physicians are saying this! To say the least, it is unacceptable and cannot be tolerated!

4. Doctors should not be allowed to disassociate themselves from a patient who doesn't approve of all that the doctor wishes him to do. Maybe if the doctor follows this type of patient, improved knowledge may come from the experience. Patients should be allowed to pursue chronic disease management (CDM) protocols or a surveillance model when appropriate. Besides, physicians generally participate with insurance plans that say nothing about complete cooperation with a physician's way of thinking as a prerequisite to seeing the doctor. Once full disclosure of the facts has been articulated by the physician, there should not be any further issues when the patient chooses a different course of action!

5. Doctors should not be repeating a biopsy on a patient previously biopsied positive for cancer when they are in a surveillance or CDM protocol. Sampling bias associated with a biopsy procedure precludes this action while doing nothing more than fostering the **biopsy 'merry-go-round'** with the patient paying the ultimate price for this indiscretion. **Google: Michael Karin, PhD from the University of California at San Diego.** He does not have a vested interest or a 'dog in the hunt'! In my opinion, patients should be scanned with a 3 T MRI scanner if more than 12 months has elapsed since the original biopsy. **This repeat scan is recommended even if the PSA is stable as it is still necessary to prove that cancer growth is not taking place (notwithstanding a stable PSA value).** Once stability of scan and PSA number is evident, confidence in the CDM protocol for the patient has been achieved. Changes in scan results or PSA value with or without additional information from other markers should be considered as the disease is monitored!

To summarize, patients must answer one question. Should I agree to a prostate biopsy procedure when it has been proven to spread prostate cancer cells or do I keep my fingers and toes crossed, hoping for the best? In two words . . ."absolutely not." To me, the decision is easy—the literature validates avoiding random biopsies and supports imaging with a 3 T magnet.

NOTES

CHAPTER SEVEN

Andropause (Male Menopause)

~The Anti-Aging Dilemma~

FEW MEN GROW old gracefully. It is often said that the most successful male, if given the choice, would choose to die in bed as an "action hero." To state more clearly, this relates to our desire to have our passing associated with sexual performance that ranks with the best of the best. Our desire has helped the pharmaceutical industry make hundreds of millions of dollars on sexual enhancement products. The success in the pharmaceutical industry has created intense interest by entrepreneurs who have created "knock-off" formulas that captivate a man's interest, but are rife with factual omissions, deception, sensationalism, and health risks. Men are so enamored with the concept of getting an erection and becoming more youthful (anti-aging), that a willingness to put themselves at health risk has become commonplace.

Biologically, as we age, testosterone decreases and estrogen increases, in association with a rise in serum hormone binding globulin (SHBG). As part of the aging process, our muscles lose strength, our bones become more fragile, weight is gained and wrinkles appear. **Our collective inability to age gracefully has spawned the anti-aging revolution.** The solution to the problem of predictable aging seems simple . . . supplement with testosterone, alter the testosterone/estrogen ratio, use growth hormone, or embrace some other less studied, but equally touted remedy, such as progesterone usage.

Testosterone supplementation would seem like the obvious elixir to turn back the hands of time. After all, who wouldn't want increased strength, vitality, youthfulness and enhanced sexual abilities. **The most significant issue is not what testosterone will do for your manhood, but rather the risk of bringing prostate cancer to life. The literature is replete with data that supports the fact that testosterone stimulates the growth of prostate cancer.** Not surprisingly, the best candidates for testosterone supplements are men who are at the greatest risk for prostate cancer. To state further, the group of men most interested in testosterone supplementation or replacement are men in their sixties. Not inconsistent with this thought pattern, prostate cancer is most commonly diagnosed in men in their sixties. Authors of non-peer reviewed articles would rather sell products that enhance sexuality than study the science behind it or continue to be confused about the relationship of testosterone to prostate cancer. **While there may be a rare prostate cancer patient who could benefit from the concomitant use of testosterone therapy, the record must show that the vast majority of men with prostate cancer need to avoid testosterone supplementation or replacement . . . period.**

To state more clearly, based on what we know, testosterone does not cause prostate cancer, but rather, testosterone causes prostate cancer to grow. Some Internet sales sites sensationalize the fact that men with prostate cancer need testosterone due to the imbalance of the testosterone/estrogen ratio as men age. Tell that to Herbie Mann, world famous jazz flutist, who died from prostate cancer, based on the use of supplemental testosterone. Tell that to the 68-year-old man from Iowa, who underwent successful radical prostatectomy, as noted by a 0 ng/ml PSA, who died from prostate cancer when the disease that he thought he had defeated came to life with testosterone replacement.

To be sure, prostate cancer is a disease of all ages. In a recent review of more than 500 autopsy specimens, Weil Sakr, M.D. and his research team from Detroit, Michigan, noted at **8 percent incidence of prostate cancer in men in their twenties.** Despite our less than complete understanding for why this may be, caution should always be used when supplementing with hormones that may initiate and/or stimulate prostate cancer. Growth hormone supplementation is a "boutique" concept that vendors offer as a solution to the problem of growing older. Unfortunately for the unwitting public, men do not understand that the use of growth hormone may be associated with stimulation of prostate cancer. Therefore, while there may be some benefit for the use of growth hormone, it pertains only to men who understand all risks, including the risk of prostate cancer acceleration. Without prior knowledge of the risk for prostate cancer, growth hormone is contraindicated. While I do not generally oppose the use of growth hormone as an anti-aging remedy, I would certainly discourage its use in men who have a PSA level of greater than 2.0 ng/ml unless an MRI scan supports an absence of disease. A basic understanding of biochemistry shows that growth hormone stimulates insulin-like growth factor (IGF), which in turn, stimulates prostate cancer. Therefore, the risks are real!

Still others, in search of the "Fountain of Youth" for men, have suggested that progesterone, an anti-estrogen, indicated for the moderation of a woman's hormonal axis, may be "just the ticket" to alter the testosterone/estrogen ratio in men. It is the expectation that alteration of this ratio will result in any combination of benefits, including an enhancement of sexual vitality, weight loss, improved physique and a more youthful appearance. Still others, including Jonathan Wright, M.D. and

John Lee, M.D., have supported the use of progesterone as a prostate cancer cure. As an objective critic, I would welcome the opportunity to review case histories that speak without bias to the successful use of progesterone as a prostate cancer cure. As a point of contradiction I have multiple clinical cases that have shown a significant rise in PSA, based on progesterone use alone, including one patient with known prostate cancer whose PSA doubled from 4.7 ng/ml to 8.38 ng/ml, following just six months of progesterone cream supplementation. Fortunately for the patient, once the cream was stopped, the PSA returned to the pre-progesterone level within four months. This is the closest I have ever come to seeing a direct "cause and effect" so clearly. Nothing else had changed in this patient's daily routine but the addition of progesterone cream. This patient had a scare, but luckily both he and his holistic physician learned considerably from this biochemical misstep.

In another case, a 45-year-old male, from Cleveland, Ohio, desperate for answers on why his PSA was rising despite a negative biopsy, tried progesterone cream, based on claims made by an Internet site. This gentleman's PSA went from 12.0 ng/ml to over 20 ng/ml in a six month time period. Based on this response, and despite the previously noted negative biopsy, this unwitting gentleman, in all likelihood, has a case of prostate cancer that has not yet been diagnosed.

Still other so-called "experts" suggest that progesterone may work as an aromatase inhibitor, thereby favorably altering the testosterone/estrogen ratio in men. It is known that testosterone is converted by an enzyme aromatase, in the peripheral tissue (to estrogen), prompting still others to blame estrogen accumulation for the high incidence of prostate cancer in men as they age. Biochemically, this does not make any sense, as estrogen is a bona fide treatment option for hormone resistant prostate cancer. In other words, prostate cancer that no longer responds to an anti-androgen (Casodex or Flutamide) and/or an LHRH Analog (Lupron, Zolodex or Trelstar—my choice as it is the least expensive) may now respond to estrogen. Estrogen, in the form of Estradiol, was the active ingredient in PC Spes, before it was pulled from the market, due to FDA infractions, while the former leader of France, Francois Mitterrand, reportedly used estrogen to treat his prostate cancer for nearly 20 years.

If the alteration in the testosterone/estrogen axis makes physiologic sense in the anti-aging dilemma, it would not be difficult to study this concept in a controlled fashion. Specifically, Arimidex, an aromatase inhibitor, could be used to enhance testosterone levels while depleting estrogen. Theoretically, an increase in the systemic level of bio-available testosterone could enhance male virility and libido. Once again, without certain knowledge of the absence of prostate cancer, as noted by a PSA of less than 2.0 ng/ml, an aging male will put himself at undue risk for the enhancement of prostate cancer with the indiscriminate use of many of these so-called "anti-aging" remedies.

Take home message #1: Progesterone usage is controversial and is shown to stimulate prostate cancer. If you intend to use it, my recommendation is to locate a homeopathic physician who understands the mechanism of action for progesterone and who will share the risk for the potential side-effect profile with you.

Take home message #2: There is no "Fountain of Youth." Despite this, I would encourage research that will provide men with safe and scientifically legitimate pathways to enhanced strength, energy and sexual performance without undue health risk.

Take home message #3: For now, testosterone supplementation or replacement remains an option for men who do not have prostate cancer or biologic markers that suggest the diagnosis is inevitable. Men are cautioned

that one of the best diagnostic tests for the presence of prostate cancer is to identify an elevation in PSA, after the use of testosterone. Despite the diagnostic implications and the short term benefit from testosterone usage, there is no guarantee that the disease stimulated can be curtailed by medical means. Men concerned about any of this should have a qualifying 3 Tesla MRI Scan prior to Testosterone replacement or supplementation. If your doctor does not understand the importance of a pre-treatment scan when the topic of Testosterone usage is discussed, you may want to consider our Diagnostic Center for Disease™ in Sarasota, Florida.

Take home message #4: "While Andropause and menopause share many similarities, the effects of androgen replacement therapy in men offer profound differences to that of estrogen and/or progesterone hormone replacement therapy in post-menopausal women. Extrapolation of effects of a hormone in one gender to another is erroneous and misleading." Alvaro Morales, M.D.—Queen's University, Kingston, Ontario

NOTES:

CHAPTER EIGHT

Testosterone Replacement or Supplementation Poses High Risk for Prostate Cancer in the Aging Male

~A Role for an MRI scan to the Anti-Aging Generation~

THE AGING PROCESS is a reality that all men must face. While we can't alter our chronological age, we can influence our physiologic age through proper diet, appropriate nutrition, adequate exercise, stress reduction and education. Speaking to this point, there isn't a man 50 years old or older who doesn't want to slow the aging process while enhancing quality of life. Who wouldn't want a body mass index (BMI) less than 25, more energy, strength and enduring sexual prowess? The secret to the "fountain of youth" may lie in testosterone supplementation or replacement. The message in the media must be making an impact, as there has been a 500 percent increase in testosterone prescription sales in the United States since 1993.

It is estimated that one in seven men suffer from Hypogonadism or decreased testosterone production. Testosterone replacement has been promoted in the literature as the panacea for hypertension, lethargy, depression, obesity, insulin resistance, cognitive dysfunction, sexual dysfunction and various other disease states. Paradoxically, the majority of men who would benefit most from testosterone are over 50 years old; an age where the risk of prostate cancer is increasingly significant. Statistics show that one in six men will get prostate cancer in their lifetime while the most prevalent decade for the diagnosis of prostate cancer is the seventh decade of life or men in their 60s. While testosterone has never been proven to cause prostate cancer, it is well accepted that this prominent male hormone causes prostate cancer to grow, when present. Therefore, with this background information, it would seem to make intuitive sense to consider testosterone usage within the context of an individual's clinical status for having prostate cancer.

According to the American Cancer Society, approximately 230,000 men are diagnosed with prostate cancer yearly. This number is expected to escalate as the "baby boomers" continue to age. **According to the Surveillance, Epidemiology and End-Results (SEER) Data more than 500,000 men will be diagnosed with prostate cancer yearly within the next 8-15 years.** While low testosterone levels are significant in an aging population, prostate cancer remains the number one risk factor that men face from a health standpoint.

PSA (prostate specific antigen), a blood test, has been shown to be the best singular marker to prove the presence of prostate disease, albeit, it is non-specific for the diagnosis of prostate cancer. Truthfully, the PSA is better utilized as **a "barometer of prostate health"** than as a prostate cancer marker. According to Johns Hopkins, the healthiest PSA value for a male aged 40-60 is less than 0.70 ng/ml. Conversely, **the Baltimore Longitudinal Data notes that a man with a PSA of 0.71 ng/ml or higher has a three to four fold increased incidence of prostate cancer when compared to the normal population.** Notwithstanding this commentary, men with a PSA value of 1-10 ng/ml have the same approximate risk of prostate cancer at 20-30 percent. To state more clearly, 70-80 percent of men with an elevated PSA will have inflammation of the prostate or **chronic non-bacterial prostatitis** as **the number one reason PSA elevates followed by any combination of inflammation, prostate enlargement (benign prostate hyperplasia-BPH) and prostate cancer.**

A reasonable PSA level under which men could confidently consider supplementation or replacement with testosterone is a number less than 2 ng/ml, provided that stability has been noted over several prior years. Not inconsistence with my beliefs, **the Society of Endocrinology recommends avoidance of testosterone usage when the PSA number is 3 ng/ml or higher.** Similarly, men should not supplement or replace with testosterone when there is a family history of prostate cancer or if the PSA number has increased by 0.75 ng/ml in consecutive years, consistence with the definition of PSA Velocity change. An exception would be made if a urologist has ruled out prostate cancer. Unfortunately, the most common method to rule out prostate cancer in traditional medicine, involves a biopsy, when the PSA is 2.5 ng/ml or higher. Historically, biopsy has been thought to be a relatively innocuous procedure associated with acceptable, albeit, temporary side effects like bleeding into the bowel, urinary tract and seminal fluid as well as the possibility of additional clinical conditions like infection, sepsis and sexual dysfunction.

While the public has been led to believe that biopsies are a reasonable solution to a rising PSA, an extensive search of the literature, exposes a more sinister and compelling reason to avoid a biopsy unless certain precautions are met and/or the procedure is deemed absolutely necessary. Specifically, there is data that proves a phenomenon called, "needle tracking" takes place routinely with prostate biopsy. This is a significant issue, whereby cells escape the prostate capsule through the biopsy procedure when cancer is present. In this scenario, 20-30 percent of men exposed to a prostate biopsy will experience needle tracking while 70-80 percent of men will be traumatized, enhance cancer development and possibly become infected. In addition to intensifying inflammation as a root cause of prostate cancer, needle tracking or seeding of prostate cancer cells beyond the prostate capsule has been identified in the perineum (the space between the scrotum and the rectum) as well as in the rectal wall.

Prostate biopsy in the traditional format is a crude diagnostic technique (at best), if not; an unacceptable means, to evaluate for prostate cancer based on inherent sampling bias and needle tracking. Sampling bias is associated with the uncertainty for what the biopsy needle will yield as a physician sticks needle after needle randomly into a prostate (up to 86 times) when a mapping procedure is performed in anticipation of treating prostate cancer definitively for cure. This may be an example of where risk does not match the intended reward. **According to Michael Karin, PhD, from the University of California at San Diego, "needle punctures of the prostate exacerbate inflammation which in turn leads to cellular mutation allowing the evolution of prostate cancer with an increased likelihood for metastasis."**

A much more sophisticated technology is now available with the arrival of the 3.0 Tesla Magnetic Resonance Imaging Scan. This technology represents the most sensitive and specific diagnostic modality for the prostate, replacing substandard scanning procedures like PET (Positron Emitting Tomography), CAT scan and Prostascint scans. As stated in an earlier chapter, Peter Scardino, M.D. (Chairman of the Departments of Surgery and Urology at Memorial Sloan-Kettering), called the 3.0 Tesla MRI scan, "the next greatest diagnostic test for prostate cancer." The MRI scan (with or without spectroscopy) creates a virtual road map enabling an evaluation of the entire organ, subsequently allowing for a determination to be made regarding the presence or absence of prostate cancer. In the event an image indicates the presence of prostate cancer; a targeted biopsy can be performed while using a specific protocol to prevent cells that escape from proliferating. Conversely, when the MRI evaluation, replete with all of its various sequences, identifies a localized area of interest that proves to be consistence with the presence of prostate cancer, a decision can be made to treat the disease conservatively with a Chronic Disease Management Protocol, referencing a peer-reviewed study published in the Journal, *Clinical Interventions in Aging* or provide the road map for a focal therapy using either cryosurgery or high-intensity focused ultrasound (HIFU). While a typical biopsy procedure has noted a yield for prostate cancer detection to be only 20-30 percent, a 3.0 Tesla MRI scan has predicted or confirmed the presence of prostate cancer in greater than 90 percent of patients scanned at the Diagnostic Center for Disease™ referencing a blinded study. **Based on these findings, we believe that the future diagnostic landscape will allow for a targeted prostate biopsy, only when preceded by an MRI scan to isolate a region of interest versus treating the diseased prostate based on a scan alone. This paradigm shift in how men qualify for a biopsy will become the new standard of care, allowing men with no evidence of prostate cancer to avoid an unnecessary procedure while treating prostatitis preferentially.** Even if doctors choose not to embrace or understand the advantage of this exceptional technology, patients will demand a change in the diagnostic model, as it is the patient who is asked to bear the scars of professional ignorance.

Presently, physicians from all over the country who have concern for the patients they treat have confidently referred patients to the Diagnostic Center for Disease™ for a 3.0 Tesla MRI scan when the PSA rises in concert with Testosterone usage. With image-guided targeted biopsies (philosophy based), the guessing game is over as no more than six selective biopsies validate the presence or absence of cancer. Every attempt is made to preclude needle tracking with the use of the generic form of Casodex (Bicalutamide). **To date, many men have been diagnosed with prostate cancer, stimulated by Testosterone. In the absence of prostate cancer as determined by an MRI scan and a subsequent reduction in inflammation as noted by a lower PSA (prostatitis resolution) with the patented Peenuts® prostate nutritional formula, it is not unexpected that Testosterone therapy can be resumed with confidence.**

A recent case of a 51-year-old male with an interest in testosterone replacement illustrates the benefits of the 3.0 Tesla MRI scan. Noting a PSA value of only 2.1 ng/ml, the digital rectal exam (DRE) identified an area of interest on the left side, consistent with isolated fibrosis or scarring possibly associated with prostatitis, albeit, it (the DRE) was not conclusive for prostate cancer. Neither the gray scale ultrasound nor Color Flow Doppler ultrasound evaluation suggested any specific abnormality consistent with the area of interest previously identified on DRE. The Mayo Clinic supported a 50% risk for prostate cancer while I predicted a 95% chance cancer was present. An MRI scan using An MRI scan using the 3.0 Tesla technology with an enhanced signal to noise ratio was suggested as the next best step in the evaluation. The scan isolated a region of interest on the left side at the Apex extending to the middle portion of the prostate gland concordant with the atypical findings on the DRE. Based upon the findings of the MRI scan, a targeted biopsy with six needle cores was recommended and implemented. An anti-androgen was initiated pre-biopsy in an attempt to preclude "needle tracking." Specifically, in this case, an anti-androgen selectively blocks the receptor on the prostate cell at the nucleus from attracting testosterone, thereby, disabling the cells in preparation for cell death or apoptosis. The pathology evaluation revealed a grade of cancer that was amenable to being treated conservatively or focally. In this case, the failure to use a 3.0 Tesla MRI scan would have exposed this patient to the possibility of missing the cancer altogether; associated with sampling bias, a very real possibility for needle tracking (assuming cancer was found), or worse yet, the go ahead to supplement with testosterone, when in fact, the cancer could have been missed. Using testosterone in this scenario would have stimulated cancer cells to grow wildly, while causing the PSA to spike abnormally, thereby, making the diagnosis of prostate cancer—a potentially uncontrollable clinical event, albeit, avoidable. Given the expertise of a urologic consultation, this case turned out well. The patient is now contemplating a focal treatment with high-intensity focused ultrasound (HIFU) with a plan to supplement with testosterone once his cancer has been cured. The inability to document the resolution of prostate cancer, however, by a repeat MRI scan and/or a stable PSA post-operatively will preclude this patient from using testosterone replacement therapy.

While studies have shown healthier men require testosterone replacement less frequently than diseased men, there is nonetheless, a generation of men who will want to try to turn back the hands of time. In men with a PSA greater than 2 ng/ml and an interest in anti-aging remedies like testosterone, I urge them to continue the educational process and consider a scan. The toll free number to call to **schedule a *free consultation* is 877-766-8400.** By doing so, an individual may avoid becoming a statistic of ignorance, as was the case with Herbie Mann, the Jazz Flutist.

NOTES:

CHAPTER NINE

Prostate Cancer Diagnosis in Chaos

PROSTATE CANCER, ARGUABLY the most dominant disease that men face, remains as much of an enigma diagnostically to the specialty of urology as it does to the professionals who practice this art form. Despite marginal technological advances over the past 50 years, we are no closer to improving our ability to diagnose prostate cancer than generations past. Proof of this is noted as we routinely schedule repeat biopsies yearly when the PSA remains elevated and of course randomly without a target or image to guide us. **Without pressure from the patient sector or the insurance industry, urologists are content to diagnose prostate cancer as their forefathers did; the "old-fashioned way."** There is no other organ in the human body where the diagnosis is dependent on sticking needles randomly and often times blindly into a delicate organ in an attempt to find cancer. **This practice is archaic, patently barbaric, unacceptable and preferentially favored by virtually all urologists.**

To set the stage, urologists have taken a blood marker called PSA (prostate-specific antigen) better suited to the diagnosis of prostatitis (inflammation) and benign prostatic hyperplasia and applied it to finding cancer. To be sure, the chaos associated with the diagnosis of prostate cancer is not diminished by the fact that an inflammatory marker representing prostatitis represents the number one clinical marker that physicians use to support the need for a biopsy procedure. Data presented at the NIH Prostatitis Collaborative in 2000 showed a PSA value of 1.0 ng/ml or higher to be associated with inflammation of the prostate or prostatitis; virtually 100 percent of the time. Validation for this statement comes from an evaluation of the EPS (expressed prostatic secretion), the proven diagnostic marker for prostatitis where the white blood cell count associated with this secretion defines the disease.

Without question, it is obvious the diagnosis of prostate cancer is anything but an exact science. **Unlike other organ cancers that use imaging excellence to identify lesions of interest, urology has eschewed this technology in favor of remaining "old school." As if stuck in a time warp, urologists have failed to show the intellectual curiosity and leadership that modern medicine demands.** Given the mismatch of applying a blood marker for inflammation to the diagnosis of prostate cancer, we should not be surprised by an abysmal and unacceptable 20-30 percent yield for prostate cancer. With the current system, men are offered random biopsies authoritatively as the "gold standard" or "standard of care." **While financial concerns are an issue in a burgeoning 2.5 billion dollar per year biopsy business, it is difficult to comprehend the tolerance of the insurance industry to accept financial responsibility for a procedure that appears to be self-perpetuated by the physicians who perform it.** More importantly, how long will patients sit quietly and remain the recipient of an invasive procedure where 70-80 percent of patients are told there is no cancer identified? Furthermore, how long will these same patients continue to get back into the line to undergo biopsy after biopsy when the disease they are seeking to find may not have the capacity to be life altering? Noting that 30-56 percent of cancer cases are over treated, suggests that urologists and radiation oncologists need to reconsider the aggressiveness of trying to find cancer at all cost. While multiple clinical models could be applied, it seems quite simple that an effective treatment of prostatitis should be the best first step to try to decrease the number of candidates currently scheduled for biopsy.

When patients begin to understand what physicians fail to commonly recognize; that biopsy procedures are not innocuous procedures but rather invasive procedures that cause scarring in the best case scenario and the spread of prostate cancer cells in the worst of circumstances, imaging should begin to gain some traction and popularity. Using a 3.0 Tesla Magnetic Resonance Imaging scanner, our team at the Diagnostic Center for Disease™ in Sarasota, Florida has been able to predict and confirm the presence of prostate cancer in approximately 90 percent of patients scanned. To be sure, this is a quantum leap from the 20-30 percent "gold standard" or 'standard of care' yield, currently being offered by a urologist near you.

In a classic case, a 67-year-old patient from Cincinnati was told by an esteemed leader in urology that random biopsies are the only way urologists diagnose prostate cancer; period . . . no questions asked. This was his attitude despite four previously negative biopsies and a rising PSA value of 8.4 ng/ml. The physician's comments, notwithstanding, the patient underwent a 3.0 Tesla MRI scan at the Diagnostic Center for Disease™. This scan identified a significant region of interest in a section of the left peripheral zone (anterior horn) from the mid-prostate to the base. The area in question noted an enhanced uptake of the injected Gadolinium (perfusion sequence) supporting the diagnosis of prostate cancer. Only after intense discussion did the urologist in question agree to go along with an image-guided biopsy; a process he called, "folly." After I had the opportunity to discuss the case with the radiologist in Cincinnati, the strategy for a targeted biopsy was set with precautions taken in an attempt to preclude "needle tracking." The biopsy session, guided by the radiologist (**not the urologist**) diagnosed prostate cancer on the left side of the prostate, where the MRI scan predicted the cancer. With the diagnosis in hand, the disbelieving Chairman of Urology in question stated that his department needed to rethink their position relevant to using imaging in the diagnosis of prostate cancer. Maybe this case will encourage more patients to challenge the system and seek the objective expertise of imaging utilizing a 3.0 Tesla MRI scan.

In another compelling case, a 49 year old from North Carolina with an elevated PSA who had experienced two previously negative biopsies underwent a scan noting a 3x12 mm lesion in the left lateral aspect of the prostate at the apex. The perfusion sequence was consistent with the presence of prostate cancer in the identical location. With the scan results in hand, the urologist was able to perform a targeted biopsy to the region of interest specified; finding the cancer. Confirmation of cancer allowed the patient to make an important decision regarding treatment options.

In both clinical cases discussed, a road map had been created allowing the physicians involved to have confidence in putting a needle into the heart of the cancer virtually every time. This is a technology that our center has employed successfully in more than a 1000 patients, thereby, changing the lives of all men we meet. This technology also allows a determination regarding organ-confinement as well as involvement of the seminal vesicles and lymph nodes; quite possibly changing the treatment course planned, assuming a positive biopsy result (www.MrisUSA. com).

Beyond the obvious benefit to being able to see a cancer and its pattern of invasion with the 3.0 Tesla MRI scan, there is no other exam or scan that competes in terms of diagnostic accuracy or predictability. Ultrasound with its gray scale and color flow power Doppler components does not have the specificity required to be considered diagnostic regardless of who administers the technology. **When the PSA continues to rise despite resolution of prostatitis and in an absence of digital findings to support cancer, 3 T MRI provides the most objective evaluation that will determine the presence or absence of prostate cancer. The discerning patient will soon recognize that guessing where a cancer is located, through random biopsies, is for the less informed.** With this in mind, the challenge remains to educate the masses so that all men will have equal advantage for what modern medicine offers while avoiding the chaos of diagnosing prostate cancer the "old fashioned way."

NOTES:

CHAPTER TEN

Controversies associated with prostate health and beyond

INCREDIBLY MORE THAN a billion dollars is spent yearly on nutrients, vitamins, minerals and herbs. The success of the nutritional industry would appear to be well founded, while based on scientific data. Unfortunately marketing genius and scientific rigor do not go hand in hand. The unwitting public at large lays prey to the slick sales staff of publications that are little more than a promotional sales piece. Often times, so-called health experts claim in a newsletter to have traveled the world seeking unique, yet little known health aids that we shouldn't live without. Most of this is hype and sales rhetoric without sound science. While a book could be written on controversial nutrients, I would like to comment on some of the more visible nutrient ingredients or concepts that have had more or less a free pass to this point relevant to objective scientific criticism.

I will begin with the five controversial ingredients that I ask patients at risk of prostate cancer to avoid. To remain fair and balanced, controversial does not mean the concept or product (ingredient or nutrient) does not have merit, but rather speaks to the need for the consumer to be cautious when the benefit perceived could be neutralized or even negated by inherent properties that are rarely if ever discussed.

In the case of Coenzyme Q10 (CoQ10), the wheels of the marketing wizards have been working overtime. CoQ10, a coenzyme that virtually all cells of our body require, is as non-essential enzyme. By non-essential, I mean the body is able to manufacture its own supply of CoQ10. While most experts agree that very little data exists to support the claims of those who would choose to have you take it, CoQ10 appears to have gained notoriety from a cardiac study from Stephen Sinatra, M.D, that showed improved cardiac output (ejection fractions) from those administered the co-enzyme. The data from this study would seem to suggest that patients with signs and symptoms of heart failure might benefit from taking this supplement. **It is my belief if ginseng or caffeine were used as the placebo versus CoQ10 in a head to head double blind study, cardiac output advantage would be negated.** Notwithstanding, the results of the study, the benefit of CoQ10 has now been elevated in status and recommended for all aging adults as we supposedly manufacture less of this co-enzyme as we grow older. That said, **no one has ever demonstrated the decrease in CoQ10 (produced naturally by the body) is insufficient for a quality life or significant to the aging process (assuming an adequate cardiac output).** For anyone to be dogmatic about the role of supplementation of coenzyme Q10 for a much broader indication, more research is required!

Men at risk for prostate cancer (all men with a PSA value of ≥ 1.0 ng/ml) should not take CoQ10 unless they have balanced the purported benefit of CoQ10 with the potential risk of causing prostate cancer to grow. In an independent study, William Fair, M.D. from Memorial Sloan-Kettering exposed various prostate cancer cell lines including DU-145, PC3 and LnCAP to CoQ10. **While some "experts" have assigned benefit of CoQ10 as a cancer cure, Dr. Fair found that prostate cancer cell growth was accelerated by CoQ10. This is referenced in**

Oncology News, September, 1998. This is pretty amazing news for a Coenzyme that heretofore couldn't do any harm. Beyond the topics discussed, CoQ10 has also been shown to elevate VLDL (Very Low Density Lipoprotein) Cholesterol in the blood stream as well. **As you can see, CoQ10 is not for everybody and is clearly controversial.**

When the topic of Flax is discussed, once again the experts are divided. Flax seed or oil is comprised of Omega 3 and Omega 6 fatty acids as well as a source of estrogen (lignan). Omega 3 fatty acids are heart healthy while Omega 6 fatty acids promote cellular oxidation, inflammation and cancer. **Data shows that Flax causes prostate cancer to grow.**

On the same note, beta carotene supplements have been implicated in osteoporosis and prostate cancer growth in independent studies, including the ATBC Study from Finland.

Lycopene, as a supplement, has been advertised as beneficial versus prostate cancer, although the studies suggest otherwise. While most studies relevant to Lycopene have been associated with tomato paste or sauce, there are studies, albeit few, that support the supplement. In a study reported on at the 2005 American Urological Association (AUA) annual meeting, Lycopene was given to men who had failed to be cured with radical prostatectomy as noted by a rising PSA consistent with treatment failure and circulating cancer cells. **The result was resoundingly clear! Lycopene failed to slow the rise in PSA, when compared to placebo, suggesting that this supplement has little to no benefit with prostate cancer.**

In an interesting study performed at Memorial Sloan-Kettering, rats were implanted with known prostate cancer cells. The rats were divided into two groups; one that ate a typical rat diet and the other who ate the identical rat diet with Lycopene added. **When tumor volume was measured,**

the rats that ingested rat diet plus Lycopene grew their tumors at an alarming rate when this data was compared to the diet-only group. As researchers, we are often reminded that rat and mice study findings are often times replicated in the human model.

Another supplement, Chondroitin, a product made from cow cartilage, is frequently found associated with Glucosamine. This combination is commonly used as an anti-arthritic or joint remedy. Unfortunately, the well-intentioned public does not realize that Versican and other specific proteins found in Chondroitin have been shown to cause prostate cancer to grow in independent studies.

As I continue to touch on ingredients, products, and/or concepts that are more about hype than hope, let us be clear about one thing... **there is no such thing as prostate health in 90 days**. The acid test that determines success or failure of any product or concept is to study that product or concept versus markers that allow a disease to be recognized or diagnosed in the first place. When prostate health is the topic, the white blood cell count (Expressed Prostatic Secretion) obtained at the time of prostate massage is the only definitive test to identify prostatitis. Without demonstrating that this marker has improved with whatever is offered, the disease process in question has not been resolved. In this instance, the product or process is worthless. To restate, until research is performed or sponsored that addresses the benefit of a particular ingredient or formula with changes in the EPS, we should discount any claims of benefit as bogus. The public needs to know that without the data, we are only guessing. Urinary symptoms are a marker that is often times incorrectly attributed to the success of an ingredient or formula versus prostatitis. Unfortunately urinary symptoms are non-diagnostic to prostate inflammation as they may be improved commonly with dietary changes or placebo with equal frequency.

Also in the hype category is Essiac tea (a product from Canada), associated with outlandish and dubious claims of benefit versus prostate cancer. While I have never professionally seen a patient who has experienced any benefit that I could attribute to Essiac Tea, I invite the company to send me valid patient data that will allow me the opportunity to assess the benefit independently. Anecdotal accounts of success are misleading to desperate individuals with disease who will commonly try various remedies without any real scientific validation; in the hope for success. **Until I see the data from the manufacturers, I encourage the public to save their money as the Essiac formula appears to be more about hype than hope.**

Graviola, allegedly, a product of a South American fruit tree, has been purported to have benefit versus prostate cancer. To this point, I have many patients who have used this formula without any appreciable benefit. More disturbing to me as I evaluate patients who were recommended by sales persons to use this formula, is that this product is associated with a worsening of prostate cancer as demonstrated by a rise in PSA (recognized worldwide as the marker or prostate cancer disease activity). **The offer remains for the manufacturers of Graviola to show me the data.** I will be happy to report on this and other findings in the next edition of this book. The gauntlet has been dropped! Now, let's see the results. **Until I am satisfied with this formula making a difference, avoid it!!**

The Health Science Institute (HSI) tries to impress its readership that its articles speak to valid medical research, while this is bolstered by a exemplary medical advisory board that appears to endorse or condone what is being written. While this may be their intention, I have seen many issues that represent blatant commercialism with little to no scientific data. I encourage this news group and others to take the higher road when educating the unwitting public-at-large; providing evidence for the benefits of all products through valid research; nothing less. Specifically, we must be accountable to a vulnerable population that wants hope; but we shouldn't promote or market products or concepts with very little science or marginal science, as this is irresponsible and unacceptable.

Antineoplastins (amino acids) popularized by Stanislaw Burzinski, M.D. for brain cancer have been suggested for other cancers including prostate cancer. While I have encouraged an interim report from Dr. Burzinski and his staff on the success of this concept versus prostate cancer, I have been told for many years that the data is not yet available. I have personally and professionally reviewed a case that fails to make a compelling argument in favor of using an expensive amino acid formulation. In my referenced case, a 64 year business executive with a Gleason 6 prostate cancer failed to show any benefit from Dr. Burzinski's formula. In fact, the patient in question, represented herein, is a test case not even outperforming patients who are benefiting from diet and nutrition alone. While one case does not make a study, this case merely suggests that this formula is not a "silver bullet" or cure for Gleason 6 prostate cancers. It is my opinion that there are many other treatment concepts that make sense without enduring the financial hardship of a costly formula that has yet to validate its claims or references for success. **As of this writing, I cannot recommend Antineoplastins for prostate cancer as I have many proven successful options to treating prostate cancer currently in the war chest. On the other hand, I applaud Dr. Burzinski and his staff for their work in brain cancer research.**

Ag Immune, an immune boosting formula popularized by Jesse Stoff, M.D. in his book, "Prostate Miracle" has not shown any benefit versus prostate cancer. **Hyped to his patients as a product that will eliminate prostate cancer, I struggle when this does not happen.** While I cannot deny a slight rise to the natural killer T cell level with its use, the T cells do not recognize the cancer cells and therefore does nothing versus prostate cancer. **The inability of this formula and other immune stimulating formulas to alter the course of prostate cancer is not new to medicine.** Vaccines are founded on the principle that an antigen(s) will be targeted through a stimulated immune system. Once again, the cancer disease process is complex, while conquering the disease is not as easy as stimulating the immune system. **Many patient case studies using Ag Immune are on file; failing to demonstrate any benefit by altering the progression of prostate cancer.**

Enzyme therapy for pancreatic cancer is intriguing. Dr. Nick Gonzalez, from New York, has been making a positive impact versus a terrible life threatening disease. While I hope we will be hearing more about his research, people with pancreatic cancer should contact him as well as consider the research of CZ Biomed (www.czbiomed.com), the research group studying the effects of oncolytic viruses versus various cancers.

A physician from the west coast of the USA has claimed at multiple cancer advocacy meetings (Cancer Control Society, as example) that her breast cancer was cured by fruits and vegetables. While the case history is complex, it is my opinion that this did not take place, but rather the benefit was gleaned from chemotherapy she had been taking concurrently. I have no doubt fruits and vegetables play a role, but it is misleading to tell a story with selective memory loss for the facts, thereby, potentially deceiving the populace in greatest need, by ignoring important and relevant treatment details. To make matters more concerning is that she sells her brand of fruits and vegetables to her listening audience without the data to support the endorsement.

The Rife Machine is advertised as having an impact on prostate cancer. I have many patients who have used this concept without success. While I am not declaring this technology as useless, someone needs to study this in earnest and show me something! Until this is done I cannot endorse something that may work and then . . . may not! Patients are cautioned about using concepts that are less than advertised. Besides, I would be happy to evaluate patients who routinely don't see doctors but still have disease that needs attention by someone like me who is open-minded to new and/or novel concepts. While I do not know all the answers, I am working on it diligently! As the former basketball coach, Jim Valvano from North Carolina State once said, referencing cancer, a disease he died from; **"don't give up, and don't ever give up"!!** While he was speaking to all people with cancer to never give up hope through his compassionate words of wisdom, he supported research and innovative thinking as well. He has been missed!

Progesterone cream, popularized by John Lee, M.D. to assist women with hormonal deficiencies as they age is currently embraced by Jonathan Wright for men with prostate cancer. More specifically, progesterone, a female hormone that modifies the impact of estradiol in women, is a precursor of androstendione and testosterone in men. Testosterone stimulation in men who have prostate cancer must be avoided excepting research models where prostate cancer cells have been deprived of testosterone for years while using an LHRH (Luteinizing Hormone Releasing Hormone) Analog like Lupron, Trelstar or Zoladex. **Regardless of what you have heard, it is imperative that you remember that in the majority of prostate cancer patients, while testosterone did not cause the prostate cancer; it causes prostate cancer to grow.** I have seen many patients in my practice who have sought my expertise in consultation relevant to prostate cancer, who have assisted their own diagnosis of prostate cancer by supplementing with testosterone or a precursor like progesterone. If you choose to ignore my advice,

I encourage you to monitor your PSA (prostate specific antigen) with vigilance, under the watchful eye of a health care advisor, while using these so-called remedies. **For the record, I do not recommend Progesterone Cream for men as I have had too many cases where the prostate cancer was stimulated to grow. End of discussion until more validated research begs to change my opinion!**

DHEA (dehydroepiandrosterone) represents a testosterone precursor and should be avoided in most cases of prostate cancer. Wild Yam, a source of DHEA should also be avoided when an elevated PSA is detected (greater than 1.0 ng/ml) or if prostate cancer had previously been diagnosed. In effect, I have not seen enough data to support its use.

Nanobacterium is a tiny microbe 1/100th the size of a typical bowel bacteria like Escherichia Coli. While it is unclear whether this microbe is a friend or a foe, it has been implicated as a source of calcium production throughout the human body. It is plausible that calcium deposition is associated with inflammation pertinent to prostate physiology or function. Research has suggested that calcium can be reduced by chelation through the use of EDTA (Ethylenediaminetetraacetic acid) and Tetracycline. At this point, we have no clue for the benefit of this concept based on response to the use of standardized biologic markers. There has only been a benefit achieved versus subjective markers like discomfort and pain attributed to the prostate. **Unfortunately, subjective markers lack the validation clarity that standardized markers provide.** The challenge to the Tampa-based company and others are to validate the benefit that they believe they are achieving versus a quantitative evaluation of white blood cells in the expressed prostatic secretion (EPS). **EPS is a marker recognized worldwide that represents prostate inflammation through the identification of white blood cells.** In studies that have been carried out in my research facility as well as others, calcium density in prostate tissue plays an unknown role. More specifically, I have been able to show resolution of white blood cells in the EPS with the Peenuts® formula, which is validation to an improvement in an inflammatory marker in prostatitis, the most dominant prostate disease. **Nowhere in my research, can the suggestion be made that a reduction in the density of calcification has anything to do with disease resolution.** Resolution of prostate disease can only be achieved with a defined reduction in white blood cells in the EPS. **Ignoring this factor while demonstrating a reduction in tissue calcium density attempts inappropriately to circumvent an obvious marker that validates inflammation. Any attempt to suggest that a decrease in calcium density has any redeeming value without the concurrent status of the white cells in the EPS, deliberately ignores more than 50 years of research associated with prostate inflammation and prostatitis.** It is for this reason, that **I cannot endorse or even consider a product or concept for my patients with prostatitis (prostate inflammation) that fails to recognize or build on what is already well established in association with prostate health.**

AMAS—(Anti-malignan Antibody in the Sera) test is a blood test popularized by George Bogash that adds nothing to my understanding of prostate cancer. **Initially, I was willing to look at the concept but my inability to enhance the information known in some meaningful manner has dropped this test from the recommended list.** For this reason, I advise men with suspicion for prostate cancer based on an elevated PSA to avoid this test and thereby **avoid the confusion that is commonly encountered when it is performed.** Specifically for prostate cancer, the sensitivity (Ability to identify true positives) and the specificity (ability to identify true negatives) with this test add nothing to the patient's diagnostic landscape. I have had a significant number of patients who received a negative cancer reading in the presence of cancer while many others had a positive result with no evidence of cancer. **While I think the individuals who developed and market this test are sincere and well intentioned, the information obtained from the test is unreliable and therefore not part of my diagnostic regimen.**

Toremifene is a SERM or selective estrogenic receptor modulator. This is a compound that our readers will be hearing more about in the future but I believe that caution must be exercised in believing the data presented. Specifically, Toremifene is a compound that supposedly has promise when prostate cancer precursor cells are identified on a biopsy. In a study where high grade prostatic intra-epithelial neoplasia (High Grade PIN; HGPIN) cells were found on a typical prostate biopsy, the addition of Toremifene showed a decrease in High grade PIN cells when compared to placebo (the sugar pill). Unfortunately, the findings were associated with random chance. In other words, **the company that markets this product is trying to convince the medical community that a biopsy with its inherent sampling bias proves something of value. Unfortunately, it does not.** Without precision diagnostics associated with improved imaging like MRI with or without enhanced perfusion agents, the research data on Toremifene amounts to little more than research bias or a guess. Relevant to this concept, a study protocol must be offered that can be validated. **An educated guess must never be construed as validation.** We hope to have an opportunity to study this important group of HGPIN patients through better imaging and precision biopsies based on mapped coordinates while controlling for prostatitis using the Peenuts® formula.

All patients with cancer deserve a measure of hope; while hype and/or sensationalism in reporting have no place in the cancer treatment arena. **While integrative medicine combines complementary medicine and traditional medicine together, it is my belief that this combination is far superior to traditional medicine in many disease models.** Nonetheless, we must not divorce ourselves from the science that validates traditional medicine. **Vulnerable prostate cancer patients must be able to find a coach who will aggressively defend fact from fiction for the individual who knows little about the disease and even less about the most appropriate treatment. As the saying goes, "if it sounds too good, it probably is."** Therefore, it is always buyer beware. With cancer in general and prostate cancer specifically, we have a long way to go before victory can be declared. Promising medications, formulas, gene therapy and vaccines in association with better imaging expects to change the landscape of prostate cancer forever. Be cautious, it's a jungle out there! There are many who choose to take advantage of you at a time of weakness or vulnerability. This is unacceptable and cannot be tolerated!

NOTES:

CHAPTER ELEVEN

Controversial Male Health Studies from the Literature

CONTROVERSY IS NOT new to the medical field. In this chapter, I have pre-selected research studies that while controversial, are nonetheless, important timely topics with implications for your health and quality of life. Clarity relevant to the take home message in these studies can only be accomplished through vigorous academic dialogue or debate. To be sure, while I expect to stimulate your interest, all that is discussed will be relevant to your journey through life. **Let's begin . . .**

> **The Prostate Cancer Prevention Trial (PCPT) sponsored by Merck appeared to make the statement that the use of a 5-Alpha Reductase Inhibitor such as Proscar (Finasteride) or Avodart (Dutasteride) could, in fact, decrease the incidence of prostate cancer**

The study conclusions documented a 25 percent decrease in the incidence of prostate cancer in men who used this drug. While such a large percentage may be controversial by itself, Peter Scardino, M.D. Chairman of the Departments of Surgery and Urology at Memorial Sloan Kettering added to the controversy when he claimed the concept of taking a drug to block the conversion of Testosterone to Dihydrotestosterone (DHT) merely created a group of more aggressive cancers when cancer was detected. In other words, if you were not one of the lucky individuals to avoid prostate cancer while taking this drug, you were likely to contract a more aggressive cancer when the use of this drug was compared to the placebo arm. **What wasn't taken into account was the reduction in size of the prostate expected with this class of drug in association with biopsy sampling bias. In other words, an element of aggressive cancer was already present (missed by the initial biopsy) and made more evident by a subsequent biopsy into a smaller prostate.**

Dr. Wheeler's commentary:

From my point of view, men who are at risk of prostate cancer based on a family history should consider a protocol to prevent prostate cancer utilizing this class of a drug. Without question, the decrease in prostate cancer detection is substantial and should not be dismissed or taken lightly in a group of individuals at high risk for prostate cancer. While my personal preference is to block type one, type two and type 3 Isoenzymes of 5-Alpha Reductase through the use of Avodart, the reduction in Dihydrotestosterone that results may play a key role in delaying or altering permanently the evolutionary path to prostate cancer. In a prevention model, I recommend patients to take Avodart at 0.5 mg weekly rather than daily as recommended by the FDA. My goal is to cut down on unwanted side effects while maximizing prevention. This recommendation is based in part on a five week half-life (the time it takes for the drug to lose half of its potency or effectiveness) for the drug, suggesting that this may be a fair compromise for a group of men who want to be proactive. This concept is currently being studied by Glaxo, the Pharmaceutical Company that manufactures Avodart. As always, men are advised to discuss this interesting concept with their trusted physician.

Testosterone supplementation is a hot topic for the "baby boomer generation"

Who among us does not want to appear and/or act younger? Who among us does not want added physical strength or enhancement to our sexual prowess? The controversy suggests that while Testosterone makes us more vital, if not virile, there is a risk with supplementation to cause prostate cancer to grow. I want to be clear about this; **Testosterone has never been shown to cause prostate cancer but has been shown to cause prostate cancer to grow.** In a small study, 41 men who had Testosterone levels identified at less than 300 ng/dl were randomized to receive 150 mg of Testosterone every two weeks into the muscle or receive a placebo delivered in the same manner. While there was no mention of baseline PSA values, biopsies were performed at baseline and at six months. The results suggested a lack of prostate cancer on biopsy supports the use of Testosterone supplementation; at least in the short term of six months. In other words, the authors theorized the intramuscular shots of Testosterone may have had a less pronounced effect on the prostate than commonly presumed. Additional lab studies that appeared to validate the conclusion included prostate tissue levels of Testosterone and Dihydrotestosterone, cell proliferation biomarkers Ki67 and MBI1, and gene expression profiles.

Dr. Wheeler's Commentary:
While I appreciate the short-term data, men who are interested in Testosterone use are not looking at the short term. **Unfortunately, men reading this commentary from other sources will mistakenly get the message that Testosterone**

supplementation appears safe and effective. For this reason, the study findings have fallen short of the intended mark and are of little value. **A point of criticism**; if prostate cancer is an issue with Testosterone usage (and it is), why wasn't the most prolific marker of prostate cancer (PSA) evaluated? If it was, why wasn't the data discussed? In my opinion, this study creates more questions than answers and frankly sends the wrong message.

If this study used MRI scanning instead of random biopsies, we could have learned something of value. Most people know and/or understand the concept that random biopsies are biased based on where the biopsy needle was placed. MRI, on the other hand, is an objective review of the entire prostate, allowing for all sequences to play a role in the identification and location of a cancer. While Jurgen Futterer, Claire Allen, Anwar Padhani, Gerald Grubbs, Thomas Fabian, Richard Goldberg, myself and others have stated **Spectroscopy, (an MRI sequence that evaluates the metabolites of cell function) is not a necessity to the diagnosis; it is nonetheless valuable information enhancing the concordance of positive data when present.** Biopsy based data based on random needles entering the prostate does little to nothing to validate an absence of prostate cancer and little to support the use of testosterone in an aging population of men with low levels of male hormone. We must never forget the lesson learned from Herbie Mann, the famed jazz flutist who died from prostate cancer after the disease was stimulated to grow wildly by testosterone supplementation/replacement. This case history and others suggest the best advice for men is to avoid testosterone or precursors like androstendione, progesterone or DHEA unless the PSA is less than 2.0 ng/ml and the prostate exam is non-suspicious. Notwithstanding what is stated above, the use of MRI with or without Spectroscopy may be used to validate a lack of suspicion for prostate cancer; enabling a role for testosterone supplementation and other youth-assisting concepts even when the PSA level is higher than 2.0 ng/ml. **While others have questioned my conservative approach, don't be fooled by the hype when you must bear the scars for what you decide! Be wise my friends!**

<h3 style="text-align:center">High grade prostatic intraepithelial neoplasia (HGPIN) is a pathologic finding associated with the evolution of prostate cancer
~A chemical compound called Toremifene claims to eradicate this precursor lesion~</h3>

According to some experts, HGPIN is a precursor lesion to prostate cancer in upwards of 40 percent of the cases. Additionally, it is not uncommon to find HGPIN in the presence of established prostate cancer. Based on the significance of this correlation, there is a keen interest in trying to delay and/or eliminate what appears to be a cause and effect process of cellular metabolic changes to prostate cancer. Toremifene, a selective estrogenic receptor modulator (SERM), has been proposed as a possible remedy for men who have had HGPIN identified on a previous biopsy in an attempt to avoid the evolution to prostate cancer.

Dr. Wheeler's commentary:

As a physician, I have seen multiple articles in various health news periodicals speaking to the potential benefit of eliminating HGPIN with the use of Toremifene. Before anyone gets too excited, it is important to note that this study suffers from the same biopsy sampling bias that has created doubt in other studies. In other words, despite the fact that professionals understand the issue of sampling bias associated with biopsy procedures, we nonetheless, continue to support findings from studies using the biopsy as definitive proof. In a phase II trial intended to evaluate the benefit of modulating estrogen receptors in the prostate with

Toremifene, 514 patients were randomized to receive various milligram doses of Toremifene or a placebo. Only men who had been diagnosed with HGPIN were permitted to enter the study. While we could debate the merits of how Toremifene interacts with prostate cells, prostate cancer cells or prostate cancer precursor cells given its estrogenic receptor modulation activity, the more important and rudimentary issue lies with trying to prove anything based on a biopsy.

To understand this concept more clearly, take a lime (the approximate size of an average prostate) and put a black dot the size of a match head on it anywhere. This will represent a precursor lesion, like HGPIN is to prostate cancer. Once the ink is dry, close your eyes and roll the lime around in your hand. With your eyes still closed tightly, place eight shirt pins in the lime without sticking your finger. This is the equivalent of what your doctor is doing when he performs biopsies on your prostate. Do this exercise 10 times over and record how many times a pin hits the black spot. If you do the experiment correctly, you will readily see the futility of trying to find a very small lesion (a common occurrence in biopsy procedures), much less, the same lesion that prompted entry into the study. **To state more clearly, depending on the amount of cancer present or precursor cells present, there is just as great a chance, if not greater, of missing cancer as finding it.** Thus, without employing sound scientific principles, there is no credibility to the data collected.

In effect, this study represents little more than a marketing exercise from the manufacturer to the doctors who participated. There was very little proven with the exception that doctors would have the same difficulty hitting the black dot on the lime as you will, as it is pretty much a blind exercise or "shot in the dark." Rather than share with the world the results of an expensive, time consuming study that proves little, we need to continue to look to improved imaging studies like MRI scans to map the entire prostate for either cancer or precursors to cancer improving the odds that subsequent objective data obtained has been validated with a reproducible location. Beyond this, a fair question might be; how did this article make it into a prestigious journal?

Brachytherapy alone is effective versus prostate cancer
~Your ability to perform sexually may depend on your treatment choice~

Patients with intermediate risk prostate cancer may be effectively treated with brachytherapy (otherwise known as seed therapy) without supplemental pelvic external beam radiation according to Javier F. Torres-Roca, M.D. (H. Lee Moffitt Cancer Center at the University of South Florida in Tampa, Fla.) **Dr. Torres-Roca and colleagues defined intermediate risk factors as a Gleason score of 7 (associated with approximately 35 percent of all prostate cancer patients), a PSA level between 10-20 ng/ml, and/or clinical stage of T2b or T2c (high volume organ-confined cancer).** According to the data, outcomes were not significantly influenced by risk factors including a Gleason score of 6 versus 7, clinical stage T1 versus T2 (non-palpable vs. palpable cancer), tumor burden (number of biopsies positive), pretreatment PSA level less than 10 ng/ml versus 10 ng/ml or greater, or one intermediate risk factor versus two or more intermediate risk factors. Furthermore, it was noted that men had an 83 percent chance to be disease free at five years when brachytherapy was performed alone. Men with perineural invasion (disease extension beyond the prostate capsule) identified on the biopsy specimen had a decreased chance of being disease-free (64 percent), demonstrating the importance of this finding. According to Dr. Torres-Roca, a recommendation should be made to perform an MRI of the prostate with an Endorectal coil to rule out any extracapsular or extraprostatic extension prior to initiating brachytherapy as a monotherapy. **These findings become more relevant to the patient as he considers his sexual abilities post-treatment. A study by Speight and colleagues showed that men who had combination therapy with brachytherapy and external beam radiation therapy had decreased quality of life (QOL) sexual performance scores when compared to men who received either brachytherapy or external beam therapy alone.**

Dr. Wheeler's commentary:

While the Moffitt data looks impressive, not all experts agree with their high yield of success. By contrast, D'Amico et. al reported only a 34 percent biochemical disease free survival rate at five years while using PSA as the disease activity marker. My professional experience would suggest the Moffitt data may not be mature and therefore, not entirely reliable. Based on this fact, patients must be carefully followed in the interim and reported on again at 7-8 years post therapy. My private practice patient experience supports a not so-glowing report consistent with the findings of nomograms (cancer prediction models) emanating with Johns Hopkins, Memorial Sloan-Kettering, and other esteemed institutions, while modestly improving on the data from D'Amico. **For this reason, patients are cautioned not to rely too heavily on five-year data.** Notwithstanding an apparent level of success at Moffitt, it is not unusual to see failure rates of 40-60 percent by 7-10 years regardless of the primary therapy performed.

Given the diversity of response, patients with prostate cancer are urged to continue to remain conservative, whenever possible, giving consideration to living with the disease through a surveillance protocol like Chronic Disease Management (CDM) discussed elsewhere in this book. It may be that MRI using a modified 1.5 Tesla magnet or a 3.0 Tesla magnet complemented by specialized software will assist us in the patient selection process while defining the relative risks associated with various objective clinical markers. Until further notice, men with prostate cancer should consider their options carefully, while keeping an open mind. That said; **the best first choice might be a choice that has not yet been considered or yet approved for use in the United States like High Intensity Focused Ultrasound (HIFU).**

NOTES

Zyflamend in men with high-grade prostatic intraepithelial neoplasia: results of a phase I clinical trial

Journal Soc Integr Oncol. 2009 Spring; Capodice JL, Gorroochurn P, Cammack AS, Eric G, McKiernan JM, Benson MC, Stone BA, Katz AE. Department of Urology, Columbia University College of Physicians and Surgeons, New York, NY 10032, USA.

Subjects diagnosed with high-grade prostatic intraepithelial neoplasia (HGPIN) at biopsy are at increased risk for developing prostate cancer (CaP). A prospective clinical trial was done to determine the safety and tolerability of a novel herbal amalgam, Zyflamend (New Chapter, Inc., Brattleboro, VT), with various dietary supplements in subjects with HGPIN. Men ages 40 to 75 years with HGPIN were eligible. Subjects were evaluated for 18 months. Every 3 months, standard blood chemistries and prostate-specific antigen (PSA) were monitored. **Rebiopsy was done every 6 months.** Tissue was evaluated for HGPIN or prostate cancer and stained for cyclooxygenase-2, nuclear factor kappaB (NF-kappaB), interleukin-6, and thromboxane. The mean PSA level was 6.0 ng/mL. Side effects, when present, were mild while gastrointestinal in nature. There were no reported serious adverse events or toxicities. No significant changes in blood chemistries, testosterone, or cardiac function were noted. Forty-eight percent of subjects demonstrated a 25 to 50% decrease in PSA after 18 months. Of subjects who had the 18-month biopsy, 60% (9 of 15) had benign tissue, 26% (4 of 15) had HGPIN in one core, and 13% (2 of 15) had CaP at 18 months. A reduction in serum C-reactive protein was observed. Immunoreactive staining demonstrated a reduction in NF-kappaB in the 18-month samples. Zyflamend alone and in combination with various dietary supplements is associated with minimal toxicity and no serious adverse events when administered orally for 18 months.

Dr. Wheeler's Commentary:

Zyflamend, a COX II Inhibitor (look alike) product from New Chapter was studied as related to its perceived effectiveness in patients with High Grade Prostatic Intraepithelial Neoplasia (HGPIN), noted on biopsy. Using random prostate biopsies with its inherent level of academic deception associated with sampling bias, Dr. Aaron Katz from Columbia University Hospital Medical Center has taken the liberty to proclaim that patients at risk for prostate cancer (based on HGPIN) lowered their risk by taking Zyflamend. In a few words, nice try but no cigar! **Intellectually, this is bad science that can never be construed as anything but that!** To be sure, Dr. Katz's conclusion cannot be supported by his diagnostic methodology! To be completely clear about this, there is zero chance that Aaron or anyone else can make their claim stand up to the scrutiny that will be given by objective research critics without a vested interest; beyond my commentary! **Unfortunately, Dr. Katz and colleagues have proven nothing more than they cannot hit the lesion previously identified on a subsequent biopsy; nothing more, nothing less!** Furthermore, **the benefits of Zyflamend have not been clearly defined as a nutritional of significant clinical value; creating more confusion than substance.**

Decreasing the number of patients who qualify for prostate biopsy—Can effect of Finasteride on prostate-specific antigen be used to decrease repeat prostate biopsy?

While I have proposed earlier in this chapter that 5-Alpha Reductase inhibitors (5-ARIs: Finasteride and Dutasteride (Avodart)) have been shown to prevent prostate cancer, Handel et. al suggest that this class of drug may prevent the need for additional prostate biopsies in men with an initial negative biopsy. Historically, men who take this class of drug in the absence of prostate cancer are expected to experience their total PSA value to be cut in half. **Those individuals, who don't decrease their PSA by at least half, should become suspicious for prostate cancer.** Noting this phenomenon, this group of authors evaluated the effect of Finasteride on PSA density (PSAD). PSA density is calculated by dividing the total PSA by the size of the prostate in cubic centimeters or grams. **Specifically, in their study using Finasteride, they noted a decrease in PSAD of 44 percent in the absence of prostate cancer while patients diagnosed with prostate cancer had a 5 percent decrease in PSAD only.**

Dr. Wheeler's commentary:

This is an important study that has the potential to reduce unnecessary secondary biopsies using a diagnostic equation, notwithstanding, a persistently elevated PSA. Unfortunately, this study also suffers from the same biopsy sampling bias discussed previously. While the authors correctly point out the need for additional studies, the process of evaluating prostate tissue integrity must become more sophisticated through imaging if we are truly going to advance the cause of selectively avoiding biopsies. Clinically, the most common risk factor that suggests the need for prostate biopsy is an elevated PSA. Regardless of the exact PSA number, studies have shown a 20-30 percent risk of prostate cancer detection when the PSA value is between 1 ng/ml and 10 ng/ml. Currently the number of men diagnosed with prostate cancer from a biopsy is approaching 250,000 a year. Even more staggering is the more than 1,250,000 men who must undergo the biopsy to find the 250,000 cancer patients at a yearly cost in excess of 2 billion dollars. Aside from the huge financial implications of putting more than 1 million men through a procedure needlessly, there is concern for trauma, side effects, time lost, misinformation and angst.

The need to develop solutions to reduce the number of biopsy candidates has never been more pronounced than now, as **"baby boomers"** age. While the future may lie in better imaging through MRI, as example, we need novel concepts today. **The inability of 5-ARIs to decrease the PSA by half is one method while PSAD reduction with this drug is yet another.** Regardless of the method, the goal is to decrease the number of men asked to wait in line for a biopsy; something they may never have needed in the first place. From a patient perspective, the side effects, no matter how minimal, associated with a medication, is, nonetheless, a deterrent to this approach.

In my opinion, the opportunity to reduce unnecessary biopsies of the prostate is not difficult but lies in the comprehension of the following conundrum. **If the number one reason prostate biopsies are performed is PSA elevation above 4.0 ng/ml, yet, the number one reason PSA rises above 4.0 ng/ml is prostatitis, why are we not paying closer attention to prostatitis? Does it not make sense intuitively, if not academically, to resolve prostatitis first while reducing PSA associated with inflammation to an acceptable level or range, thereby, possibly avoiding a biopsy?** Am I missing something here? Resolution of prostatitis with its inherent reduction in PSA value will allow men to predictably step out of line and avoid what appears to be an unnecessary, if not, premature biopsy. Relevant to prostatitis, we have learned from history that antibiotics are ineffective in the vast majority of cases. **To be sure, according to the National Institutes of Health or other reputable sources, in excess of 95 percent of cases of prostatitis are non-bacterial.** Effectively, if there is an absence of fever, chills or rigors (uncontrollable shaking) in association with signs and symptoms consistent with prostatitis, we have a non-bacterial event most of the time. **So why not try an all-natural prostatitis formula called Peenuts®; a product that is patented all over the world?** Not only does PSA decrease on this formula with continuous usage in the absence of cancer; urinary symptoms improve, while inflammation resolves. Critics may argue that this sounds too logical. While additional studies are always encouraged, **I submit to you, resolving prostatitis, and the concurrent rise in PSA is the best first step in avoiding unnecessary biopsies.** In my practice, biopsy is only viable with insisting patients who fail to lower the PSA dramatically or to normal levels. The lower PSA number correlates to a decrease in the white blood cell count in the EPS (expressed prostatic secretion), obtained at the time of prostate examination.

I had a Urologist from the prestigious Watson Clinic in Lakeland, Florida tell me he diagnosed a patient with prostate cancer while taking the Peenuts® formula. **This is not unusual as this formula does not mask prostate cancer or falsely lower the PSA.** In a small study, men who failed to lower their PSA dramatically to less than 4.0 ng/ml, (while using the formula for minimally one year), were subjected to a traditional random 8 core biopsy. What I found was more than 90 percent of men in this group had prostate cancer. **In effect, the inability of this prostatitis formula to decrease the PSA over time appears to be sine qua non to the diagnosis of prostate cancer.** While the news is exciting, a larger study is suggested to validate the findings. In the short term, there is literally no down side for the use of an all-natural formula without any known side effects. Interested men are encouraged to learn more by visiting www. Peenuts.com.

While there is no shortage of skeptics, without a randomized, double blind, placebo-controlled study to validate the efficacy of this formula clinically and statistically; how many men in their

40s, much less their 50s, can boast of a PSA of 0.3 ng/ml? More importantly, my PSA value has been flat-lined at 0.3 ng/ml for more than 10 consecutive years, following a drop in PSA of 40 percent after the first year while on the Peenuts® formula only. While I encourage others to offer their novel ideas or solutions for avoiding future biopsies, I equally expect scientific data to validate their claims based on biologic markers that include EPS, PSA and urinary symptoms.

When should 80-year-old men with prostate cancer consider Radical Prostatectomy?

According to Houston Thompson, M.D. and a few of his colleagues at the Mayo Clinic, Radical prostatectomy for prostate cancer in a man in his 80s is quite reasonable. The article provides data that healthy well-informed octogenarians will request radical prostatectomy for prostate cancer treatment. The article goes on to suggest that doctors should not stand in the way of men who have made up their mind regarding how they choose to manage their disease. **The take-home message from the article is that 80-year-old men can tolerate a radical prostatectomy and that the procedure can be performed safely and effectively in this group of men.**

Dr. Wheeler's commentary:
Just when I am about to close this chapter, another article comes across my desk that is screaming for my commentary. **While most of the articles discussed in this chapter have merit, this article seems to bend all the rules.** As far as I know, no one has ever said that doing surgery successfully on an 80-year-old man cannot be done. The question is not when to do the surgery but why do the surgery? The article points out that patients should not be denied their right to choose a radical

prostatectomy if their mind is made up. It is not necessarily the patients' understanding of prostate cancer treatment that I am concerned about, but rather, the rationalization of some of my esteemed colleagues who see nothing irregular with the process, thereby **claiming discrimination of the elderly or ageism.** What are the criteria for knowledge prior to a patient being able to make this decision regardless of age? What constitutes informed consent? Can we assume that the good doctors at Mayo told the men that they would live 15 years (on average) regardless of what was done for prostate cancer? Did they inform their patients that living with prostate cancer could be far more appealing than wetting their pants? Protocols that encourage conservative management for prostate cancer include Chronic Disease Management (CDM) or active surveillance. Did we tell this noble group of risk takers that the chance of dying from heart disease was likely greater than dying from a Gleason 6 cancer? Don't we at least owe this group a level of confidence that the cancer is organ-confined prior to prostatectomy, when in fact it was not?

While the risks from any surgery can be significant, how many of these patients realized this disease had virtually no chance of killing them, if left alone? How many of these patients would have gone through with the procedure if the doctor who presented the facts in a fair and balanced manner insisted on an additional opinion. How many patients would have gone through with the surgery had they realized the percent chance their cancer was already outside the prostate (extracapsular) was minimally 26 percent. If they had known, would they still agree to a procedure that promised to alter their quality of life matters not, as it only seems to make the determined participants even more adamant that what they were doing made perfect sense. **No one can deny the influence of a physician sitting in front of a less than educated patient speaking the virtues**

of a possible cure even if the natural history of the disease is not well understood by the doctor or the disadvantaged patient. Clearly, there are more questions than answers in this "world-class study." **I had to laugh when the authors claimed the "patients would likely suffer psychologically if the prostate wasn't removed."** This suggests we are not reading the same journals or practicing on the same planet. This study should not be about why we should perform a surgery or whose rights have been violated if we don't; but rather to try to understand why it is important to try to convince others that the actions of a few patients and a few doctors justifies others to follow suit based on a research article that validates little more than it is physically possible for 80-year-old men to survive the surgery. Wow!!!!

NOTES:

CHAPTER TWELVE

Pathology of Prostate Cancer

THIS CHAPTER, LARGELY presented by David Bostwick and Isabelle Meiers, is accompanied by my editorial commentary. Patients are increasingly mindful of my position on biopsy and the changes needed in the urology profession relevant to the importance of imaging to the diagnosis of prostate cancer.

Epidemiology

The incidence of prostate cancer has risen dramatically in the past decade, probably owing to early detection programs that employ digital rectal examination, serum PSA, transrectal ultrasonography and MRI. In 2010, 27,350 Americans died of prostate cancer, and 234,460 new cases were diagnosed. As competing causes of mortality, such as lung cancer and heart disease decline, men are living longer and increasing their risk of developing clinically apparent prostate cancer. Despite an autopsy prevalence of up to 80% by age 80 years, the clinical incidence is much lower, indicating that most men die *with* prostate carcinoma rather than *of* prostate cancer. The incidence of prostate cancer is higher in blacks (100 per 100,000) than in whites (70.1 per 100,000), and is low in American Indians, Hispanics, and Orientals. Interestingly, the prevalence of latent cancer is similar in different geographic groups despite wide variation in clinical incidence.

When are suspicious results not a diagnosis of prostate cancer?

Prostate cancer has no specific presenting symptoms (such as urinary problems), and is usually clinically silent, although it may cause lower urinary tract symptoms (weak urination or inability to urinate) mimicking benign prostatic hyperplasia (BPH). Most cases today are found during screening or routine physical examination in men over 40 years of age; digital rectal examination shows a nodular or diffusely enlarged prostate, or serum PSA concentration is elevated, usually greater than 2.5 ng/ml. Other clinical manifestations include incidental carcinoma in transurethral resection specimens and metastatic cancer of unknown primary.

Fortunately, in a majority of cases, when the PSA is noted to be greater than 2.5 ng/ml, men are examined and determined to have benign (non-cancerous) conditions. The two most common prostate conditions, BPH and prostatitis, may cause symptoms men fear are due to prostate cancer. But the symptoms are rarely caused by prostate cancer and by themselves do not increase the risk of developing prostate cancer. Notwithstanding this comment, when the discussion turns to the importance of a disease state to prostate cancer, BPH does not lead to prostate cancer. On the hand, most experts agree chronic inflammation associated with a non-bacterial prostatitis has been noted to be associated with the evolution of prostate cancer.

Sometimes screening and other tests result in a misdiagnosis of prostate cancer. The process of accurately diagnosing prostate cancer can be tricky. (This is one reason why second opinions—having your biopsy slides reread—are so valuable for men diagnosed with prostate cancer). For example, the PSA test is valuable in indicating that a problem might exist and require additional testing. But because both benign and malignant conditions may cause a rise in PSA levels, the PSA test by itself doesn't show whether cancer is present or absent (see below). It is also possible that rare microscopic findings may be mistaken for prostate cancer, including normal parts of the anatomy, such as the seminal vesicles (glands at the base of the bladder that release fluid into the semen during orgasm), as well as a wide variety of other prostate changes. Additionally, other prostate conditions may look like prostate cancer under a microscope and may be mistakenly identified as cancer; this is what is referred to as a "false positive" result.

Suspicious Test Results

Benign prostatic hyperplasia (BPH) is the noncancerous enlargement of the prostate. Like prostate cancer, BPH may cause the prostate specific antigen (PSA) level in the blood to rise. BPH may be diagnosed when a man reports urinary symptoms such as weak urination, difficulty urinating, or an inability to urinate, or because of a rise in his PSA. Because a larger percentage of PSA tends to circulate in the "free" or unbound form when due to BPH than when due to prostate cancer, doctors may be able to differentiate BPH from prostate cancer through more specific PSA testing. We are not sure what causes BPH to develop. Symptoms can be monitored and treated with medications or surgery if necessary.

Prostatitis

Like BPH, a diagnosis of prostatitis is usually made when a patient has frequent urination, urgent urination, and discomfort in the prostate area. Most men have areas of mild inflammation, or swelling, in their prostate glands. However, when the inflammation is severe, is extensive, or causes a rise in PSA, it is referred to as prostatitis. (The suffix "itis" indicates an inflammatory condition; "arthritis" is inflammation of the joints, for example.) There is a wide spectrum of prostatitis, much of which is rare and poorly understood.

Further testing, such as cultures of urine and any prostatic secretions, may allow for diagnosis. Prostatitis may be caused by bacteria or other infections, tissue disruption after a biopsy, or other factors. **The cause of some types of prostatitis is not known but the majority is non-bacterial.** (Antibiotics help treat some types of prostatitis including acute bacterial prostatitis. Other potential treatments include medications like anti-inflammatories and sitz baths, which involves sitting in warm water.)

Severe Prostatitis

Severe prostatitis disrupts the microscopic architecture of the prostate, obscuring usual landmarks and making interpretation difficult for a pathologist. Rarely, severe prostatitis is incorrectly diagnosed as high-grade prostate cancer. Pathologists may use special stains, such as prostate specific antigen (PSA) and prostatic acid phosphatase (PAP), when examining severe prostatitis under the microscope to differentiate virtually all cases of prostatitis and cancer.

Prostatic Intraepithelial Neoplasia (PIN)

Prostatic Intraepithelial Neoplasia (PIN) is a diagnosis made by a pathologist when a biopsy shows certain changes in the microscopic appearance (for example, size and shape) of prostate gland cells. These changes are classified as either low grade, meaning they appear almost normal; or high grade, meaning they look abnormal, although the term "PIN" is usually used to indicate high grade PIN. High grade PIN is considered the pre-invasive stage of invasive cancer and represents the putative precancerous end of the morphologic continuum of cellular proliferations within the lining of prostatic ducts, ductules, and acini. PIN is defined as an abnormal epithelial proliferation within the pre-existing ducts and ductules with nucleomegaly and nucleolomegaly involving at least 10% of the cells.

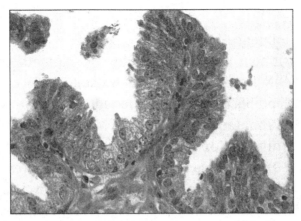

(**Figure 1**) High Grade Prostatic Intraepithelial Neoplasia

The condition begins to appear in men in their twenties, and almost half of all men have PIN by the time they reach age 50. The only method of detection is biopsy; PIN does not significantly elevate total and free serum PSA concentration and cannot be detected by ultrasonography.

PIN coexists with cancer in more than 85% of cases and early invasive carcinoma occurs at sites of acinar outpouching and basal cell disruption. Such microinvasion is present in about 2% of high power microscopic fields of PIN. In such equivocal cases, we prefer the term PIN+ASAP to avoid over-diagnosis of tangential cutting of PIN as cancer (see below). High grade PIN, patient age, and serum PSA concentration were jointly highly significant predictors of cancer, with PIN providing the highest risk ratio (14.9).

PIN is sometimes misinterpreted as prostate cancer. It is not a cancerous condition, but a man who has had high-grade PIN diagnosed through a prostate biopsy has a 30 to 50 percent chance of also being diagnosed with prostate cancer at some point. If all procedures fail to identify coexistent cancer, close surveillance and follow-up appear to be indicated. Follow-up is suggested at six-month intervals for two years, and thereafter yearly for life. The identification of PIN in the prostate should not influence or dictate therapeutic decisions. Currently, routine treatment is not available for patients who have high-grade PIN. Prophylactic radical prostatectomy or radiation is not an acceptable treatment for patients who have high-grade PIN only. **Dr. Wheeler's commentary: Men who have HGPIN as a predictor disease for the concurrent presence of prostate cancer in 30-50% of cases should be candidates for High Intensity Focused Ultrasound (HIFU) when the clinical scenario is associated with a progressively rising PSA!**

Chronic therapy, however, would most likely be required to prevent new high-grade PIN lesions from becoming cancerous. New agents with better safety and lower side effect profile are needed since patients may be taking the agent at least until they attain 70 years of age. Toremifene (Acapodene™) is a selective estrogen receptor modulator that supposedly eliminates high-grade PIN and reduces the incidence of prostate cancer. After 4 months of toremifene (60 mg/day orally for 4 months), 72% of men treated (vs. 17.9% of controls) had no high-grade PIN on subsequent prostate biopsies. **Dr. Wheeler's commentary: As stated earlier, this study suffers from 'sampling bias'.**

Green tea catechins (GTCs) also may reduce the incidence of prostate cancer. Catechins are antioxidants in the class of polyphenols called flavonols. After 6 months of green tea catechins (600 mg/day orally), 3.3% of the men with PIN had cancer compared with 30% of those who took placebo. Selenium and Vitamin E are also under investigation as putative chemopreventive agents.

Recently, some investigators conducted a chemoprevention trial assessing the efficacy of Flutamide (anti-androgen) in reducing the rate of prostate cancer development in men with PIN. Men with biopsy proven PIN but no evidence of prostate cancer were randomized in a double-blind manner to either

Flutamide 250 mg/d or a placebo. Treatment was continued for 1 year. Repeat biopsies were obtained at 1 and 2 years. This study showed no evidence of benefit from Flutamide as a chemoprevention agent in men with PIN.

Atypical Small Acinar Proliferation (ASAP)

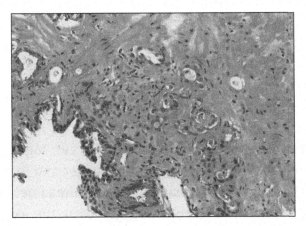

(**Figure 2**) Atypical Small Acinar Proliferation

The concept of atypical small acinar proliferation (ASAP) suspicious for but not diagnostic of malignancy was only introduced approximately a decade ago, identified in about 2% of biopsies. ASAP represents our inability and "absolute uncertainty" to render an incontrovertible diagnosis of cancer in a needle biopsy. The most frequent reasons why the pathologist is unable to preclude a definitive diagnosis of malignancy are the small size of the focus (70% of cases), disappearance on step levels (61%), lack of atypical cells within the small glands (55%), and associated inflammation (9%), raising the possibility of one of many conditions that mimics prostate cancer.

Similar to high-grade prostatic intraepithelial neoplasia, ASAP holds a significant predictive value for cancer on repeat biopsy.

In a recent provocative report, the investigators recommended immediate radical prostatectomy in patients with the biopsy diagnosis of ASAP. They suggested that the risk of subsequent cancer is 100% in radical prostatectomy specimens. We urge caution in recommending expansion of the indications for prostatectomy to include patients with ASAP. **ASAP is best considered as a diagnostic risk category and not a true entity.**

We routinely use Immunohistochemical techniques in the diagnostic workup of atypical prostate lesions in needle biopsies, thereby decreasing the incidence of ASAP and reducing the risk of false negatives and the need for additional biopsies.

Atypical small acinar proliferation lesions and high grade prostatic intraepithelial neoplasia can occur together in the same biopsy set without concomitant cancer and is referred as "PIN+ASAP" when the two lesions coexist in the same high-power microscopic field. The predictive value of the combination diagnosis of PIN+ASAP is similar to that of ASAP alone.

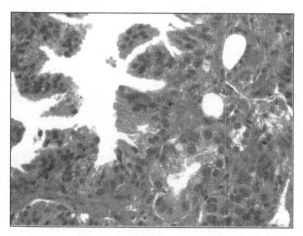

(Figure 3) PIN + ASAP

The presence of ASAP or PIN+ASAP in a biopsy is a significant predictor for concurrent or subsequent cancer compared to the cohorts of patients lacking these lesions. Repeat biopsy of the entire prostate is indicated.

Dr. Wheeler's Commentary:

With this type of presentation, I generally recommend an MRI scan and treatment with a non-surgical procedure like HIFU as the threshold for treatment has been met from my point of view. Remember, in women, HIFU is used for uterine fibroids, a benign disease. Why should men have to present with documented cancer when women do not? The qualifications should be the same or we suffer from a double standard! In men with a progressively rising PSA while controlling for inflammation; there is only one disease that meets this criteria; prostate cancer!

Atrophy and Postatrophic Hyperplasia

Atrophy, or gradual cell damage, is a near-constant microscopic finding in adult prostates. Damage to the prostate becomes more common and more extensive with age, particularly after the age of 40. Atrophy can be seen in portions of healthy men's prostates. (More extensive atrophy can also be seen in the prostates of men who have had hormone therapy or radiation.) A pathologist may confuse atrophy with adenocarcinoma (cancer that starts in glandular tissue, such as the prostate gland). Clusters of atrophic acini that display proliferative epithelial changes are referred to as postatrophic hyperplasia (PAH) and PAH is at the extreme end of the morphologic continuum of acinar atrophy that most closely mimics prostate cancer.

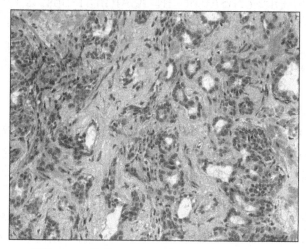

(**Figure 4**) Postatrophic Hyperplasia

Table 1 summarizes the differential diagnosis of prostate cancer. **Figures 5-8** represent some mimics of prostate cancer listed in **Table 1**.

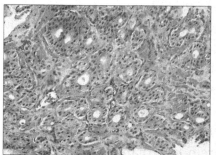

(**Figure 5**) Basil Cell Hyperplasia

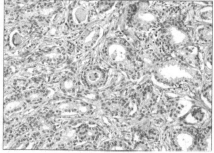

(**Figure 6**) Atypical Adenomatous Hyperplasia (AAH)

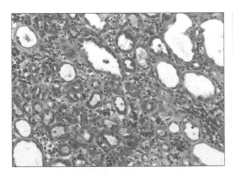

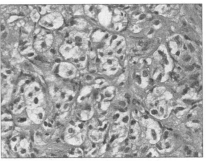

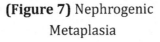

(Figure 7) Nephrogenic
Metaplasia

(Figure 8) Mesonephric
Remnants

Table 1 (pages 209-210) summarizes the **Differential Diagnosis of Prostate Cancer. Figures 5-8** represent tissue types that mimic prostate cancer; listed in **Table 1** (page 209) **and explained in the Figure Legend** (pages 208-209).

Understanding the role of the pathologist in the diagnosis of prostate cancer

How biopsies are handled by the pathologist . . .

While the healthcare system may one day move to embrace preferentially other less common diagnostic tools like imaging, it is likely targeted biopsies will gain some attention worldwide in the meantime. When a biopsy is performed, each biopsy specimen is submitted in separate carefully labeled formalin-filled bottles by the urologist and rapidly sent for processing. In the laboratory, each specimen is individually placed into a separate labeled plastic cassette for processing. The processing cycle usually involves fixation, dehydration, clearing, and embedding through sequential immersion in formalin, alcohol, xylene, and, ultimately, paraffin wax. Then the tissue technologist thinly slices the tissue surrounded by wax, places the thin slice on a labeled microscope slide, stains the tissue with hematoxylin (purple) and eosin (red) to give the specimen contrast, and submits all of the slides to the pathologist for light microscopic review. There is often a small amount of residual tissue remaining in the tissue block for further studies at the discretion of the pathologist. The process is remarkably similar in laboratories around the world, and usually requires no more than a few days for completion.

The pathologist who examines the specimens is a licensed physician who is usually certified by the American Board of Pathology as having special advanced training and experience in gross and microscopic examination of specimens. He or she issues a report based on the findings on the slides, sometimes after obtaining special stains to assist with difficult diagnoses. When the pathologist encounters a diagnostically challenging specimen owing to the small size of the area of concern under the microscope or the unusual nature of the finding, he or she resorts to examining additional slices through the remaining tissue block, obtaining special stains that may aid diagnosis such as Immunohistochemical studies, consultation with colleagues within the Pathology department, or consultation with extramural colleagues who have a special interest in prostate pathology. A final report is issued only after the pathologist is satisfied that the diagnosis is certain.

The Biopsy Pathology Report

The pathologist issues a report outlining the cell type and extent of the cancer. A pathology report for a biopsy will include the information shown in **Figure 9**, although the format may vary from laboratory to laboratory. A pathology report shows the type of cancer, the cancer grade, and whether the cancer has grown outside the prostate and into surrounding tissue, in addition to other information.

This information is essential in assuring that your report doesn't get confused with that of another patient with a similar or identical name and that it gets delivered to your doctor. Every specimen is given a pathology number. The number "BL03-200005" means that 200,004 other surgical pathology specimens have already been analyzed in your hospital's pathology department during the year (in this case, 2003). At the end of the year, numbering starts again, beginning with "BL04-000001".

This information identifies from where the biopsy was taken. This is especially important for patients that may have biopsies from more than one area during the same operation. The size of biopsies is also described here in centimeter (cm).

This image documented the histology of prostate cancer identified in one biopsy. It allows pathologist show the surgeon what areas of the sample contained cancer and the appearance of cancer cells.

This is the most important section of the report—its "bottom line." Prostate, right mid (biopsy): This indicates the type of cancer, its grade, the size of cancer (indicated by percentage of specimen involvement), and the number of biopsy core containing cancer. Good news—the cancer is low-grade (well differentiated).

Other findings in pathologic report:
High-grade prostatic intraepithelial neoplasia—A premalignant lesion of the prostate, which co-exists with cancer in more than 80% cancer cases. Acute or chronic inflammation is also called "prostatitis". Atrophy—decreased size of glands, height and number of epithelium.

A final report is issued only after the pathologist is satisfied that the diagnosis is certain. However, if you want a second opinion, your pathologist will send the biopsy slides themselves for review and interpretation, not his or her report.

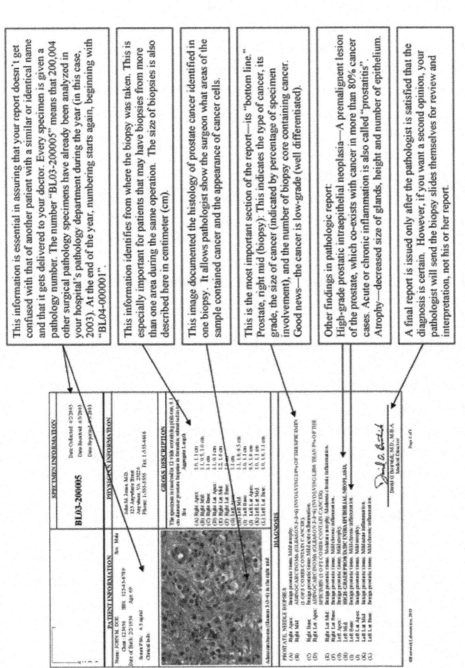

(Figure 9) Biopsy Pathology Report

Location and Multicentricity of Cancer

The urologist usually documents for the pathologist the sites within the prostate from which the biopsy cores were obtained. Often more than one needle core specimen was taken from the same site, and the pathologist reports each specimen separately to provide information about the location and multiple sites of cancer (multicentric cancer), if they exist.

Cancer Grade and its Importance

GRADE: Grade remains one of the most powerful prognostic factors in prostate cancer and it predicts pathological stage, margin status, local recurrences, biochemical failure, lymph node, disease progression, or metastatic status after radical prostatectomy. The grade is evaluated by *Gleason Score* (**Figure 10-Table 2**).

The Gleason Grading System was devised by Dr. Donald F. Gleason. It is based on the microscopic appearance of cancer cells present in the prostate biopsy. The pathologist examines the cancer cells under the microscope and assigns grade by studying the shape and architecture of tumor cells. The extent to which cancer cells and the glands formed by them resemble normal prostate cells and glands is called *differentiation*. The cancer that closely resembles normal prostate cells and glands is well-differentiated. Well-differentiated cancer tends to be the slowest growing and least dangerous. Poorly differentiated cancer does not form identifiable glands and is often very aggressive and fast growing and it can be deadly. See **Figure 10** (page 199)for photos of well differentiated cells and poorly differentiated cells.

Interobserver and intraobserver variability have been reported with the Gleason grading system. The subjective nature of grading precludes absolute precision, no matter how carefully the system is defined, yet the significant correlation of prostate cancer grade with virtually every outcome measure attests to the predictive strength and utility of grading in the hands of most investigators. Gleason himself noted exact reproducibility of score in 50% of needle biopsies and + 1 score in 85%, similar to the findings of others. Yet the interobserver reproducibility of Gleason grading has improved in the past few years, it can be improved by educating physicians via meetings, courses, website tutorials and publications focused on this topic.

Dr. Wheeler's Commentary:
I recommend Bostwick Laboratories for a primary assessment as well as a second opinion when warranted. A significant percentage of other pathologists are equally expert!

GLEASON SCORE: In assigning Gleason score, the pathologist carefully studies biopsy slides and identifies the two most common patterns present: the *primary* and *secondary* patterns. Gleason grade between 1 (for well-differentiated) and 5 (for undifferentiated) is then assigned to each of these two patterns. The two grades are added to produce *Gleason Score*, also sometimes called *Gleason Sum*.

For example, if the most common (primary) pattern of cancer in a biopsy is Grade 3 and there is a small cancer focus (secondary pattern) with Grade 2, the combined Gleason Score would be 3+2=5. Accordingly, the lowest possible score is 2 (1+1) and the highest possible score is 10 (5+5).

We also report the relative amount of Gleason patterns 4 and 5 whenever they are present, recognizing that the *amount of high-grade cancer* (poorly-differentiated or undifferentiated cancer) is information that you and your urologist should have available to make the most informed decisions regarding your treatment.

The lower your Gleason score, the better you are *likely* to do. But please remember that ultimately how well you do depends upon several additional factors. For example, the cancer STAGE (the extent of spread of tumor within the body) is also important in determining your outcome. Other factors include DNA ploidy, p27 expression, bcl-2 expression, and others (see biomarkers below). Moreover, **the possibility remains that a higher grade tumor may be present in your prostate that has not been sampled by the needle biopsy.**

Prostate Cancer: Understanding Gleason Grading System

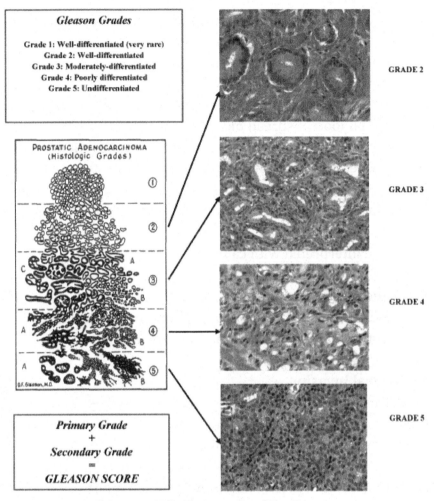

(Figure 10) Gleason Grading System

Dr. Wheeler's Commentary:

Based on biopsy bias, imaging must precede any invasive needle placement allowing for targeted biopsies when biopsy is the agreed upon as the preferred diagnostic modality of the advising urologist and consenting patient.

Tumor Volume

There are several ways of measuring the volume of cancer in needle biopsies, including the number of positive cores and the percentage of biopsy cores affected by cancer. The amount of cancer in the needle biopsy is predictive of the volume of tumor in the prostate only for those with a great amount of cancer in multiple needle biopsies. A large amount of cancer indicates a higher likelihood of spread outside the prostate and metastasis to lymph nodes. **However, a low tumor presence on a needle biopsy does not reliably predict low-volume tumor in the prostate.** Usually if more than 30 percent of biopsy cores show tumor involvement, the tumor is considered high volume, though this criterion in not official. Therefore, the volume of cancer should be interpreted with caution.

Dr. Wheeler's Commentary:

Again, the need for MRI Imaging preferentially in a diagnostic setting has never been more apparent!

Perineural Invasion

Perineural invasion is defined as the presence of cancer in intimate contact or surrounding nerves; this usually refers to small nerves that are in abundance within the prostate, but can also refer to cancer abutting large nerve trunks or even the neurovascular bundles. **The finding of perineural invasion is thought to be an adverse prognostic factor, but not all studies agree with this conclusion.**

Extraprostatic Extension (EPE; Capsular Invasion; Capsular Penetration (ECE) or Capsular Perforation)

Cancer within adipose tissue is indicative of extraprostatic extension; this is a rare finding in biopsy specimens. Similarly, tumor within the muscular wall or near the epithelium of the seminal vesicles indicates extraprostatic extension, which should be documented in the biopsy report. Some biopsies target the seminal vesicles in an effort to document unequivocal extraprostatic extension, recognizing that this may alter treatment decisions. For example, many physicians would recommend against having a patient with extraprostatic extension undergo surgery to remove the prostate because all the cancer is not likely to be removed during the surgery.

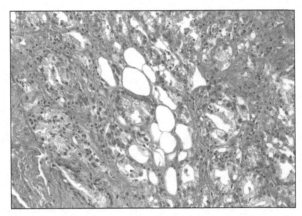

(Figure 11) Extraprostatic Capsular Extension (ECE)

DNA Ploidy Analysis (DNA Content Analysis)

A tumor is classified as either diploid or aneuploid. The ploidy is a measure of how much DNA (deoxyribonucleic acid, the genetic "blueprint" found in the nucleus of each cell that holds genetic information on cell growth, division, and function) is contained in each cell. DNA ploidy analysis of prostate cancer provides important prognostic information which supplements light microscopic examination. **Patients with diploid tumors (normal amount of genetic material, or DNA) have a more favorable outcome than those with aneuploid tumors (excessive amount of genetic material,** or DNA; for example, among patients with lymph node metastases treated with radical prostatectomy and androgen deprivation therapy, those patients with diploid tumors may survive 20 years or more, whereas those with aneuploid tumors usually don't survive more than 5 years). However, the ploidy pattern of prostate cancer is often mixed, creating potential problems with sampling error. DNA ploidy is a separate analysis and usually does not appear on the same pathology report. A sample report of abnormal DNA ploidy analysis is found in **Figure 12**.

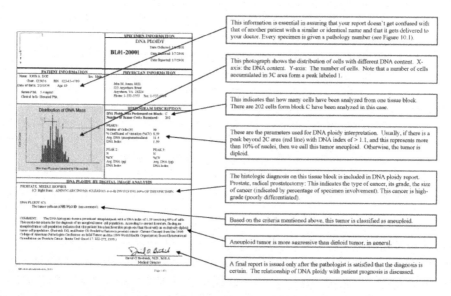

(Figure 12) Sample DNA Ploidy Report

Ten Questions to Ask Your Doctor about
Your Pathology Biopsy Report (if positive for cancer)

1. *What is the type of cancer that I have?*
2. *What is the Gleason score of my cancer?*
3. *How many needle biopsies were taken, and how many had cancer in them and how much cancer did they contain?*
4. *Who did the pathologic examination of my biopsies, and should we obtain a second opinion?*
5. *Was there any evidence of cancer extending outside of the prostate?*
6. *Where was the cancer within the prostate?*
7. *Did the pathologist provide you with a photograph of the cancer to document its appearance?*
8. *Was there any inflammation or other important findings in the biopsies?*
9. *Was there any evidence of perineural invasion?*
10. *Should we obtain special studies such as DNA ploidy to further assess the aggressiveness of the cancer?*

Dr. Wheeler's Commentary:

In addition to the top 10 Bostwick questions to ask your doctor; equally important is the location of the cancer. Gone are the days when urologists can label specimens 'Left' and 'Right' in anticipation of performing a radical prostatectomy. It is important to note; the number one reason radical prostatectomy fails to cure is based on cancer left behind at the apex of the gland as doctors try to preserve continence of urine. If you are a patient willing to risk 'needle tracking', you must know the comprehensive assessment of all areas of the prostate including the apex before you agree to a radical prostatectomy!

Grade and Stage after Androgen Deprivation Therapy

One of the most popular forms of treatment for prostate cancer—androgen deprivation therapy (hormonal treatment)—has been in use for more than five decades. Hormonal treatment is used for preoperative tumor shrinkage, symptomatic relief of metastases, cancer prophylaxis, and treatment of hyperplasia.

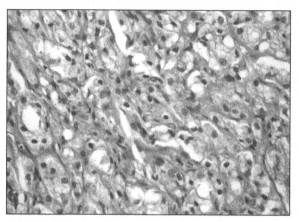

(Figure 13) Androgen Deprivation Treatment Effects

Androgen deprivation therapy (an LHRH-Analogue) causes an apparent increase in the Gleason grading of the tumor (**Figure 13**). Therefore Gleason grading after hormonal therapy is potentially misleading and is not recommended. The volume of prostate cancer is reduced by more than 40% after treatment, and there is a 20-25% decline in positive margins at radical prostatectomy. Pathologic stage is similar in untreated and treated prostate cancer, according to retrospective reports of radical prostatectomies, although there is a trend toward lower stage in treated cases. **Occasional cases after therapy display the "vanishing cancer phenomenon" in which no residual cancer was found in the radical prostatectomy specimen.** Finasteride and Dutasteride are 5 alpha-reductase inhibitors that decrease the androgen drive to hyperplastic and malignant prostate cells while maintaining testosterone levels. The Prostate Cancer Prevention trial (PCPT) was the first large-scale study to provide significant evidence for the role of 5 alpha-reductase inhibitors in the prevention of developing prostate cancer. PCPT demonstrated that treatment with Finasteride in a 7-year period was associated with a 24.8% decrease in the prevalence of prostate cancer vs. placebo. Another study reported that the incidence of prostate cancer was 51% lower with dutasteride compared to the placebo group at 27 months.

Grade and DNA Ploidy after Radiotherapy

Post irradiation Gleason grade and DNA ploidy are independent prognostic factors in patients with prostate cancer who fail radiotherapy. There is a slight shift after therapy toward non-diploid cancer, higher Gleason grade, and high tumor stage, indicating increasing biologic aggressiveness and cancer dedifferentiation after radiation. Particularly in grade 4 cancer, radiotherapy may cause disappearance of glandular lumina, resulting in grade 5 morphology.

Some investigators recommend grading of cancer in specimens after radiotherapy, recognizing that the biologic significance of grade may be different from that in untreated cancer. We believe that Gleason grading after radiation therapy is potentially misleading, particularly the risk of overestimation and in daily practice, we do not report it when requested with appropriate disclaimer (*"Grading of adenocarcinoma after radiation therapy is not validated and may create spurious and misleading higher grade, so these results may not be predictive of patient outcome and should be interpreted with caution"*) despite suggestions to the contrary.

Current and new biomarkers in prostate cancer

Determine the risk of prostate cancer: the role of PSA and PCA3 tests.

In recent years the discovery of cancer biomarkers has become a major focus of cancer research. A biomarker is defined as a molecular test that provides additional information to available clinical and pathological tests.

PSA is the most important, accurate, and clinically useful biochemical marker in the prostate because it is, for all practicality, produced by and specific for prostatic tissue. Immunohistochemical expression of PSA is diagnostically helpful for the pathologist in distinguishing high grade prostate cancer from bladder cancer, colon cancer, prostatitis, lymphoma, and other histologic mimics. It also allows identification of site of tumor origin in metastatic cancer. PSA expression is generally greater in low grade tumors than in high grade tumors, but there is significant heterogeneity from cell to cell. Up to 1.6% of poorly differentiated cancers do not express PSA or prostatic acid phosphatase. At present, serum PAP has little or no clinical utility, but this marker is valuable for staining when used in combination with stains for PSA.

Although serum PSA is currently used to screen for prostate cancer, recently, a new urine-based test called PCA3 test has been shown to be more accurate for detecting prostate cancer.[33] When PCA3 was used with PSA, only PCA3 contributed significantly to the predictive accuracy of the model for predicting cancer, which suggests that performing both tests is not useful. Furthermore, the sensitivity, specificity, positive and negative predictive value of PCA3 was consistently more accurate than serum PSA.[33]

Other current markers with potential prognostic value include p53, Bcl-2, p16INK4A, p27Kip1, c-Myc, Androgen Receptor, E-cadherin and vascular endothelial growth factor (VEGF).

Proteomics is the future of diagnostic pathology

In years to come, we predict that molecular biology will revolutionize the field of diagnostic pathology. Genomic and proteomic methodology has recently been used to discover more than 200 putative new markers for prostate cancer like alpha-methylacyl CoA racemase (AMACR), hepsin, glutathione S-transferase pi, EZH2 and PCA3. Proteomics has distinct advantages over genomic and ribonucleic acid (RNA) expression studies because it is the proteins that are ultimately responsible for the malignant features.[34] With the advent of new and improved genomic and proteomic technologies, it is possible to develop biomarkers that are able to reliably and accurately predict outcomes during cancer management and treatment.

Dr. Wheeler's Commentary:

PSA is an incredibly accurate blood marker as a 'barometer of prostate health'! While not specific to the type of prostate disease present, any PSA value of 1.0 ng/ml or higher indicates prostate disease; while prostatitis is the leading disease causing PSA elevation.

About Bostwick Laboratories

Our mission is to help physicians and patients make informed treatment decisions when faced with the diagnosis of cancer and other urologic diseases by providing the best in technical and scientific expertise. We focus on diagnosis of cancer of urologic organs (prostate, urinary bladder, kidney, and testis) with a special interest in prostate cancer. Other laboratories deal with all 24 organs in the body and its incredible diversity of laboratory studies and their interpretation; instead, we restrict study to a small group of urologic disorders that allows us to uphold the highest standards of care.

Our mission is fulfilled by providing a reliable, accurate, and prompt interpretation of outpatient biopsies. We offer complete histologic services, including tissue processing with routine and special stains. DNA ploidy analysis is offered on prostate biopsies with cancer. We also render second opinion on challenging cases referred to us by physicians and patients from around the world. Our laboratory is actively involved in clinical and basic research, continuing medical education of our pathology colleagues, and patient education.

Figure Legend Explained

1. High Grade Prostatic Intraepithelial Neoplasia (PIN) involving a single gland. The epithelial cells (cells lining the gland) show moderate enlargement of the nucleus and the nucleolus (nucleolomegaly).
2. Atypical small acinar proliferation (ASAP) suspicious for but not diagnostic of cancer. Small focus has glands that cannot be diagnosed as cancer with certainty.
3. PIN+ASAP. Small glands with architectural distortion and abnormal cells in association with High Grade Prostatic Intraepithelial Neoplasia. An unequivocal diagnosis cannot be rendered due to the small size of this focus and full complement of architectural and cells abnormalities.
4. Postatrophic hyperplasia (PAH) is at the extreme end of the morphologic continuum of glandular atrophy that most closely mimics prostate cancer.
5. Basal Cell Hyperplasia is another mimic of prostate cancer.
6. Atypical Adenomatous Hyperplasia (AAH) is a localized proliferation of small glands within the prostate arising in intimate association with nodular hyperplasia. The epithelial cells appear normal, unlike epithelial cells in cancer.

7. Nephrogenic metaplasia is another pitfall that can be misdiagnosed as prostate cancer.

8. Mesonephric remnants. Rarely this entity may be misinterpreted as prostate cancer.

9. Pathology report for low grade prostate cancer (with explanatory comments). (*From American cancer Society's Complete Guide to Prostate Cancer. Bostwick DG, Crawford ED, Higano CS, et al. (Eds), Atlanta, Georgia, 2005; with permission.*)

10. Understanding the Gleason Grading System. (*From American cancer Society's Complete Guide to Prostate Cancer. Bostwick DG, Crawford ED, Higano CS, et al. (Eds), Atlanta, Georgia, 2005; with permission.*)

11. Extraprostatic extension of prostate cancer. Note the fatty cells (centrally, optically "empty/transparent" cells) surrounded by the cancer.

12. Sample DNA Ploidy report. (*From American cancer Society's Complete Guide to Prostate Cancer. Bostwick DG, Crawford ED, Higano CS, et al. (Eds), Atlanta, Georgia, 2005; with permission.*)

13. Androgen deprivation treatment effects. Note almost all the infiltrative glands are compressed and have lost their lumen.

Table 1: DIFFERENTIAL DIAGNOSIS OF PROSTATIC ADENOCARCINOMA

- Atrophy
- Postatrophic Hyperplasia
- Basal Cell Hyperplasia
- Atypical Adenomatous Hyperplasia (AAH)
- Sclerosing Adenosis
- Nephrogenic Metaplasia

- Verumontanum Mucosal Gland Hyperplasia
- Hyperplasia of Mesonephric Remnants
- High Grade Prostatic Intraepithelial Neoplasia (PIN)
- Atypical Small Acinar Proliferation (ASAP)

Table 2 FIVE GLEASON GRADES

- **Grade 1:** Cancer is well-differentiated and consists of uniformly-spaced glands forming a circumscribed mass. This pattern is virtually never seen in needle biopsies.
- **Grade 2:** Cancer is still well differentiated, but the glands are arranged more loosely and are slightly more irregular in shape. The cancer no longer forms a compact circumscribed mass.
- **Grade 3:** Cancer is moderately-differentiated. This is the most commonly seen grade. The cancer glands vary in size in shape and size and they invade the surrounding prostate.
- **Grade 4:** Cancer is poorly-differentiated. The cancer glands are highly distorted and no longer recognized as separate units. They merge into one another and invade the surrounding prostate.
- **Grade 5:** Cancer is undifferentiated and bears no resemblance to normal prostate. The cancer cells form solid clusters and necrosis may be present.

NOTES:

CHAPTER THIRTEEN

Is it Necessary to Cure Prostate Cancer when it is Possible?

~ (Understanding the role of prostate inflammation resolution to prostate cancer evolution) ~

Published in the Peer-Reviewed Journal,
"Clinical Interventions in Aging"
Volume 2, Number 1-2007 (Dove Press)
Author: Ronald E. Wheeler, M.D.
(The following patient data collection represents an update from the original study of 23 patients published in Dove Press in 2007)

Abstract

OBJECTIVE—DEFINITIVE THERAPY WITH radical prostatectomy, cryotherapy, radiation therapy, or HIFU generally follows the initial diagnosis of prostate cancer, particularly when men have at least 10 additional years of life expectancy. There is growing concern regarding the optimal conservative treatment for patients who decline or do not otherwise qualify for such definitive curative treatment. For those patients who choose a watchful waiting approach, it would be beneficial to know what specific dietary and nutritional methods could potentially slow the progression of their disease. In this prospective study, it was our goal to analyze the efficacy and safety of treating prostate cancer conservatively using the principles of a modified Mediterranean diet in association with a specific prostate nutritional supplement.

Method—Thirty men aged 43-84 (median age: 64) with biopsy proven, organ-confined prostate cancer who had already declined immediate hormonal therapy and attempts at a curative cancer treatment agreed to participate in a Chronic Disease management (CDM) protocol highlighted by a diet with a specific prostate nutritional supplement. The diet recommended was a modified Mediterranean diet while a patented nutritional prostatitis formula (Peenuts®) was the supplement common to all patients. PSA, a recognized marker of prostate disease and prostate cancer activity, was the primary indicator to validate exacerbation or suppression of disease. All men were followed with serial PSA testing, a digital rectal exam, an International Prostate Symptom Score index (IPSS-Index) and an expressed prostatic secretion (EPS) examination. The primary Gleason sum/score represented in this study was 6 (n = 17), while Gleason sum patterns 5, 5/6, 6/7 and 7 were also evaluated. Referencing the Partin Tables, organ confinement was predicted to be 66 percent.

Results—93% of men (n = 28) noted a 58 percent reduction (range of improvement: 16-95%) in PSA over an average of 49 months (range: 12-91 months). The remaining 7% of men represented two men who experienced a mild elevation n PSA of 0.5 and 1.3 ng/ml over 34 months and 75 months, respectively. 18 men had completed an initial and secondary IPSS-Index while 17 men had undergone an initial and secondary EPS. The mean percentage reduction in IPSS-Index was 67 percent (range: 20-100 percent with a median of 62.5 percent), while men evaluated with EPS examinations noted a mean percentage reduction in white blood cells of 77.5 percent (range: 33-99 percent with a median of 82 percent). These results were evaluated using the t-Test, Wilcoxon Analysis and the Null Hypothesis and found to be statistically significant.

Conclusion—Clearly there is a need to develop effective alternative conservative therapies for the increasing numbers of prostate cancer patients who will not tolerate definitive curative measures or simply choose a conservative approach. Although this prospective study had no control arm, was limited in duration and included only 30 participants, it did appear to show significant benefit to the majority of prostate cancer patients treated with selective nutritional and dietary therapy alone. Such treatments may provide a safe and effective long-term treatment alternative for some patients. Further study is encouraged.

This study data was presented as a 'poster' in Bariloche, Argentina to the SIU (Society of International Urology) meeting in October, 2003 and at the Prostate Cancer Symposium Research Meeting sponsored by the American Society of Clinical Oncology (ASCO) February 23-26, 2006—San Francisco, California while the original work with 23 patients was published by Dove Press in the (peer reviewed Journal), 'Clinical Interventions in Aging', April—2007, Volume 2, Number 1.

Introduction

Prostate cancer is the most commonly diagnosed malignant neoplasm among men in North America. Notwithstanding the strides that have been made related to diagnosis and treatment, prostate cancer still poses a significant health risk. In 2005, the incidence of prostate cancer was noted to be in excess of 232,000 new cases while prostate cancer death currently ranked as the second most common male cancer death with approximately 32,000 men dying from the disease. According to the SEER (Surveillance, Epidemiology & End Result) data and the age-specific population projections in association with the United States Census Bureau, it is estimated that 99,000 men will die from prostate cancer in the year 2045. Besides the inherent health risk, there is also concern regarding the best way to pay for expensive prostate cancer detection. Despite our best efforts to cure, failure rates for prostate cancer may be as high as 40-60 percent in high-risk cases (Gleason scores: ≥ 7)

Epidemiological studies suggest that diets rich in grains, specific vitamins, fruits and vegetable are associated with lower prostate cancer rates than high-fat diets associated with red meat, dairy product intake and high-dose calcium. High-temperature cooking and/or well-done or charred meats contains heterocyclic amines, nitrosamines and polycyclic aromatic hydrocarbons that have been shown prospectively to increase prostate cancer risk in the prostate, lung, colorectal and ovarian cancer screening trial. Dairy products and diets with high calcium content have also been found to increase the risk of prostate cancer possibly through an increase in phytanic acid levels which are also elevated in high protein meat diets. A number of studies have found an association between saturated fat (Palmitic Acid, as example) and prostate cancer although the precise mechanisms are not clear. We, therefore, selected **a modified Mediterranean diet which includes a high intake of cereals, grains, vegetables, fruits, olive oil, beans, garlic, fresh herbs and seafood or poultry (white meat) with an avoidance of red meat and dairy products.**

We know that many prostate cancer patients; up to 73 percent in one study, will take nutritional supplements on their own and **the typical patient averages about three separate supplements daily**. Animal studies, epidemiological data and other evidence suggests that plant-based dietary supplements providing indoles, isothiocyanates, phenolics, monoterpenes, flavonoids, phytosterols, lignan precursors, lycopenes, and soy proteins as well as zinc, selenium, Vitamin E and various other anti-oxidants may serve as natural inhibitors of prostate carcinogenesis and growth. The Peenuts® product is a standardized, certified and patented nutritional supplement that contains appropriate levels of beneficial ingredients from plant-based sources. **The formula has been shown to suppress and help resolve non-bacterial prostatitis in a randomized, placebo-controlled double blinded study and is readily available commercially.** Reductions in white blood cell count in the expressed prostatic secretions of prostatitis patients were reported at **66-77 percent**, when only using this nutritional supplement.

A number of recent studies have suggested that nutritional therapies alone could possibly lower the aggressiveness of prostate cancer and prevent its progression but randomized clinical trial data so far is limited and no prospective studies have yet identified an optimal combination of dietary measures and nutritional supplementation that can effectively control prostate cancer growth.

There are many experts who question whether we are over treating prostate cancer. The poignant words of the late Willet Whitmore, M.D. may prove most prophetic. To paraphrase, his oft-quoted rhetorical question asks, "Is it possible to cure prostate cancer when it is necessary?" and "Is necessary to cure prostate cancer when it is possible?" If we accept that a cure is not always possible or even desirable in some cases due to complications, surgical risks, side effects, morbidity, cost and patient choice, this leads us to the next logical question; **"Is it possible to significantly suppress or slow prostate cancer growth for prolonged periods using only nutritional and dietary measures?"** The goal of this study was to attempt to begin to answer this important question by prospectively treating prostate cancer patients exclusively with conservative measures including optimal dietary modification and standardized complex nutritional supplementation to determine the feasibility and effectiveness of such an approach as a possible alternative to traditional prostate cancer treatments.

Methods and Materials

Between 1998 and 2007, 30 men (mean age: 64 years) with biopsy proven prostate cancer who had declined attempts at curative cancer treatment or hormonal therapy, were given appropriate informed consent and offered the opportunity to try a strictly dietary and nutritionally oriented conservative protocol. The diet used was a Modified Mediterranean Diet (**prostate diet/Wheeler Diet**) while a patented prostatitis formula (Peenuts®) was the nutritional supplement common to all patients. By study design, none of the patients had ever been exposed to anti-androgen therapy, a Luteinizing Hormone-Releasing Hormone LHRH) analogue, LHRH antagonist or definitive therapy with surgery, radiation, cryosurgery or HIFU. All men were followed at varying time intervals with a PSA (prostate specific antigen) blood test, while many of the men were also followed with the International Prostate Symptom Score (IPSS) index and the Expressed Prostatic Secretion (EPS) examinations. With the exception of 3 men with Gleason 6/7 components, three men with Gleason 5/6 components and one male with a Gleason 7 pattern, all men exhibited either a Gleason 5 (n = 6) or a Gleason 6 (n = 17) pathological pattern. All men were clinically diagnosed as T1c (n = 21), T2a (n = 3), T2b (n = 2), or T2c (n = 4). Interestingly, all of the men, except one, who met the entry criteria outlined above, enthusiastically chose to treat their disease through a dietary and nutritional supplement protocol represented by the term Chronic Disease management (CDM) rather than undergo definitive therapy. The one male who initially qualified dropped out after seven successful months, opting for a radical prostatectomy. CDM therapy is a unique cancer concept, but not dissimilar to the conservative holistic treatment of diabetes, hypertension, or arthritis whereby patients learn to live with the disease based on lifestyle changes consistent with improved diet, nutritional supplementation, stress reduction, exercise and enhanced education.

While the PSA level is a recognized marker of disease activity worldwide, it is noted that PSA levels may rise based on any combination of prostatitis (non-bacterial inflammation in ≥ 95 percent of cases), BPH (benign prostatic hyperplasia), and/or prostate cancer. The IPSS-index is a recognized marker associated primarily with BPH and prostatitis, while the EPS (expressed prostatic secretion) represents the diagnostic biological marker for prostatitis. All men were evaluated at varying intervals of surveillance ranging from 12 months to 91 months (mean: 49 months). Two study subjects had a slight increase in their PSA levels of 0.5 and 1.3 ng/ml at 34 months and 75 months, respectively. **Excepting these two patients, who experienced a small rise in PSA, the remaining 28 patients (93%) decreased their PSA levels during the study period an average of 58%.**

Statistical Analysis

A performance analysis was carried out for 30 patients relative to any change in PSA; noting statistical significance using the null hypothesis, t-Test and Wilcoxon Analyses. There was a significant decrease in PSA levels (ng/ml) after treatment with dietary modification and the specific herbal supplement taken at two capsules daily. The P value was statistically significant.

Statistical Assessment: there was a significant decrease in PSA levels (ng/ml) after treatment with dietary encouragement and herbal supplementation, two capsules daily.

These nutritional variables had a statistically significant effect in reducing PSA levels in the subject group.

Results

All men within an age range of 43-84 years with a diagnosis of prostate cancer (Gleason Score: 5, 5/6, 6/7, 7) who declined standard curative and/or hormonal therapy were offered an opportunity to participate in a conservative quality of life protecting study with the understanding that diet and nutrition could play a significant role in disease proliferation or control. With the exception of excluding men with a Gleason Score of 8, 9, or 10 as a qualifying entry category for prostate cancer, there was no bias inherent in the entrance process. It is my opinion; patients with Gleason scores of 8-10 are not appropriate candidates for a CDM protocol as a means to defer other treatment options.

30 men qualified for study evaluation using the PSA levels from the date of diagnosis (biopsy date) or the initial clinic appointment date (whichever was higher) as the reference PSA value for the starting point for data collection. 28 of the 30 men experienced a positive response (decrease in PSA levels) relevant to the conservative therapy, while two men noted a mild increase in their PSA values. Specifically, 93% of men (n = 28) noted a 58 percent reduction (range of improvement: 16-90 percent) in PSA levels over an average of 49 months (range: 12-91 months). Using a mean PSA starting point of 6.4 ng/ml, 93% of men in the study experienced a mean reduction in PSA of 3.83 ng/ml (range: 0.6-13.7 ng/ml) over the identified time frame, while the median reduction was 3.1 ng/ml. The two men,

who experienced a mild elevation in PSA, noted an increase of 0.5 ng/ml and 1.3 ng/ml over 34 months and 75 months, respectively. **Overall, the effectiveness of CDM therapy to suppress prostate cancer was 93 percent using the PSA level as the disease activity marker.**

A urinary assessment with a voiding symptom score (IPSS-Index) and prostatitis evaluation utilizing the expressed prostatic secretion (EPS) examination was conducted at the time of baseline (initial visit) and follow–up evaluations on the majority of the participants. 18 men completed an initial and secondary IPSS-Index while 17 men had undergone an initial and secondary EPS. **All men reduced their voiding symptom score with an average 4.9 points (range: 1.5-11), while noting an average starting score of 8.6 points (range: 2.5-19.5 with a median of 8).** The mean percentage reduction in IPSS-Index was 57% (range: 20-100 percent with a median of 62.5%). Relevant to the EPS, a patient with an average starting point of 247 white blood cells (WBC's) per high-powered field (HPF) (400X) demonstrated an average decrease to 57 WBC's/HPF. **To state further, a mean reduction was noted in the prostatitis marker of 190 white blood cells (range: 70-495) with a mean percentage improvement of 77.5% (range: 33-99 percent with a median of 83 percent). The reduced number of white blood cells on the EPS examinations as well as the improvement in urinary symptoms as documented by the average reductions in IPSS-Index scores in this group of men treated with nutritional means alone was statistically significant.**

Study Analysis and Discussion

The possibility of treating prostate cancer conservatively has always been intriguing to the patient and a concern for the clinician. Previous studies have commonly grouped Gleason 7 scores with Gleason 5 and 6 scores within the designation of moderately well differentiated cancers. Ostensibly, this would give patients with Gleason 7 scores improved odds for cure while decreasing the chance for success in patients with Gleason 5 and 6 scores. **This assumes the higher the Gleason score, the lower the chance for cure.** Increasing evidence through analysis now suggests that Gleason 7 prostate cancer responds better than a Gleason 8-10 but not as well as a Gleason 5 or 6. **Additionally, it is believed that Gleason scores of 5-7 may comprise almost 90 percent of all cancers encountered as 35-62 percent of men in most study groups analyzed are identified in the Gleason 6 category.**

Qualification for this study included men with the diagnosis of prostate cancer who had not been exposed previously to anti-androgen therapy, LHRH therapy or any other definitive process of prostate cancer manipulation. Of the 30 patients evaluated, 17 men were diagnosed with a Gleason 6 score, 6 men had a Gleason 5 score, 3 men had a Gleason 5/6 score, 3 men were noted with a Gleason 6/7 score, while one man had a Gleason 7 pattern. The clinical stage assessment noted 21 men with a T1c, 4 men with a T2c, 2 men with a T2b and 3 men with a T2a stage classification. Pathologically, the biopsy diagnosis ranged from T1a-T2c. While the number of biopsy cores positive for cancer and the percentage of cancer per core varied widely the percentage of cores positive for cancer (identified at the biopsy procedure) ranged from 12.5% to 73% (mean: 33 percent; median 20 percent) associated with a range of biopsy samples from 2-18. **This suggests the presence of significant disease in the study group.**

In an interesting, albeit, unique study, Dean Ornish and colleagues at the University of California—San Francisco evaluated the ability of the vegan diet (n = 44) to alter the PSA in a comparative analysis with a non-restrictive diet (n = 43) over a period of one year, in men documented with a documented Gleason 6 prostate cancer. All men in this study, as in ours, had declined definitive curative treatment and/or hormonal therapy. While the merits of the vegan diet cannot be disputed as a benefit in heart disease prevention, it was less clear what effect this diet would have on men with known prostate cancer. An average decrease in PSA of 0.25 ng/ml (4%) identified in the vegan group was statistically significant when evaluated in concert with a 0.38 ng/ml (6%) rise in the placebo group. **While statistically significant, the difference was nonetheless modest at one year. This study result does not suggest a lack of benefit to the vegan diet, but rather demonstrates that the impact of diet alone on prostate cancer may be modest.**

In our prospective study, we evaluated the benefit of a modified Mediterranean diet on known prostate cancer patients with Gleason scores of 5-7. The Mediterranean diet is recognized worldwide for its health benefits systemically but more specifically its promotion of cardiovascular health and cancer avoidance (colorectal, breast, pancreas, prostate and endometrial) properties. By design, men were asked to avoid red meat and dairy products including egg yolks in an effort to decrease saturated fat. It is commonly recognized that animal fat and dairy fat may play a role in prostate cancer proliferation. Unlike the Ornish cohort, men did not use soy in their diets. Fresh fruits and cruciferous vegetables belonging to the Brassica classification were highlighted while the oil of choice was olive oil.

Beyond the modified Mediterranean diet, our study group used a complex nutritional supplement called Peenuts® that was originally developed to treat prostatitis. This formula represents a unique, synergistic blend of vitamins, minerals, amino acids and herbs. These ingredients have been shown individually to affect cellular oxidation, inflammation and immune function, while less clearly offering additional potential benefits from beta-sitosterols. While using this formula, previous clinical investigations have shown an improvement in the expressed prostatic secretion (EPS) and voiding symptoms. The EPS is the recognized marker for prostatitis as seen through the historic work of Stamey, Meares, and others while voiding symptoms are common to the diagnosis of benign prostatic hyperplasia and prostatitis.

The concept of looking at prostatitis within this study group was prompted by previous research from the American Association of Cancer Research (AACR) that supports a role for prostatitis in the evolution of prostate cancer. It is postulated that the cellular oxidative stress associated with a chronic inflammatory process leads to proliferative inflammatory atrophy with subsequent evolution of free radicals through oxidative change. This eventually results in DNA alteration (cellular mutation), prostatic intra-epithelial neoplasia (PIN) and cancer. While it is beyond the scope of this article to review these findings in greater depth, it is well known that the process of inflammation is commonly associated with organ-specific cancers including but not limited to cancer of the esophagus, colon, stomach, liver, lung and cervix.

Within our study group, the mean PSA at the time of diagnosis was 6.4 ng/ml (range: 2.1-14.4 ng/ml). A statistically significant reduction in mean PSA of 3.5 ng/ml was validated using the t-test, Wilcoxon analysis and the null hypothesis. **The mean percentage reduction in PSA was 55 percent, while the likelihood for organ confinement in this group was 66 percent referencing the Partin Prediction tables.**

While the topic of prostatitis and its role in prostate cancer evolution is likely to remain controversial for the immediate future, the topic's relevance may be best left for the health care provider and the patient to decide. **Based on an average percent reduction in the white blood cells (a universal marker for inflammation) of 77% associated with the EPS, there appears to be sufficient clinical indication to support the addition of a scientifically validated prostatitis therapy to any long-term prostate cancer management protocol.** The relative failure of the vegan diet in the Ornish study to significantly suppress prostate cancer (based on PSA analysis) supports this hypothesis.

Additionally, it is not unreasonable to suggest the noted reduction in PSA in our study is based mainly on the improvement in prostatitis, as it is well known that prostatitis is a common cause of PSA elevations. However, **the long average duration of the reduction in PSA levels at over five years in patients with known prostate cancer receiving no other therapy would suggest that the treatment is acting directly on the prostate cancer.** Only further study will be able to determine if this conclusion is accurate. **At the very least, we can say that the nutritional component complements the diet and may well enhance the durability of response seen in the study patients.**

There is a clear indication that the nutritional treatment evaluated had an impact on voiding symptoms, as there was a mean percentage reduction in the International Prostate Symptom Score Index (IPSS-Index) of 57 percent. This is consistent with findings from a previously performed randomized, double blind, placebo controlled study. **This response exceeds that of any prostate or prostatitis nutritional formula such as saw palmetto described in the world's medical literature suggesting a synergistic effect from the particular blend of nutrients selected.**

One gentleman, age 54, who had initially qualified for the study decided on a radical prostatectomy despite performing quite well at seven months. The delay in surgery had no adverse effect on the outcome, as his PSA was < 0.2 ng/ml, one year post-prostatectomy. While further research could evaluate the potential benefit of this protocol to an outcome, the delay in definitive treatment allowed for improved awareness and decision making on the part of the patient and his family. Alternatively, research may demonstrate the use of the Peenuts® formula or similarly validated supplements to be a reasonable first step in avoiding additional biopsies in patients where prostatitis is present.

While the use of the modified Mediterranean diet and a prostate nutritional supplement has been shown to be effective; additional ingredients and/or products may be added to enhance the collective benefit in the prostate cancer disease suppression process. Beyond the modified Mediterranean diet and the Peenuts® nutritional formula that were used by all patients, 17 patients used an active form of Vitamin D, 13 patients used an anti-cholesterolemic agent, 14 patients used omega-3 fatty acids, 13 patients used a 5-alpha reductase inhibitor (5-ARIs), 7 patients used a COX II inhibitor and 4 patients used an alpha-blocker. When the men using 5-ARIs were studied versus the men who didn't use them, there was a 52 percent reduction in PSA in the 5-ARIs group (n = 13) over 32 months versus a 43 percent reduction in the cohort not on 5-ARIs (n = 10) over 48 months. This suggests a relatively insignificant benefit in PSA reduction relevant to the men on the 5-ARIs at this point in the study. Interestingly, when the nutritional supplement formula was evaluated alone (n = 4), a reduction in mean PSA of 53.8 percent was noted over 41.3 months of surveillance. While this finding is potentially quite significant, it would be premature to draw any conclusions from such a small sample size. A larger study is encouraged as this all important question of PSA reduction using this supplement alone can be addressed.

Conclusions

Prostate cancer is recognized as the number one male cancer health risk with a new case diagnosed every three minutes. With baby boomers aging and health care costs rising, an opportunity to examine novel concepts for the care of patients diagnosed with prostate cancer could not be more relevant. **When a radical prostatectomy is successfully performed for a cure, consideration should be given to the potential average benefit of adding three years, 1.5 years and 0.4 years to the life of a typical man in his 50s, 60s or 70s, respectively.** When this benefit is weighed against the possibility of failure to cure and the associated morbidity, pain, surgical risks, complications, side effects and costs, an effective dietary and nutritional protocol may present a reasonable alternative.

When all of these factors are considered in our aging population together with the risks for a significant decrease in quality of life even in successful cases of definitive, curative therapy, a conservative approach may be welcomed as a viable first choice in Gleason 5 and 6 prostate cancer patients by governmental agencies such as Medicare, the Health Care Insurance Industry and patients alike. Critical to research regarding the concept of living with the disease is to locate and allocate funding to study this protocol and similar programs in greater depth with adequate patient populations followed over a longer period of time. **This study has perhaps provided the first step in our improved understanding of the concept of nutritional therapy for prostate cancer.** Beyond the issue of prostate cancer treatment is the potential role of prevention. Ultimately through this research effort and that of others, the landscape of prostate cancer treatment will become better defined.

NOTES:

CHAPTER FOURTEEN

High-intensity Focused Ultrasound for Prostate Cancer: 2006 Technology and Outcome Update

JOHN C. REWCASTLE, Ph.D. has provided insight into High Intensity Focused Ultrasound (HIFU); a very effective, patient friendly treatment for organ confined prostate cancer in a fair and balanced manner for all to appreciate. In the past 15 years, thousands of men have had their prostate cancer treated with high-intensity focused ultrasound (HIFU). Most patients have been treated in Europe. The National Institute for Clinical Excellence is a government body in the United Kingdom that evaluates new treatments. It has reviewed the clinical data associated with HIFU and concluded that the evidence is sufficient and recommend its use to the UK's National Health System. Despite these facts, HIFU is new to North America. It has yet to be approved by the U.S. Food and Drug Administration (FDA) but the procedure is available in Canada, the Bahamas, Dominican Republic and Mexico. Although not reimbursed by any public or private health insurers, many men from these countries, as well as the United States, have been treated.

The purpose of this report is to explain, from a fundamental prospective, how HIFU works as well as to review the technologies used to perform HIFU and the published clinical literature regarding the procedure. The motivation behind this update is twofold: First, there is currently a void in the literature regarding a simple explanation of what HIFU is and the thought processes used in the development of commercially available technologies. Second, there is an availability of newly published important clinical data, which allows for a better clinical outcome evaluation.

HIFU Fundamentals

Sound is vibration. Vocal chords vibrate the air near you when you speak and sound waves (air vibrations) travel away from you. When these vibrations reach another person, they cause their eardrum to vibrate creating a signal that is processed by the brain. Vibrations are measured in units called hertz (Hz), which are the number of vibrations per second. Typically, the human ear can hear frequencies between about 20 and 20,000 Hz. Higher frequency sounds have a higher "pitch." Sounds with frequencies higher than the range that humans can hear are called "ultrasound." Medical ultrasound uses frequencies so high that they are measured in millions of hertz or "megahertz" (MHz).

Ultrasound waves can be created by a special type of crystal that vibrates at a specific frequency when an electric current passes through it. The reverse is also true; the crystal will create electricity when vibrated. Both effects are important for medical ultrasound. When a pulse of electricity is passed through one of these crystals a group of sound waves is created and travels away from the crystal. As the sound passes through the tissue, some of it will be reflected back to the crystal as it encounters different tissue structures. This is an "echo" and is exactly the same effect as when you yell into a canyon and some sound is bounced back. Now, when the echo comes back to the crystal it vibrates the crystal creating an electric current. By analyzing the current created by all the echoes it is possible to construct an image that leads to the most common medical application of ultrasound: imaging. It is also important to note that air is the enemy of ultrasound imaging and causes near complete reflection of the signal destroying the ability to image. This is why a gel is put on the skin before imaging occurs. This creates an air-free path for the ultrasound waves to travel through. When gel is applied correctly, there is no air between the ultrasound crystal and the patient and the image is readable. Air also compromises the ability to perform HIFU but that will be discussed later.

Ultrasound waves deposit energy as they travel through tissue but the amount deposited during ultrasound imaging is completely insignificant. Ultrasound imaging is harmless and is so safe that it is used to image unborn babies. The premise behind HIFU is the destruction of tissue by depositing huge amounts of energy into it. This is accomplished by doing two things: increasing the intensity of the waves (similar to turning up the volume) and focusing the waves on a single point (like a magnifying lens). If done in the right conditions it will raise the temperature of tissue to a level sufficient to cause irreversible tissue damage (ablation).

The deposit of energy during HIFU can result in two mechanisms of tissue damage. Elevation of tissue temperature leads to the melting of lipid membranes and protein denaturation. This is the desired effect of HIFU. If large deposits of energy occur, mechanical damage may result in the form of cavitation. Cavitation is the formation of gas bubbles within the tissue. It is difficult to create discrete ablation zones in the presence of cavitation as the gas strongly reflects sonographic waves. Thus, cavitation should be avoided during the procedure.

During HIFU, a reproducible but small volume of ablation is created for each pulse of energy. The geometry of each ablation volume is an ellipsoid (it is shaped like a cigar), and is roughly the size of a few grains of rice stacked end to end. Treatment of prostate cancer accomplished by systematically pulsing energy throughout the target volume at different locations until the entire tumor has been ablated.

Table I: Changes in cavitation probability, temperature rise, penetration and image quality that result from changes in intensity and frequency.

Change	Net Effect			
	Cavitation probability	Temperature rise	Signal Penetration	Image resolution
Increase the frequency	↑	↑	↓	↑
Reduce the frequency	↓	↓		

Commercially Available HIFU Technologies

There are currently two commercially available HIFU technologies for the treatment of prostate cancer. The first to be available was the Ablatherm® (Edap-Technomed, Lyon, France). Subsequently, Focus Surgery (Indianapolis, Ind., U.S.) developed a system called the Sonablate® 500. The foundation HIFU technology of both systems is identical but there are several technological differences between the two machines. These differences, for the most part, arise from different schools of thought with regards to how best design the most effective HIFU treatment system. Specifically, the differences arise in how the manufacturers went about choosing operating frequencies and intensities. This is an optimization based on the effects that modifying these parameters have on image quality and ablation quality. The different approaches have resulted in the development of two commercially available HIFU devices for the treatment of prostate cancer.

The amount of energy deposited in tissue during HIFU is dependent upon both the transducer operating frequency and intensity. Increasing the intensity increases the energy incident on, and absorbed by, the tissue and therefore also increases the probability of inducing cavitation (Table I). However, reducing the intensity reduces the temperature rise of the tissue, which results in a lower temperature increase and consequently decreased injury. Increasing the frequency increases the incidence of cavitation, increases image resolution near the ultrasound crystal, but reduces ultrasound penetration. It is the different strategies used to manage these interactions that have led to the development of different commercially available HIFU devices.

Imaging and Treatment Probes

The Ablatherm uses separate crystals for imaging (7.5Mhz) and treatment (3MHz). Thus, the dependence of image resolution is removed from the equation when ablation is occurring. Imaging probes for prostate applications tend to range from 5Mhz to 7.5Mhz with probes creating higher quality images having higher frequencies. The real-time 7.5MHz probe used by the Ablatherm creates a very high quality image throughout the prostate and a 3Mhz treatment probe is the best frequency for treatment. Thus, optimal values are used for both imaging and treatment. The most recent Ablatherm model has both the imaging and treatment crystals contained within a single probe. This allows not only for optimal operating frequencies for both treatment and imaging but also allows for real-time imaging during the procedure.

The Sonablate 500 uses a single crystal for both imaging and treatment, which also allows for real-time imaging. This is accomplished by using a concave rectangular element cut from a spherical crystal surface that has a central 10mm diameter segment used for imaging. As with the newest Ablatherm device, there is no need to change probes between imaging and treatment. Unfortunately, this constrains the probe to be of only one frequency as probe frequency is characteristic of the crystal. An operating frequency of 4MHz was determined to provide both sufficient image quality and effective treatment although not optimal for either. The 4MHz resolution probe allows for excellent imaging of the anterior part of the prostate but has decreased resolution and image quality in the posterior margin of the gland and the rectal wall in comparison to higher frequency ultrasound probes.

Treatment Planning

HIFU allows for the creation of an accurate geometrical ablation volume. With both technologies, treatments are planned based on the anatomy of the individual patient. Pretreatment ultrasound images are captured and the user defines on them, with computer assistance, the regions to be ablated. The program then controls the ablation probe which treats exactly where the user specifies. The Sonablate uses a single treatment program in which the power can be adjusted manually. Conversely, the Ablatherm uses three treatment algorithms, each designed for specific applications: HIFU as a primary treatment, HIFU following failed radiation therapy and HIFU retreatment. This is critical as the thermal property of a prostate that has never undergone a treatment is vastly different than one that has. When treating a gland that has been irradiated, care must be taken as the dissipation of energy will now be slower due to decreased blood flow throughout the prostate. This is a result of radiation damage to the prostate's blood supply. The same will be true, but to a different extent, for a prostate that has previously been treated with HIFU. The reason this is important is that if not enough time is given for energy to dissipate, a buildup can occur which could lead to rectal injury and other complications.

Real-time Monitoring

If a patient moves during the procedure, the treatment must be stopped immediately and the treatment plan must be rechecked with plan adjustments made. The strategy used to detect movement is different for the two technologies. Although real-time imaging is available with the Ablatherm, it does not use it to detect patient movement. Rather, it relies on an automated infrared detection system to ensure that the patient has not moved. This removes human error from the equation. The real-time imaging available with the Ablatherm is used to detect the rectal wall position and compares this position to the one measured during treatment planning. The probe position is automatically adjusted to compensate any difference between these two measurements. The Sonablate utilizes its real-time imaging comprised of a reference image to a treating image to detect patient movement. The physician must watch the entire procedure to ensure that the images line up indicating no patient movement has occurred. If the patient does move, the treatment plan is no longer valid and must be redone. This is the same for both technologies.

Ablation Volume Geometry and Transducer Size

The fundamental physical constraint in the physical constraint in the physical design of a transducer is the fact that it must be inserted into the rectum during treatment. The physical size and shape of the ultrasound transducer determines where the energy is focused. Each pulse of a HIFU crystal will induce a discrete and consistent volume of tissue necrosis.

The Ablatherm uses a single treatment probe that has a focal point 45mm from the crystal. The 3MHz probe creates an ablation volume that's size is adjustable from 26 mm (anterior to posterior) x 1.7mm x 1.7mm (total volume = 36mm^3) down to 19mm x 1.7mm x 1.7mm (total volume = 29mm^3). The intent is that a single pulse will result in an ablation that extends the entire anterior to posterior height of the prostate. This strategy has the advantage that only one focus is needed to treat the entire height of the gland but given that prostates are not uniform in height (the base is taller than the apex) it can result in the ablation of some tissue beyond the prostate. However, such additional treatment beyond the anterior margin of the prostate will **not lead** to complications.

The Sonablate probe is comprised of two different crystals with different focal lengths. This is accomplished by having two crystals placed back to back within the probe, one with a 3cm focal length and the other 4cm. The discrete ablation volume of both these crystals is 10mm (anterior to posterior) x 2mm x 2mm (total volume = 21mm^3) when operated in normal mode and 10mm x 3mm x 3mm (total volume = 47mm^3) when operated in split-beam mode (see discussion on split beams below). Due to the decreased height of the focal areas, complete anterior to posterior ablation is not usually possible with a single pulse of energy necessitating extra pulses to treat the whole gland. The advantage to this strategy is that the reduced ablation volume allows for better conformation on the ablation zone to the anterior margin of the prostate. The disadvantage is time. Most every prostate has an anterior/posterior height in excess of 10mm and when this is the case, multiple passes will be required. This means that to treat the prostate from top to bottom, the first 10mm will be treated with the first pass. The next 10mm will then be treated with a second pass. **If the prostate is greater than 20mm high, a third pulse of energy would be required. This results in more treatment time, which is undesirable for any treatment in which the patient is under anesthesia.**

That being said, both technologies are limited in their ability to treat *very* large glands. It is, however, possible to perform either a pretreatment **transurethral resection of the prostate** or ablate the posterior portion of the gland, then perform a subsequent HIFU treatment another day after allowing sufficient time for debulking to occur.

Treatment of the posterior margin of the gland can be difficult and unintentional ablation of the rectal wall will lead to fistula formation. Thusly, the physical proximal truncation of the discrete ablation volumes must not include any of the rectal wall. Both manufacturers, erring appropriately on the side of caution, have ablation zones that will not usually encroach on the rectal wall. However, it may be the case that the posterior margin of the prostate will not be ablated due to a small rectal wall to prostate distance. To get around this with the Sonablate, additional water can be added to the condom surrounding the HIFU probe to increase its separation from the rectal wall. This facilitates full ablation of the posterior margin. The treatment crystal within the Ablatherm probe is mounting such that it can be mechanically and automatically moved in three dimensions to fine-tune its position relative to the rectal wall, which is detected on the real-time images.

Safety Features

1. Patient Position

The two technologies use different patient positions during treatment. Several urologic procedures are performed with the patient in the lithotomy position (patient lying on their back with their feet in stirrups). This is the position utilized during treatment with the Sonablate and allows for easy access. However, if bubbles are present in the fluid surrounding the treatment crystal or are created during treatment, they will rise and end up between the crystal and the prostate. This can compromise the treatment quality (both in terms of ablation and targeting) as air sharply reflects ultrasound. Treatment by the Ablatherm is performed with the patient in a right lateral decubitus position (lying on their right side). This is done as a safety precaution. If there are any bubbles in the fluid surrounding the treatment probe, they will rise upwards. With the patient on his side and the treatment aimed laterally, bubbles will not end up between the HIFU treatment crystal and the prostate.

2. Rectal Wall Monitoring

During HIFU, temperatures increase not only at the zones of ablation created by the deposit of sonographic energy, but also throughout and adjacent to the prostate due to thermal conduction. The rectal wall is sensitive to temperature changes. Both manufacturers recognize the need for precise rectal monitoring. To maintain acceptable temperatures throughout the rectal wall, both Sonablate and Ablatherm use the following strategy:

1. Active cooling of the rectal wall during treatment,
2. Continuous monitoring of the temperature of the rectal wall and,

3. Continually measuring the distance between the rectal wall and the prostate.

Combined, these measures have reduced the occurrence of rectal fistulas with both the Ablatherm and Sonablate to essentially zero. Additionally, the infrared system used by the Ablatherm to monitor patient position will cause the device to shut off instantly if any movement is detected. **Of note, there have been no reports in the literature of fistula formation in patients treated with the Ablatherm since 2003.**

3. Reflectivity Measurement

Although cavitation should not occur during HIFU regardless of the choice of treatment frequencies, Sonablate does incorporate an additional safety measure regarding reflectivity measurement. Tissue changes resulting from increased temperatures can be detected by analyzing reflected ultrasound signals and comparing them to images taken prior to the commencement of therapy. As the temperature increases, the reflectivity index (ratio of the two signals) changes. This allows for a real-time feedback indicating that an excessive buildup of thermal energy may be imminent. If significant reflectivity index changes are observed in a region, the device will automatically pause until sufficient energy has dissipated and therapy continues.

Split beams

HIFU transducers can be comprised of one of more arrays of piezoelectric crystals. A flat central element can serve dual purposes as it can be used for both imaging and treatment.

Table II: Outcome observed following HIFU. Multicenter trials are marked with an *.

Study	Device	n	PSA (ng/ml)	Gleason	Stage	Median f/u (months)	Negative biopsy	Long term Efficacy (definition)
Chaussy 2001	A	184	12		T1-2 Nx		80%	
Gelet 2001	A	102	8.38 Mean	54% 2-6 46% 7-10	T1-T2	19	75%	66% @ 5 years (ASTRO)
Poissonnier 2003	A	120	5.67 Mean 100% < 10	64% 2-6 36% 7-10	T1-T2	27	86%	76.9% @ 5 years (ASTRO)
Thüroff 2003*	A	402	10.9 Mean	13.2% 2-4 77.5% 5-7 9.3% 8-10	T1-T2	13	87.2%	
Blana 2004	A	146	7.6 Mean	5 ± 1.2	T1-T2 N0M0	22	93.4%	84% @ 22 months (PSA < 1.0)
Uchida 2005*	S	72	8.1 Median		T1c-T2b N0M0	14	68%	
Uchida 2006	S	63	11.2 Mean	21% 2-4 73% 5-7 15% 8-10	T1c=T2b	23.3	87%	74% @ 3 years (ASTRO)

f/u = follow-up, **A = Ablatherm, S = Sonablate**

Surrounding elements are utilized only for treatment. During treatment, if all arrays are incorporated and active during the therapy mode (single beam) then a sharply demarcated ablation zone will be created. By not including the central element, ultrasound wave interference occurs and the resultant focal zone of ablation is approximately three times the size for the same energy and focal length. This is referred to as a split beam and has the possibility of reducing treatment time somewhat.

Efficacy Comparison and Update

Several papers have been published since my last outcome review of HIFU. Specifically, an update of Dr. Thomas K. Uchida's patient series, as well as a report from the Japanese multicenter trial is now available. Both of these papers report outcomes with the Sonablate. The following summary is based on all papers published in all languages in the peer-reviewed medical literature from 2001 to 2006. Only full medical journal articles are included. Conference abstracts, as they do not undergo thorough peer review to assess validity and accuracy, were not included.

Table II summarizes all papers published regarding HIFU from the past 5 years. One paper was excluded from this table, which was Dr. Uchida's 2002 report. This was done because it is replaced by his 2006 report, which is an update of his personal experience with HIFU, which includes the patient from the 2002 report. This was done because it is replaced by his 2006 report, which is an update of his personal experience with HIFU, which includes the patients from the 2002 report. The two most important studies in the table are those of Thüroff et al. 2003 (Ablatherm) and Uchida et al. 2005 (Sonablate). These two studies report outcomes of multicenter clinical trials utilizing the Ablatherm and Sonablate, respectfully. They both have similar patient populations and similar lengths of follow-up. They (as well as all other studies listed in table II) use negative biopsies as a fundamental endpoint. Those patients with negative biopsies show no clinical evidence of untreated or recurrent disease: a higher value indicates better cancer control. The negative biopsy rates of the two multicenter studies are quite different at 87 percent for the Ablatherm and 68 percent for the Sonablate. It is inappropriate to draw solid conclusions based solely on these two reports due to their short-term follow-up. When the negative biopsy rates of all published studies are compared, a different picture emerges. Figure I is a comparison of all negative biopsy rates.

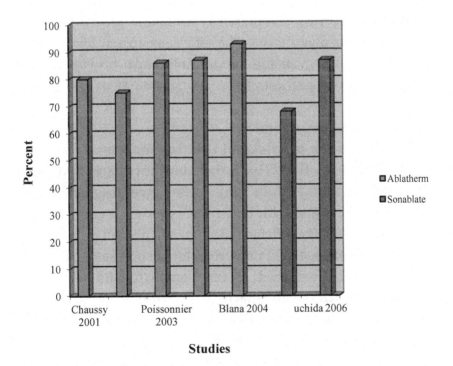

Figure I: Comparison of negative biopsy rates between the Ablatherm and Sonablate device. Multicenter trials are marked with an *.

Based on this comparison is appears that the efficacies of the two technologies are somewhat similar. A more definitive comparison will not be possible until more articles appear in the medical literature.

What can be concluded now is that there is less uncertainty regarding the long-term outcomes of the Ablatherm device. The Ablatherm publications have significantly more patients and the follow-ups are longer.

Conclusions

High-intensity focused ultrasound is a technologically advanced noninvasive therapy for prostate cancer. There currently exist two commercially available treatment units each with their own merits. The efficacies appear similar with long-term results available for the Ablatherm providing more certainty regarding efficacy.

Dr. Wheeler's Commentary:
I have had the privilege of treating more male patients successfully with HIFU (both the Ablatherm and Sonablate 500 technologies) than any other treating physician (urologist) in the world. Given my experience and expertise in both technologies, I believe Ablatherm (EDAP) provides the best opportunity for the most predictable successful treatment outcome when compared to the Sonablate 500 technology (International HIFU). Ablatherm, a true robotic procedure, has a safety and treatment outcome profile that exceeds that of the Sonablate 500, given the fact that physician decision making based on ultrasound recognition with the Sonablate 500 is the dependent variable to success or failure of the operation! To be certain, many very qualified urologists in areas of genitourinary medicine (other than HIFU) are unable to grasp the methodology

including detail of procedure and concepts for success with the Sonablate 500. **To state more clearly, there are so many more critical decisions (that need to be addressed) during the Sonablate 500 procedure that only the most skilled and focused urologists can comprehend. Unfortunately, there are no more than a handful or two of Urologists worldwide who can navigate the Sonablate 500 technology comfortably and accurately after more than 5 years of exposure.** As I have stated often times, many urologists have trained with the Sonablate 500 but only a very few can achieve a skill level commensurate with expert status. Ablatherm on the other hand, allows the physician to set the parameters of treatment prior to the procedure based on his ultrasound skill set without the need to make intra-operational adjustments! Ablatherm is a technology that all interested urologists can learn provided the motivation to learn is present. Time of treatment is important and varies from 3-4 hours with the Sonablate 500 while commonly less than 2 hours with the Ablatherm technology. I believe the greater number of times a physician is asked to make a critical decision during a procedure relates to a greater chance for error or failure in a 3-4 hour visually intensive procedure. Ultimately, this puts the patient at risk for complication including a less than adequate opportunity for cure necessitating a second HIFU procedure or alternative procedure in an effort to achieve success as defined by cure!

Beyond what has been stated above, there are additional variables that relate to success or failure of any HIFU procedure including but not limited to: physician patient selection, a comprehensively informed patient with full disclosure in consent, patient expectation, physician selection by patients, physician outcome data based on a minimum of 100 cases performed, a total PSA value and highest PSA value prior to treatment, a comprehensive ultrasound skills including color 'Power Doppler', biochemical adjustments for needle tracking, discrimination of disease volume, location and extension based on imaging with Magnetic Resonance Imaging (MRI) as opposed to guessing with random biopsies or ultrasound, understanding of stricture disease and how best to handle it (pre or post treatment) as well as an expected absence of incontinence of bowel and bladder with a reasonable and acceptable minimal impotency rate.

My data becomes 5 year data in May 2012. I encourage all treating urologists to present their data as I will my own while allowing other interested and non-biased physicians to independently inspect and scrutinize the data gathered from all performed cases at their discretion. Minimally, the 3 most prolific urologists in the USA must compare their data openly in a fair and balanced manner for the consumption of the future male participants.

A Glossary of Prostate Cancer Related Terms & Abbreviations

3 dimensional conformal radiation therapy (3DCRT): an external radiation treatment approach that focuses on directing the radiation energy to the tumor target while sparing the surrounding normal tissues; see conformal

5-alpha-dihydrotestosterone: usually known as dihydrotestosterone or DHT

5-alpha reductase (5AR): enzymes that convert testosterone to dihydrotestosterone

5-alpha reductase inhibitor: A drug used to block the conversion of testosterone to dihydrotestosterone. Examples: finasteride (Proscar®) and dutasteride (Avodart®).

5-FU: 5-Fluorouracil; (Adrucil®); a drug in the group of cancer-fighting medicines known as *antineoplastics*, which interferes with the growth of cancer cells. It is approved for palliative management of colon, rectum, breast, stomach and pancreatic cancer

17,20 lyase: an enzyme important in the adrenal androgen pathways that converts 17 alpha hydroxyprogesterone to *androstenedione* and also converts 17 alpha hydroxypregneneolone to *DHEA*

A

a1-antichymotrypsin (ACT): one of the many serine protease inhibitors or serpins (short for serine protease inhibitor) which are proteins that inhibit peptidases (old name: proteases). Serine proteases are defined by the presence of a serine (an amino acid) residue in their active domain.

AAT: androgen ablation therapy; preferred terms might be androgen deprivation therapy (ADT) or hormone therapy.

AAWR: **antiandrogen withdrawal response**; a decrease in PSA seen upon stopping an antiandrogen such as Flutamide® or Casodex®; it is believed that this occurs because the antiandrogen has induced a mutation in the *androgen receptor (AR)* which is allowing the antiandrogen to stimulate PC growth rather than inhibit it

abdomen adj. **abdominal**: the part of the body below the ribs and above the pelvic bone that contains organs like the intestines, the liver, the kidneys, the stomach, the bladder, and the prostate

ablation: relating to the removal or destruction of tissue or a system; androgen ablation refers to blocking the effects of androgens by surgical or chemical mean

acinus: pl. ACINI: any of the small sac-like structures that terminate the ducts of some glands, also called alveolus; ACINAR: of, relating to or comprising an acinus

acronym: an abbreviation formed from the initial letters of a name; e.g. see *ARM*

ACTH: adrenal corticotrophic hormone; a pituitary hormone that stimulates the outer portion of the adrenal glands to secrete various hormones including cortisol, *DHEA* and *androstenedione*

active objectified surveillance: active observation and regular monitoring of a patient without actual treatment ; also called 'watchful waiting'

acute: beginning quickly and sharp or severe

acute urinary retention: the sudden inability to urinate, causing pain and discomfort. Causes can be related to an obstruction in the urinary system, stress, neurologic problems, or certain medications.

adenocarcinoma: a form of cancer that develops from a malignant abnormality in the cells lining a glandular organ such as the prostate; almost all prostate cancers are adenocarcinomas

adenoma: a benign tumor of a glandular structure

adenovirus: a (20 sided) virus that contains DNA; there are over 40 different adenovirus varieties, some of which cause the common cold. Modified versions have shown some ability to cause apoptosis in laboratory testing

adipose: tissue made of fat cells

adjuvant: an additional treatment used to increase the effectiveness of the primary therapy; radiation therapy is often used as an adjuvant treatment after a radical prostatectomy if the surgical margins are involved by PC

ADPC (androgen-dependent PC): PC cells that depend on androgens for continued cell growth and vitality

adrenal androgen (AA): a male hormone produced by the adrenal glands; actually, the adrenal makes AA precursors such as *DHEA* and *androstenedione* that are metabolized to androgens within the prostate.

adrenal cortex: the outer portion of the adrenal gland; it secretes various hormones.

adrenal glands: the two adrenal glands are located above the kidneys; they produce a variety of different hormones, including cortisol, adrenal androgens and hormones important in blood pressure control and electrolyte balance

adrenalectomy: the surgical removal of one or both adrenal glands

Adriamycin® (doxorubicin): a genotoxic drug, a chemotherapy agent that affects DNA and alters its function

ADS (androgen deprivation syndrome): a number of side effects associated with low levels of androgen associated with _ADT_

ADT: see _androgen deprivation therapy_**adverse reaction**: a harmful or unexpected effect of a medication or treatment

aerobic: in biochemistry, reactions that need oxygen to happen or happen when oxygen is present

AG: aminogluthethimide; a drug that blocks the production of _adrenal hormones_ such as _DHEA, androstenedione_ and also cortisol

age-adjusted: ndividual or group of individuals; for example, it has been suggested that normal PSA values can be adjusted according to age groupings of men:

Age	PSA "cutoff"
40-49	up to 2.5 ng/ml
50-59	up to 3.5
60-69	up to 4.5
70-79	up to 6.5

agonist: A drug or other chemical that can combine with a _receptor_ on a cell to produce a physiologic reaction typical of a naturally occurring substance

AIPC (androgen-independent PC): PC cells that do not depend on androgen for growth

Akt: a _protein kinase_ which is one of the key _enzymes_ for regulating anti-_apoptotic_ events

albumin: A class of simple, water-soluble proteins that can be coagulated by heat and precipitated by strong acids and are found in egg white, blood serum, milk, and many other animal and plant juices and tissues

alendronate sodium: a drug that affects bone metabolism used in treating _osteoporosis_ and being studied in the treatment of _hypercalcemia_ (abnormally high levels of calcium in the blood) and in treating and reducing the risk of bone pain caused by cancer; active ingredient in Fosamax®

algorithm: procedure or formula for solving a problem; for a set of computer programs that provide algorithms relating to prostate cancer, see the software section of www.pcri.org

alkaline phosphatase (ALP): an enzyme in blood, bone, kidney, spleen, and lungs; used to monitor bone or liver metastasis when elevated

alk phos: alkaline phosphatase

alopecia: loss of hair

alpha-blockers: pharmaceuticals that act on the prostate by relaxing certain types of muscle tissue; these pharmaceuticals are often used in the treatment of BPH; examples are lomax®, Cardura® and Hytrin®

alpha receptors: a cell site that responds to adrenaline (epinephrine) or adrenaline-like substances, causing various physiological changes related to blood vessels getting smaller

alprostadil: a prostaglandin that relaxes the smooth muscles of the penis, enhancing blood flow, and producing erection; first produced as Caverject®, an injectable *Prostaglandin* E1

amino: Containing NH2; used in the context of "amino group"; see *polyamine*

aminoglutethimide (Cytadren®): an aromatase inhibitor that blocks the production of adrenal steroids. It also blocks the conversion of androgens to estrogens

amplicon: the DNA product of a PCR reaction, usually an amplified segment of a gene or DNA

anaerobic: an organism, such as a bacterium, that can live in the absence of atmospheric oxygen

analgesia: pain relief without loss of consciousness

analgesic: a drug that alleviates pain without causing loss of consciousness

analog: a synthetic chemical or pharmaceutical that behaves like a normal chemical in the body, e.g., LHRH analogs such as Lupron® or Zoladex®

Anandron®: trade or brand name for nilutamide, an <u>antiandrogen</u>; in the USA this is called Nilandron®.

anastomosis: (pl. **anastomoses**)—the connection of separate parts of a branching system to form a network, as of blood vessels; also the surgical connection of separate or severed tubular hollow organs to form a continuous channel, as the severed <u>urethra</u> in <u>radical prostatectomy</u>.

anastrozole (Arimidex®): an <u>aromatase</u> inhibitor that reduces the level of <u>estrogen</u> in the body

Androcur®: trade name for cyproterone, an antiandrogen with progestational activity; also called CPA for cyproterone acetate (not available in U.S.)

androgen: a hormone which is responsible for male characteristics and the development and function of male sexual organs (e.g., testosterone) produced mainly by the testicles but also in the *cortex* of the *adrenal* glands; androgens have far reaching effects on blood formation, muscle and bone mass, *cognitive* function, emotional *lability*, skin and hair, etc

androgen dependent PC (ADPC): PC cells that depend on androgens for continued cell growth and vitality

androgen deprivation syndrome (ADS): a number of side effects associated with elimination or blockage of androgens from ADT

androgen deprivation therapy (ADT):(also called <u>hormone therapy</u>) or testosterone inactivating pharmaceuticals (TIP)) a prostate cancer treatment that eliminates or blocks androgens to the PC cell; includes diverse mechanisms such as surgical or chemical castration, antiandrogens, *5 AR inhibitors*, <u>estrogenic</u> compounds, agents that interfere with adrenal androgen production, agents that decrease sensitivity of the <u>androgen receptor</u> (AR)

androgen independent prostate cancer (AIPC): PC cells that do not depend on androgen for growth

androgen receptor (AR): A structural entity that is the site of interaction of a chemical substance called a ligand as is a lock and key; a docking site for a ligand

androgen receptor mutation (ARM): a mutation in the gene located on the <u>androgen receptor</u> that allows the <u>antiandrogen</u> to stimulate PC growth rather than block growth; a paradoxical effect usually occurring in about 30% of patients on long-term antiandrogen therapy in the setting of a rising PSA with a <u>castrate testosterone</u> level

androstenedione: an adrenal androgen precursor that is transformed to testosterone by 3 beta hydroxysteroid dehydrogenase within the prostate cell; testosterone can also be oxidized to androstenedione by 17 beta hydroxysteroid dehydrogenase

anemia: A disorder characterized by a decrease in hemoglobin in the blood to levels below the normal range. Symptoms include fatigue, weakness and difficulty breathing.

anesthetic, anesthesia: a drug that produces general or local loss of physical sensations, particularly pain; a "spinal" is the injection of a local anesthetic into the area surrounding the spinal cord

aneuploid: having an abnormal number of sets of <u>chromosomes</u>; for example, <u>tetraploid</u> means having two paired sets of chromosomes, which is twice as many as normal; aneuploid cancer cells tend not to respond well to <u>androgen deprivation therapy</u>; aneuploidy refers to the state of being aneuploid; (see also <u>diploid</u>)

angiogenesis: the growth of new blood vessels; a characteristic of tumors; angiogenesis is normal biologic process that occurs in both healthy and disease states; "angiogenesis factor" or "tumor angiogenesis factor" refers to a substance that tumors produce in order to grow new blood vessels

anorexia: loss of appetite

antagonist: a drug that has an opposite reaction or competes for the same thing

anterior: the front; for example, the anterior of the prostate is the part of the prostate that faces forward

anterolateral: situated or occurring in front and to the side from the midpoint

antiandrogen: a compound (usually a synthetic pharmaceutical) that blocks or otherwise interferes with the normal action of androgens at cellular receptor sites

antiandrogen monotherapy (AAM): the use of an antiandrogen to block the androgen receptors of the cancer cells as a single therapy to reduce the side-effects normally associated with androgen deprivation therapy

antiandrogen withdrawal response: PSA alteration based on elimination of an antiandrogen; commonly favorable

antibiotic: a pharmaceutical that can kill certain types of bacteria

antibody: _protein_ produced by the immune system as a defense against an invading or "foreign" material or substance (an _antigen_); for example, when you get a cold, your body produces antibodies to the cold virus

anticholinergic: an agent that blocks certain receptors on the nerves, lessens muscle spasms and reduces release of liquids by the stomach, mouth, sweat glands, etc.

anticoagulant: a pharmaceutical that helps to stop the blood from clotting

antiemetic: a medicine that prevents or alleviates nausea and vomiting

antiestrogen: a substance capable of preventing full expression of the biological effects of an estrogen

antigen: "foreign" material introduced into the body (a virus or bacterium, for example) or other material which the immune system considers to be "foreign" because it is not part of the body's normal biology (e.g., prostate cancer cells); a substance that elicits a cellular-level immune response or causes the formation of an antibody

antigen-presenting cell (APC): A type of cell that provokes an immune response from _T-cells_ by binding foreign antigens to its own surface and then interacting with the T-cells. Also known as antigen-processing cell

antineoplastic: Inhibiting or preventing the development of abnormal tissue growth, checking the maturation and proliferation of _malignant_ cells

antioxidant: a substance that inhibits oxidation or reactions promoted by oxygen or peroxides. Antioxidant nutrients protect human cells from damage caused by "free radicals" (highly reactive oxygen compounds).

anus: the opening of the _rectum_ through which solid waste leaves the body

apex, apical: the tip or bottom of the prostate, e.g., the part of the prostate farthest away from the bladder; the top of the prostate is called the base

apoptosis: programmed cell death due to an alteration in a critical substance or chemical necessary for cell viability; the lack of male hormones causes apoptosis of _androgen dependent PC_

arachidonic acid: an omega-6 fatty acid that has been shown to be a stimulator of PC growth; found in egg yolk, animal red meat and organ meats as example; has free-radical generating properties

Arimidex®: the trademarked name for _anastrozole_

ARM (androgen receptor mutation): a mutation in the gene located on the _androgen receptor_ that allows the antiandrogen to stimulate PC growth rather than block growth; a paradoxical effect usually occurring in about 30% of patients on long-term antiandrogen therapy in the setting of a rising PSA with a _castrate_ testosterone level

aromatase: an _enzyme_ that converts _testosterone_ to _estrogen_ (estradiol or estrone)

arteriosclerosis: a chronic disease characterized by abnormal thickening and hardening of the arterial walls

ASCO: American Society of Clinical Oncology

aspiration: the use of suction to remove fluid or tissue, usually through a fine needle (e.g., aspiration biopsy)

assay: a method of performing a standard test for the quality or quantity of a substance (ex: PSA). Assay results may vary depending on the methods, reagents and equipment used.

ASTRO: American Society for Therapeutic Radiation and Oncology

asymptomatic: having no recognizable symptoms of a particular disorder

ATF (amino terminal fragment): highly active part of the uPA molecule

atherosclerosis: a disorder of the arteries leading to reduced blood flow caused by the narrowing of blood vessels due to the accumulation of plaques composed up of cholesterols and fats

atrophic: undergoing atrophy or shrinkage in size and usually function

atrophy: a wasting or decrease in size of a body organ, tissue, or part owing to disease, injury, or lack of use: *muscular atrophy of a person affected with paralysis.* a wasting away, deterioration, or diminution: *intellectual atrophy.*

attentive DRE: a DRE described for PCA3 test as "applying firm digital pressure to the prostate from base to apex and from the lateral to the median line for each lobe with exactly three strokes per lobe" (Dr. Yves Fradet—AUA 2006)

atypical hyperplasia (atypia): non typical enlargement of an organ or tissue

AUA (American Urological Association): the official society of American urologists

AUA Symptom Score: an evaluation of the lower urinary tract symptoms (*LUTS*) based on questions published by the American Urological Association

autocrine: of, relating to, promoted by, or being a substance secreted by a cell and acting on surface receptors of the same cell

autologous: one's own; for example, autologous blood is a patient's own blood which is removed prior to surgery in case a patient needs a transfusion during or after surgery

auxotroph, auxotrophic: mutant that differs from the wild—type (normal) in requiring a nutritional supplement beyond the minimum required for metabolism and reproduction

Avodart®: dutasteride

axial: extending in a direction essentially perpendicular to the plane of a cyclic structure

axial spin-echo T1 weighted image: an image acquired in the axial plane using a pulse-sequence that weights the signal intensity of each pixel to the T1 (the time it takes for water protons to return to thermal equilibrium) relaxation of water

azotemia: elevation in blood nitrogen level due to dehydration or kidney dysfunction; in laboratory tests this manifests as elevation in BUN and/or creatinine

B

base: the base of the prostate is the wide part at the top of the prostate closest to the seminal vesicles and bladder

baseline PSA (bPSA): the PSA level before a new treatment has begun; used to establish efficacy of a therapy based on response of the PSA to the treatment; can also be used in principle with any other marker, radiologic imaging study or any finding that shows pathology relating to PC

BAT: B-mode acquisition and targeting; an ultrasound evaluation of the prostate localizing it prior to each and every RT therapy treatment; currently used in conjunction with IMRT and mechanically integrated into the treatment program

Bcl-2: an anti-apoptotic protein that protects cells from programmed cell death by preventing the activation of pro—apoptotic proteins

Benadryl®: antihistamine often used to treat allergic reactions involving the nasal passages (hay fever) and also to treat motion sickness

benign: relatively harmless; not cancerous; not malignant

benign prostatic hyperplasia or hypertrophy (BPH): A noncancerous condition of the prostate that results in the growth of both glandular and stromal (supporting connective) tumorous tissue, enlarging the prostate and obstructing urination

benign prostatic hypertrophy (BPH): similar to benign prostatic hyperplasia, but caused by an increase in the size of cells rather than the growth of more cells

beta particle: a charged particle (electron or positron) that is emitted by the decay of certain radioactive atoms

bevacizumab (Avastin®): an anti-angiogenesis drug used in treatment of cancer. It is used in combination with standard chemotherapy drugs in patients with metastatic colorectal cancer.

bicalutamide (Casodex®): a nonsteroidal antiandrogen available in the USA and some European countries for the treatment of advanced prostate cancer

bid or b.i.d.: to be taken twice a day (morning and evening); stands for "bis in die" (in Latin, 2 times a day)

bilateral: both sides; for example, a bilateral orchiectomy is an orchiectomy in which both testicles are removed and a bilateral adrenalectomy is an operation in which both adrenal glands are removed

bimix, bi-mix: usually refers to a mixture of papaverine and phentolamine that is injected into the penis to cause an erection.

biochemical: involving chemical processes in living organisms

biochemical control: control of a *biochemical marker*, such as an antigen (ex: PSA), antibody, abnormal enzyme (ex: PAP), or hormone that is sufficiently altered in a disease to serve as an aid in diagnosing or in predicting susceptibility to the disease.

biochemical failure: loss of biochemical control

biomarker: A specific biochemical in the body which is useful for measuring the progress of disease or the effects of treatment

biopsy (Bx): sampling of tissue from a particular part of the body (e.g., the prostate) in order to check for abnormalities such as cancer; in the case of prostate cancer, biopsies are usually carried out under ultrasound guidance using a specially designed device known as a prostate biopsy gun; removed tissue is typically examined microscopically by a pathologist in order to make a precise diagnosis of the patient's condition. See our paper <u>Understanding Your</u> <u>Biopsy Results</u>.

bisphosphonates (BPs): any of a group of carbon—substituted analogs (as <u>etidronate</u>) of <u>pyrophosphate</u> that are potent inhibitors of <u>osteoclast</u>-mediated bone <u>resorption</u>

bladder: the hollow organ in which urine is collected and stored in the body

blastic: having a dense appearance on a plain x-ray; associated with increased density of bone involved by prostate cancer and looking whiter on an ordinary x-ray; prostate cancer bone metastases are usually blastic; breast cancer <u>metastases</u> are usually lytic (showing evidence of less bone density in areas of cancer)

blood chemistry: measured concentrations of many chemicals in the blood; abnormal values can indicate spread of cancer or side effects of therapy

blood count: analysis of blood cells including white blood cells, red blood cells and <u>platelets</u>; abnormal values can indicate cancer in the bone or side effects of therapy. See our paper <u>Laboratory Tests Defined</u>

blot: a nitrocellulose (cotton-like polymer) sheet that contains spots of immobilized macromolecules (as of <u>DNA</u>, <u>RNA</u>, or <u>protein</u>) or their fragments and that is used to identify specific components of the spots by applying a suitable molecular probe (as a complementary <u>nucleic acid</u> or a <u>radiolabeled</u> <u>antibody</u>)

Ronald E. Wheeler, M.D.

Bluestein tables: tables containing algorithms which use the variables clinical stage, Gleason grade, and PSA to predict high vs low risk for lymph node involvement with prostate cancer. See our paper Bluestein Tables.

BMD: See bone mineral density.

bombesin: an amino acid peptide which stimulates gastrin release

bone marrow: soft tissue in bone cavities that produces blood cells

bone mineral density (BMD): a measure of the strength of bones, androgen deprivation can cause the loss of BMD resulting in osteoporosis, usually BMD is tested by dual-energy absorption x-ray (DEXA) or quantitative CAT scan (qCT) methods

bone scan: a technique more sensitive than conventional x—rays which uses a radiolabelled agent to identify abnormal or cancerous growths within or attached to bone; in the case of prostate cancer, a bone scan is used to identify bony metastases which are definitive for cancer which has escaped from the prostate; metastases appear as "hot spots" on the film; however the absence of hot spots does not prove the absence of tiny metastases

bound PSA: PSA molecules in the blood that are attached to other proteins

bowel preparation: the cleaning of the bowels or intestines that is normal prior to abdominal surgery such as radical prostatectomy

BPH: see benign prostatic hyperplasia

brachytherapy: A form of radiation therapy in which radioactive seeds or pellets which emit radiation are implanted within the prostate in order to destroy PC. See our paper Seed Implantation for Prostate Cancer

BRM (bone resorption marker): a laboratory test that quantifies the bone loss (resorption) occurring usually from *ADT* or PC; examples include Pyrilinks-D (Dpd) and N—telopeptides

BUN: blood urea nitrogen; a reflection of kidney function;

C

CAB (complete androgen blockade): see <u>CHT</u>

cachexia: physical wasting with loss of weight and muscle mass caused by disease

calcification: impregnation with calcium or calcium salts. Also called *calcareous infiltration*

calcitriol: (1,25-dihydroxycholecalciferol) a <u>hormone</u> related to vitamin D that is synthesized in the liver and kidney and stimulates the intestinal absorption of calcium and phosphorus

calcitonin: a <u>hormone</u> produced by the thyroid that plays a role in regulating calcium levels

cancer: the growth of abnormal cells in the body in an uncontrolled manner; unlike benign tumors, these tend to invade surrounding tissues, and spread to distant sites of the body via the blood stream and lymphatic system

CaP: cancer of the prostate; also <u>PC</u>, <u>PCa</u>

capecitabine (trade name Xeloda®): a drug first used to treat <u>metastatic</u> breast cancer in patients who had not responded well to <u>chemotherapy</u>. In some patients, capecitabine helps shrink tumor size by killing cancer

capsular penetration: tumor extends through the wall of the prostate

capsule: the fibrous tissue that acts as an outer lining of the prostate

CaPSURE™: (Cancer of the Prostate Strategic Urologic Research Endeavor) is a longitudinal observational study of prostate cancer patients nationwide.

carboplatin: a platinum based compound that is used as a cancer <u>chemotherapeutic</u> agent

carcinoembryonic: relating to a <u>carcinoma</u>-associated substance present in embryonic tissue, as a carcinoembryonic antigen

carcinogen, adj. carcinogenic: a cancer-causing substance or agent

carcinogenesis: the process by which normal cells are transformed into cancer cells

carcinoma: a form of cancer that originates in tissues that line or cover a particular organ; See <u>adenocarcinoma</u>

cardiovascular: referring to the heart and blood vessels

carotenoid: orange, yellow or red-colored accessory photosynthetic pigments, related to vitamin A, found in higher plants and photosynthetic bacteria

Casodex®: brand or trade name of <u>bicalutamide</u> in the USA, a non-steroidal <u>antiandrogen</u>

castrate: a level associated with what occurs after castration; traditionally surgical removal of the testicles; a castrate testosterone is defined by most physicians as less than 20 ng/ml or less than 0.69 nM/L; (nM/L x 28.8 = ng/dl)

castration: the use of surgical or chemical techniques to eliminate <u>testosterone</u> produced by the <u>testes</u>

CAT Scan (CT or computerized axial tomography): is a method of combining images from multiple x-rays under the control of a computer to produce cross-sectional or three-dimensional pictures of the internal organs which can be used to identify abnormalities; the CAT scan can identify prostate enlargement but is not always effective for assessing the stage of prostate cancer; for evaluating <u>metastases</u> of the lymph nodes or more distant soft tissue sites, the CAT scan is significantly more accurate

catalyst: a substance that increases the rate of a chemical reaction, without being consumed or produced by the reaction

catheter: a hollow (usually flexible plastic) tube which can be used to drain fluids from or inject fluids into the body; in the case of prostate cancer, it is common for patients to have a <u>transurethral</u> catheter to drain urine for some time after treatment by surgery or some forms of radiation therapy

CBC: complete blood count; includes the white blood count (<u>WBC</u>), <u>hematocrit</u> (HCT) and the <u>platelet</u> count (PLT).

CDK-1 (cyclin-dependent kinase inhibitor): a regulator of cell growth; an <u>enzyme</u> inhibitor

CDUS (color-flow Doppler ultrasound): an <u>ultrasound</u> method that more clearly images tumors by observing the Doppler shift in sound waves caused by the rapid flow of blood through tiny blood vessels that are characteristic of tumors

CEA (<u>carcinoembryonic</u> antigen): a fetal <u>antigen</u> or <u>protein</u> that may be expressed by PC that is aggressive and often androgen independent

celecoxib (Celebrex®): an FDA-approved drug for the treatment of rheumatoid arthritis, osteoarthritis and pain; it has also been reported to block <u>Akt</u> function and cause the death of human prostate cancer cell lines.

cell-mediated immunity: Immunity dependent upon <u>T-cells'</u> recognition of an antigen and their subsequent destruction of cells bearing the antigen

centigray (cGy): 1/100 of a <u>Gray</u>

CGA: chromogranin A; a <u>small cell prostate cancer</u> or <u>neuroendocrine</u> cell marker; a progressive increase in CGA indicates an aggressive clone of PC cells that often metastasizes to lymph nodes, liver and lungs

CHB (combination hormone blockade): also referred to as <u>CHT</u>, MAB, TAB or <u>ADT</u> (androgen deprivation therapy); therapy usually involving an <u>LHRH agonist</u> and an <u>antiandrogen</u>; may involve other agents such as Proscar® or <u>prolactin</u> inhibitors such as Dostinex®; preferred term is <u>ADT</u> with number attached to show number of agents e.g. ADT3 (Flutamide®, Lupron®, Proscar®) or ADT3 (FLP)

chemoprevention: the use of a pharmaceutical or other substance to prevent the development of cancer

chemotherapeutic: related to the use of <u>chemotherapy</u>

chemotherapy: the use of pharmaceuticals or other chemicals to kill cancer cells; in many cases chemotherapeutic agents kill not only cancer cells but also other cells in the body, which makes such agents potentially very dangerous

cholesterol: substance found in animal fats and in the human body that helps absorb and move fatty acids: cholesterol deposits can clog blood vessels leading to atherosclerosis

choline: a B-complex vitamin that is a constituent of lecithin; essential in the <u>metabolism</u> of fat

chromatin: the material in the center of the cell (nucleus) that forms <u>chromosomes</u>

chromosome: a threadlike linear strand of <u>DNA</u> and associated proteins in the nucleus of cells that carries the <u>genes</u> and functions in the transmission of hereditary information

chronic: referring to a disease or condition that develops slowly and persists over a long period of time

CHT (combined hormonal therapy): the use of more than one variety of hormone therapy; especially the use of <u>LHRH analogs</u> (e.g., Lupron®, Zoladex®) to block the production of <u>testosterone</u> by the <u>testes</u>, plus <u>antiandrogens</u> (e.g., Casodex® (bicalutamide), Eulexin® (flutamide), Anandron® (nilutamide), or Androcur® (cyproterone)) to compete with <u>DHT</u> and with T (testosterone) for cell <u>androgen receptors</u> thereby depriving cancer cells of DHT and T needed for growth; also referred to as <u>CHB</u>, MAB, TAB; the preferred term is <u>ADT</u>

ciprofloxacin (trade name **Cipro®)**: an <u>antibiotic</u> used in various infections including urinary tract infections (<u>UTI</u>) and <u>prostatitis</u>

circadian rhythm: a daily rhythmic activity cycle based on a 24 hour interval

citrate: a salt or <u>ester</u> of citric acid

clinical, clinically: involving or based on direct observation of the patient

clinical stage: <u>staging</u> of prostate cancer as determined by the <u>digital rectal examination</u>.

clinical trial: a carefully planned process by which researchers evaluate experimental new therapies and drugs through an orderly series of phases. **Phase I** trials evaluate how a new therapy or drug should be given, how often, and what dose is safe. **Phase II** trials continue to test safety but also begin to evaluate how well it works. **Phase III** trials test a new therapy or drug in comparison to the current standard of care. Participants are randomly assigned to the standard or new therapy. A placebo is only used when there is no standard therapy for comparison. Placebos are not used in Phase I or II. **Phase IV** trials are required when a drug manufacturer wishes to test an approved therapy for a different condition or with a different formulation.

clinicopathological: relating to or concerned both with the signs and symptoms directly observable by the physician and with the results of laboratory examination

cognitive: of, relating to, or being conscious intellectual activity (as thinking, reasoning, remembering, imagining, or learning words)

cohort: a group of individuals having a statistical factor (as age or risk) in common

collagen: a protein consisting of bundles of tiny fibers that form connective tissue such as tendons, ligaments, bones and cartilage

collimator: A device used to define the size and shape of a radiation beam in <u>radiation therapy</u> treatment machines; A collimator typically consists of large blocks of heavy metals, such as steel or tungsten, moved by mechanical motors to define rectangular fields; see *IMRT*

colon: the part of the large intestine that extends to the <u>rectum</u>

color Doppler ultrasound (CDU): an <u>ultrasound</u> imaging technology utilizing sound waves that can simultaneously show blood flow superimposed on detailed gray scale anatomic images—"power Doppler" and "tissue harmonic" are enhancements to basic CDU.

colorectal: relating to the <u>colon</u> and <u>rectum</u>, or to the entire large bowel (large intestine) **combined therapy**: see *CHT* or *CHB*; *ADT* with designation ADT1 vs ADT2 or ADT3 is preferred since this communicates the number of drugs used in the androgen deprivation therapy; ADT also more clearly communicates the mechanism of this form of treatment

comorbidity: a condition that exists along with and usually independently of another medical condition

complete response (CR): total disappearance of all evidence of disease using physical examination, laboratory studies and radiologic imaging; a criterion for evaluating the efficacy of a particular anti-cancer therapy; also see partial response

complexed PSA: PSA molecules which are bound to a protease inhibitor such as a1-antichymotrypsin

complication: an unexpected or unwanted effect of a treatment, pharmaceutical or other procedure

concordance: the agreement in findings that support the accuracy of a particular investigation or treatment; concordance is a critical concept in studies to diagnose, stage and treat PC

conformal therapy: the use of careful planning and delivery techniques designed to focus external radiation on the areas of the prostate and surrounding tissue which need treatment and protect areas which do not need treatment; three—dimensional conformal radiation therapy (*3DCRT*) is a sophisticated form of this method

conformality: see "Conformal Therapy"; pertaining to the ability to achieve conformal therapy.

contracture: scarring which can occur at the bladder neck after a radical prostatectomy and which results in narrowing of the urethra coming from the bladder; same as stricture

contraindication: any condition which renders some particular line of treatment improper or undesirable

control group: participants in a clinical trial who are receiving placebo or current standard of care for comparison to those receiving the new therapy being evaluated

COQ10 (coenzyme Q10): important in cardiac function; a substance that energizes the *mitochondria* within the heart cells and allows them to function better; an anti-oxidant that protects LDL cholesterol from oxidation

core: a tissue sample removed during biopsy

coronal: an imaging plane bisecting the body into top and bottom parts perpendicular (rotated 90°) to the long axis of the human body

corpora cavernosa: two cavities in the upper portion of a man's penis that fill with blood when he is sexually excited, giving the organ the stiffness required for intercourse

corpus spongiosum: a spongy chamber in the lower portion of a man's penis that surrounds the urethra and fills with blood when he is sexually excited, providing additional stiffness required for intercourse

cortex: the outer layer of an organ, usually surrounding an inner section; the cortex of the prostate gland is also called a capsule

crtisol: a hormone from the outer layer of the adrenal glands

Cowper's glands: A pair of pea-sized glands that lie beneath the prostate gland, named after the English surgeon William Cowper (1660-1709). Cowper's glands secrete an alkaline fluid that forms part of the semen. This fluid neutralizes the acidic environment of the urethra, thereby protecting the sperm

creatine: a compound which is made by the body and is used to store energy in the form of phosphate molecules

creatine kinase: any of three enzymes found especially in skeletal and heart muscle and the brain that accelerate the transfer of a high-energy phosphate group and typically occur in elevated levels in the blood following injury to brain or muscle tissue

creatinine: a chemical substance resulting from the metabolism of creatine, that is found in muscle tissue and blood; creatinine is normally excreted in the urine as a metabolic waste; when elevated in the blood it indicates impairment of kidney function

Chronic Disease Management (CDM): an active surveillance Protocol utilized that includes diet, nutrition, exercise, stress reduction and education as patients learn to live with prostate cancer; See study: 'Is it necessary to cure prostate cancer when it is possible', Google: Journal, Clinical Interventions in Aging, Dove Press, Volume 2, Number 1, 2007

cryoablation: see cryosurgery; tissue destruction as the result of freezing typically by Argon gas

cryoprobe: a surgical instrument used to apply extreme cold to tissues during cryosurgery

cryosurgery: the use of liquid nitrogen probes to freeze a particular organ to extremely low temperatures to kill the tissue, including any cancerous tissue; When used to treat prostate cancer, the cryoprobes are guided by transrectal ultrasound (TRUS).

cryotherapy: see cryosurgery

CT scan: computerized or computed tomography; See CAT Scan

curcumin: a biologically active substance derived from the curcuma longa plant; found within the Indian spice called turmeric; curcumin and its curcuminoid *polyphenols* have anti-prostate cancer activity against both AIPC and ADPC

cyproterone: an antiandrogen with progestational activity; see progesterone.

cystitis: inflammation of the bladder that may be caused by infection or chemical injury or radiation; characterized by increased urinary frequency, discomfort on urination and often red blood cells, white blood cells and/or bacteria in the urine

cystoscope: an instrument used by physicians to look inside the urethra and the bladder

cystoscopy: the use of a cystoscope to look inside the urethra and the bladder

cystosol: the soluble components of the fluid matter enclosed within the cellular membrane

Cytadren®: the trademarked name for aminogluthethimide

cytochrome C: a protein that carries electrons released from the mitochondria to initiate cell death

cytochrome P-450 dependent 14-demethylation: an enzyme system that is important in the <u>endocrine</u> pathways of hormone production and activation

cytokines: any of several regulatory proteins, such as the *interleukins* and lymphokines, that are released by cells of the immune system and act as intercellular mediators in the generation of an immune response

cytology: science that deals with the structure and function of cells

cytoplasm: the material of a cell between the cell membrane and the nucleus

cytoskeleton adj. **cytoskeletal**: the internal scaffolding of cells which determines cell shape, and organizes structures within cells

cytotoxin, cytotoxic: chemicals that have direct <u>toxicity</u> to cancer cells, preventing their reproduction or growth. Cytotoxic agents can, as a side effect, damage healthy, non—cancerous tissues or organs which have a high proportion of actively dividing cells, for example, bone marrow and hair follicles

Cytoxan®: a genotoxic drug, a <u>chemotherapy</u> agent that affects <u>DNA</u> and alters its function

D

D1 or D2 disease: <u>metastatic</u> disease; see <u>Staging</u>; see also <u>Whitmore-Jewett Staging</u>

de novo: in a new form or manner

debility: the state of being weak or feeble; infirmity

debulking: reduction of the volume of cancer by one of several techniques; most frequently used to imply surgical removal

definitive local treatment: generally that treatment which includes generally accepted procedures necessary to ultimately produce recovery of the patient. For prostate cancer this is usually considered to include <u>radical</u> <u>prostatectomy, radiation therapy,</u> and <u>cryosurgery.</u>

dendritic cells (DC): cells that process <u>antigens</u> (proteins) and present them to immune lymphocytes called <u>T cells</u> playing a major role in the initiation of the immune response against tumor and other types of abnormal cells; antigen presenting cells; e.g. Provenge® is an investigational therapy employing DC

Denonvillier's fascia: thin layer of connective tissue that separates <u>prostate</u> and <u>seminal vesicles</u> from <u>rectum</u>

DES: see <u>diethylstilbestrol or estradiol</u>

DEXA (dual energy X-RAY absorptiometry): a type of bone mineral density radiologic examination using x-ray absorption; see also <u>qCT</u>

dexamethasone (DXM): a synthetic <u>glucocorticoid</u> used primarily in the treatment of inflammatory disorders. It can have both an <u>antiemetic</u> and an anti-prostate cancer effect.

dextrans: a group of glucose polymers made by certain bacteria

DHEA (dehydroepiandrosterone): an <u>adrenal androgen</u> precursor produced in the adrenal cortex and transformed into <u>testosterone</u> within prostate cells

DHEA-S: the sulfated form of <u>DHEA</u>; sulfation is a chemical process that alters the molecule by adding a sulfur-type group; sulfation occurs in the liver; DHEA-S is a more reliable laboratory test than DHEA

DHT: see <u>dihydrotestosterone</u>

diabetes: a condition in which the body either cannot produce insulin or cannot effectively use the insulin it produces

diabetes mellitus: a severe, chronic form of diabetes caused by insufficient production of insulin and resulting in abnormal metabolism of carbohydrates, fats, and proteins.

diagnosis (Dx): the evaluation of signs, symptoms and selected test results by a physician to determine the physical and biological causes of the signs and symptoms and whether a specific disease or disorder is involved

Diagnostic Center for Disease™ (DCD): A comprehensive prostate cancer diagnostic and treatment center in Sarasota, Florida specializing in non-invasive diagnostics (MRI/MRIS) without biopsy as an integral part of the diagnostic evaluation of prostate cancer. Center also specializes in High Intensity Focused Ultrasound (as a world leader) utilizing all technologies available in non-invasive prostate cancer treatment.

diethylstilbestrol (DES): also called stilbestrol—a synthetic hormone with estrogenic properties; a treatment of prostate cancer with activity against AIPC as well as ADPC

differentiation: the use of the differences between prostate cancer cells when seen under the microscope as a method to grade the severity of the disease; well differentiated cells are easily recognized as normal cells, while poorly differentiated cells are abnormal, cancerous and difficult to recognize as belonging to any particular type of cell group

digital rectal examination (DRE): the use by a medical provider of a lubricated and gloved finger inserted into the rectum to feel for abnormalities of the prostate and rectum **dihydrotestosterone (DHT or 5 alpha—dihydrotestosterone)**: a male hormone more potent than testosterone that is converted from testosterone within the prostate by 5 alpha reductase

dimethyl sulfoxide (DMSO): a colorless solvent, used to penetrate and convey medications into the tissues

diploid: having one complete set of normally paired chromosomes, i.e., a normal amount of DNA; diploid cancer cells tend to grow slowly and respond well to hormone therapy; a diploid number of chromosomes would equal 46, a haploid set would equal 23; see also haploid

dissection: the cutting a part of an organism to examine its structure

distal: away from a point of reference, compare to proximal

distensibility: The ability to enlarge or distend

diurnal: pertaining to the day; having a cyclic nature involving the 24-hour day; prolactin levels are at their peak in the early morning—they have a diurnal variation; calcium utilization appears highest in the evening close to bedtime

DMSO: dimethyl sulfoxide

DNA (deoxyribonucleic acid): the basic biologically active chemical that defines the physical development and growth of nearly all living organisms; a complex protein that is the carrier of genetic information

docetaxel (Taxotere®): one of a type of chemotherapy agents called taxanes that block microtubule formation during cell division

Doppler: a method in ultrasound imaging to monitor a moving structure or fluid (esp. blood)

dose volume histogram (DVH): A graph that displays the distribution of the absorbed radiation dose in tissue resulting from the delivery of a particular treatment plan.

dosimetry: Relating to the doses of radiation employed in treating a tumor

double-blind: a form of clinical trial in which neither the physician nor the patient knows the actual treatment which any individual patient is receiving; double-blind trials are a way of minimizing the effects of the personal opinions of patients and physicians on the results of the trial

doubling time: the time that it takes a value (like PSA) to double

down-regulation: the process of reducing or suppressing a response to a stimulus; specifically reduction in a cellular response to a molecule (as insulin) due to a decrease in the number of receptors on the cell surface

downsizing: the use of hormonal or other forms of management to reduce the volume of prostate cancer in and/or around the prostate prior to attempted curative treatment

downstaging: the use of hormonal or other forms of management in the attempt to lower the <u>clinical stage</u> of prostate cancer prior to attempted curative treatment (e.g., from stage T3a to stage T2b); this technique is highly controversial

doxorubicin (trade name Adriamycin®): an anticancer drug that belongs to the family of drugs called anti-<u>tumor</u> <u>antibiotics</u>. It is an <u>anthracycline</u>.

Dpd: deoxypyridinoline (Pyrilinks-D®); a bone <u>resorption</u> marker reflecting breakdown of bone collagen

DRE: see <u>digital rectal examination</u> **dry orgasm**: ejaculation without the release of <u>semen</u>

ductal: a tubular bodily canal or passage, especially one for carrying a glandular secretion: *a tear duct.*

dutasteride (trade name Avodart®): an inhibitor of the <u>enzyme</u> (<u>5 alpha-reductase or 5AR</u>) that stimulates the conversion of <u>testosterone</u> to <u>DHT</u>; used to treat <u>BPH</u>

Dx: standard abbreviation for diagnosis

dysfunction: abnormal or impaired functioning, especially of a bodily system or organ

dysplasia: abnormal development or growth of tissues, organs, or cells; see also <u>PIN</u>

dysuria: painful urination

E

EBRT (external beam radiation therapy): external beam radiation treatment that can include conventional <u>photons</u>, or use protons, neutrons, or electrons. This may be given conventionally or with 3D conformal techniques; see also <u>IMRT</u>.

ECE: an abbreviation for <u>extra-capsular extension</u>

ECOG: Eastern Cooperative Oncology Group; one of the clinical trials groups

ECOG Performance Status: criteria used by doctors and researchers to assess how a patient's disease is progressing, assess how the disease affects the daily living abilities of the patient, and determine appropriate treatment and prognosis. See also: Karnofsky Performance Status

ED: erectile dysfunction

edema: swelling or accumulation of fluid in some part of the body

efferent: moving or carrying outward or away from a central part. Refers to vessels, nerves, etc. For example: blood vessels carrying blood away from the heart or nerves carrying signals from the brain

efficacy: the greatest ability of a drug of treatment to produce a result, regardless of dosage

EGCG (epigallocatechin gallate): the active ingredient of green tea that relates to the potency of the green tea product

EGF: epidermal growth factor; a polypeptide hormone that stimulates cell proliferation by binding to receptor proteins on the cell surface

eicosanoid: any of a class of compounds derived from polyunsaturated fatty acids (as arachidonic acid) and involved in cellular activity

ejaculation: the release of semen through the penis during orgasm; ejaculation may be termed "dry" if there is scanty or no fluid component to the ejaculate resulting from radiation therapy or surgery.

ejaculatory ducts: The tubular passages through which semen reaches the prostatic urethra during orgasm

EKG: electrocardiogram; a study showing the electrical activity of the heart

ELISA: enzyme-linked immunosorbent assay; a sensitive immunoassay that uses an enzyme linked to an antibody or antigen as a marker for the detection of a specific protein, especially an antigen or antibody; often used as a diagnostic test to determine exposure to a particular infectious agent, such as the AIDS virus, by identifying antibodies present in a blood sample; see immunoassay

embolus, embolic: a mass, such as an air bubble, a detached blood clot, or a foreign body, that travels through the bloodstream and lodges so as to obstruct or occlude a blood vessel.

EMCYT: see estramustine phosphate

endocrine: pertaining to ductless glands that secrete hormones into the blood stream

endocrinology: the study of hormones, their function, the organs that produce them and how they are produced

endogenous: inherent naturally to the organism; originating or produced within an organism, tissue, or cell, e.g. *endogenous secretions.*

endorectal: (inserted) within the rectum

endorectal coil: a device that is inserted into a patient's rectum beneath the prostate and is used to acquire spectroscopy for prostate MRI/MRSI exams

endorectal MRI: magnetic resonance imaging performed with a coil placed in the rectum, may be combined with endorectal magnetic resonance spectroscopy (developed at University of California at San Francisco and Memorial Sloan Kettering in New York City)

epididymis: tightly coiled, thin-walled tube that conducts sperm from the testes to the *vas deferens* and provides for the storage, transmission, and maturation of sperm; inflammation of the epididymis is called epididymitis

epidural: outside the outer membrane surrounding the brain or spinal column

epinephrine: a hormone and neurotransmitter (Also called adrenaline); one of the secretions of the adrenal glands. It helps the liver release glucose (sugar) and limit the release of insulin; it also makes the heart beat faster and can raise blood pressure

epithelial cell: in PC the cells within the prostate that line the ducts and functionally secrete chemicals such as PSA into the blood stream or into the duct openings or lumen

epithelium, epithelial: the covering of internal and external surfaces of the body, including the lining of vessels and other small cavities. It consists of cells joined by small amounts of cementing substances. Epithelium is classified into types on the basis of the number of layers deep and the shape of the <u>superficial</u> cells.

epothilones: a new class of natural and potent agents that stabilize <u>microtubules</u> to inhibit the growth and spread of <u>malignant</u> cells

ER (estrogen receptor): the docking site on the cell or in the cell for <u>estrogen</u>

erectile dysfunction (ED): an inability to get or maintain an erection; see impotence.

erythropoietin: a <u>glycoprotein</u> hormone that stimulates the production of red blood cells by stem cells in <u>bone marrow</u>

endoscope: an instrument for examining visually the interior of a bodily canal or hollow organ such as the colon, bladder, or stomach

endothelin-1 (ET-1): a prostate cell product that stimulates <u>osteoblasts</u>, acts as a vasoconstrictor (narrows blood vessels) and may be responsible for bone pain in <u>metastatic</u> prostate cancer; blockers of the receptor for ET-1 are in clinical trials and showing promise e.g. Atrasentan®

endotoxin: a toxin produced by certain bacteria and released upon destruction of the bacterial cell

enzyme: any of a group of chemical substances which are produced by living cells and which cause particular chemical reactions to happen while not being changed themselves

EOD (extent of disease): part of what should be a standard approach to staging the bone scan; after work by Soloway

EPA (eicosapentenoic acid): a fish oil supplement, an omega 3 fatty acid that inhibits the delta 5 desaturase enzyme that converts DGLA (dihomo-gamma-linolenic acid) to arachidonic acid

epidemiology: the branch of medicine that deals with the study of the causes, distribution, and control of disease in populations

ester: any of a class of organic compounds corresponding to the inorganic salts and formed from an organic acid and an alcohol, usually with the elimination of water

estradiol: the most potent naturally occurring estrogen. In men it is naturally produced in small amounts.

estramustine: A nitrogen mustard linked to estradiol, usually as phosphate (see EMCYT); used to treat prostatic neoplasms; also has radiation protective properties.

estramustine phosphate sodium (EMCYT): a chemotherapeutic agent; a hybrid drug combination of nitrogen mustard and estrogen that disrupts cytoplasmic microtubules

estrogen: a female hormone or estrogen (e.g., diethylstilbestrol) used in the treatment of PC

estrogen receptor (ER): the docking site on the cell or in the cell for estrogen

etidronate: a white disodium bisphosphonate salt $C_2H_6Na_2O_7P_2$ used to treat osteoporosis called also *etidronate disodium*

etiology: the study of all of the factors involved in the development of a disease

etoposide: a genotoxic drug, a chemotherapy agent that affects DNA and alters its function

eukaryotic: a single-celled or multicellular organism whose cells contain a distinct membrane-bound nucleus

Eulexin®: the brand or trade name of flutamide in the USA

exogenous: developed or originating outside the organism, as exogenous disease

experimental: an unproven (or even untested) technique or procedure; note that certain experimental treatments are commonly used in the management of prostate cancer

expression: the process by which a gene's coded information is converted into the structures present and operating in the cell. Expressed genes include those that are transcribed into mRNA and then translated into protein and those that are transcribed into RNA but not translated into protein.

external beam radiation therapy (EBRT): a form of radiation therapy in which the radiation is delivered by a machine directed at the area to be radiated as opposed to radiation given within the target tissue such as brachytherapy, see also IMRT

extra-capsular extension (ECE): cancer extending beyond the prostate capsule

extracellular: outside a cell or cells **extraprostatic**: located outside the prostate *ex vivo*: outside the living organism

F

false negative: an erroneous negative test result; for example, an imaging test that fails to show the presence of a cancer tumor later found by biopsy to be present in the patient is said to have returned a false negative result

false positive: a positive test result mistakenly identifying a state or condition that does not in fact exist

fast echo spin (FSE): in MRI, echo sequence is characterized by a series of rapidly applied 180° rephasing pulses and multiple echoes

FDA: United States Food and Drug Administration

ferritin: an iron-containing protein complex, found principally in the intestinal mucosa, spleen and liver that functions as the primary form of iron storage in the body

Feulgen stain: a histology stain used in microscopy to identify chromosomal material or DNA

FGF: fibroblast growth factor (contributes to blood vessel development

fibril: a small thread-like structure that is often part of a cell

fibroblast, fibroblastic: a connective-tissue cell that secretes proteins and especially molecular collagen from which the extracellular matrix of connective tissue forms

fiducial: used as a fixed standard of reference for comparison or measurement

finasteride (Proscar®): an inhibitor of the enzyme (5 alpha—reductase or 5AR) that stimulates the conversion of testosterone to DHT; used to treat BPH

fistula: an abnormal passage between two organs

flare reaction: the transient increase in serum testosterone for the first few weeks after starting an LHRH agonist. This increase in testosterone can potentially worsen the signs and symptoms of disease, especially in those patients with vertebral metastases and/or urinary obstruction; may be prevented by taking an antiandrogen (Casodex® or Eulexin®) several days before starting an LHRH agonist or by the use of an LHRH antagonist such as abarelix (Plenaxis®). See our paper Clinical Flare: A Crisis That Can Be Avoided.

flow cytometry: a measurement method that determines the fraction of cells that are diploid, tetraploid, aneuploid, etc

fluence: Particles per unit time; similar to current only the particles are photons

fluoroscope: a device consisting of a fluorescent screen, used in conjunction with an X-ray tube, that shows the images of objects between the tube and the screen

fluorouracil: an antineoplastic chemotherapy agent that inhibits certain DNA building blocks, used especially in the treatment of cancers of the skin, breast, and digestive system

flutamide (Eulexin®): an antiandrogen used in the palliative hormonal treatment of advanced prostate cancer and in the

<u>adjuvant</u> and <u>neoadjuvant</u> hormonal treatment of earlier stages of prostate cancer; normal dosage is 2 capsules three times a day

focal therapy: a more localized treatment directed at the cancerous foci within the gland, rather than removing or destroying the entire prostate

focus: pl. foci: Group of (frequently <u>neoplastic</u>) cells, identifiable by distinctive distribution or structure.

Foley: a transurethral (Foley) catheter

follicle stimulating hormone (FSH): in the male, stimulates the Sertoli cells of the <u>testicle</u> to make sperm

fossa: a cavity, or depression; as the location from which the prostate was removed

fraction: The portion of a fractionated <u>radiation treatment</u> that is delivered in a single session

free PSA: <u>PSA</u> molecules in the blood stream that are not "bound" to other proteins

free PSA %: reports the percentage of free-PSA and usually expressed as a percentage based on free PSA divided by total <u>PSA</u> x 100; one study showed that men with free PSA % > 25% had low risk of PC while those with < 10% free PSA % were more likely to have PC.

free radical: An atom or group of atoms that has at least one unpaired electron and is therefore unstable and highly reactive. In animal tissues, free radicals can damage cells and are believed to accelerate the progression of cancer, cardiovascular disease, and age-related diseases

frequency: (as relates to the prostate) the need to urinate often

frozen section: a technique in which removed tissue is frozen, cut into thin slices, and stained for microscopic examination; a <u>pathologist</u> can rapidly complete a frozen section analysis, and for this reason, it is commonly used during surgery to quickly provide the surgeon with vital information such as a preliminary pathologic opinion of the presence or absence of prostate cancer (usually in the <u>pelvic</u> lymph nodes)

FSH: See <u>follicle stimulating hormone</u>

fusion: combining two or more inputs of data so that they can be overlaid one upon another to provide a sense of agreement or <u>concordance</u>; fusion imaging studies such as ProstaScint-CT-PET are examples

G

G-CSF: <u>granulocyte</u> colony-stimulating factor

G0G1 growth phase: with G0 being the relatively dormant phase of the cell growth cycle and G1 the phase just preceding <u>DNA</u> synthesis or S-phase

G1 arrest: arrest or halting the cell cycle at the stage of G1; the normal sequence is G1-S-G2-M

gantry: <u>Radiation therapy</u> hardware from which the linear accelerator delivers its energy; the multileaf collimator <u>MLC</u> is attached to the gantry and modulates the radiation beam as it exits

gastrin: <u>hormone</u> released after eating, which causes the stomach to produce more acid

gastrointestinal (GI): related to the digestive system and/or the intestines

gefitinib (Iressa®): a drug that blocks cancer cell growth signals caused by an <u>enzyme</u> called <u>tyrosine kinase</u>. Iressa® blocks several of these tyrosine kinases, including one associated with <u>Epidermal Growth Factor Receptor</u> (EGF)

gene, adj. **genetic**: the unit of <u>DNA</u> that carries physical characteristics from parent to child

genital system: the biological system that, in males, includes the <u>testicles</u>, the *vas deferens*, the prostate and the <u>penis</u>

genitourinary system (GU system): In the male, pertaining to the organs comprising the genital and urinary system. This includes the <u>testicles, penis, seminal vesicles, urethra, bladder, ureters</u> and <u>kidneys</u>

genome: the total genetic content contained in a <u>haploid</u> set of <u>chromosomes</u> in single or multi-celled organisms, in a single chromosome in bacteria, or in the <u>DNA</u> or <u>RNA</u> of viruses; an organism's genetic material

genomic instability: the instability of genetic material as a result of destructive chemical processes that lead to mutation

GH (growth hormone): a <u>pituitary</u> <u>hormone</u> shown to stimulate <u>amino</u> acid uptake into tissues, promote <u>DNA</u> and <u>RNA</u> and protein synthesis, have a role in cell division and <u>hypertrophy</u> and increase bone growth and lean body mass

gland: a structure or organ that produces a substance which is used in another part of the body

gland volume (GV): the size in cubic centimeters or grams of the prostate gland

glans penis: cap-shaped expansion at the end of the <u>penis,</u> having the <u>urethral</u> opening at the center.

Gleason: name of physician who developed the Gleason grading system commonly used to grade prostate cancer

Gleason grade: a widely used method for classifying prostate cancer tissue for the degree of loss of the normal glandular architecture (size, shape and <u>differentiation</u> of glands); a grade from 1–5 is assigned successively to each the two most predominant tissue patterns present in the examined tissue sample and are added together to produce the <u>Gleason score;</u> high numbers indicate poor differentiation and therefore more aggressive cancer.

Gleason score: two <u>Gleason Grade</u> numbers are added together to produce the Gleason Score. The first Gleason Grade number indicates the Gleason Grade of the cancer cells found most commonly within the sample, the second number the second most commonly found grade. For example, a Gleason Score of 4+3=7 means that Gleason Grade 4 is the most commonly found type of cell, Gleason Grade 3 the second most commonly found, producing a total Gleason Score of 7.

glia: supportive tissue of the brain. There are three types of glial tissue: astrocytes, oligodendrocytes and microglia. Glial cells do not conduct electrical impulses, as do neurons.

glucocorticoid: any of a group of anti-inflammatory steroid like compounds, such as hydrocortisone, that are produced by the adrenal cortex, are involved in carbohydrate, protein, and fat metabolism, and are used as anti-inflammatory agents

glucose: an optically active sugar; the usual form in which carbohydrate is assimilated by animals

glutathione: a compound of the amino acids glycine, cystine, and glutamic acid occurring widely in plant and animal tissues and forming reduced and oxidized forms important in biological oxidation-reduction reactions

glutathione S-transferase: a protein which plays an important role in inactivating chemicals that are able to cause gene damage and promote genetic instability. A recent study has shown that this protein is deactivated very early in the development of prostate cancer.

glycemia, glycemic: the concentration of glucose in the blood. It is usually expressed in milligrams per deciliter (mg/dl).

glycolysis: a set of ten chemical reactions that is the first stage in the metabolism of glucose

glycoprotein: any of a group of conjugated proteins that contain a carbohydrate as the nonprotein component

GM-CSF: granulocyte-macrophage colony-stimulating factor

GNRH: gonadotropin-releasing hormone, see LHRH

goserelin acetate (Zoladex®): a luteinizing hormone releasing hormone (LHRH) analog used in the hormonal treatment of advanced prostate cancer and in the adjuvant and neoadjuvant hormonal treatment of earlier stages of prostate cancer

GP: general practice physician

grade: a means of describing the potential degree of severity of a cancer; see Gleason Grade

granulocyte: any of a group of white blood cells having granules in the cytoplasm

gray (Gy): The SI (Systeme International) unit of absorbed radiation dose:

1 Gy = 1 joule/kg = 100 rads

1/100 Gy = 1 **centigray (cGy)**

GTP: green tea polyphenols, the active substances within green tea

gynecomastia: enlargement or tenderness of the male breasts or nipples; a possible side effect of hormonal therapy which leads to increased levels of estrogens as seen with DES, antiandrogen monotherapy (Flutamide® or Casodex®) or the combination of the latter with Proscar®

H

H-2 blockers: blockers of histamine, a substance responsible for gastric acidity among other functions

half-life: the time it takes for half of the nuclei of a radioactive substance to decay or the amount of time required to reduce a drug level to one half of the initial value

haploid: having the same number of sets of chromosomes as a germ cell (sperm or egg) or half as many as a somatic cell (all remaining cells having to do with the body); having a single set of chromosomes; see diploid

HC: hydrocortisone

HDK: high dose ketoconazole; Nizoral®

HDL cholesterol: high density lipoprotein cholesterol; a beneficial cholesterol composed of a high proportion of protein (with little triglyceride and cholesterol) and that is associated with decreased probability of developing atherosclerosis

HDR (high dose radiation): radiation delivered by temporary insertion of radioactive Iridium wire into flexible needles placed in the prostate through the perineum.

hematocrit (HCT): a measure of the number of red cells found in the blood, stated as a percentage of the total blood volume

hematology: a medical science that deals with the blood and blood-forming organs

hematopoietic: pertaining to tissues such as the bone marrow, spleen and lymph nodes where blood cell formation and destruction occur

hematospermia: the occurrence of blood in the semen **hematuria**: the occurrence of blood in the urine **hemiprostate**: the left or right side of the prostate

hemoglobin (HGB): a complex protein-iron compound in the blood that carries oxygen from the lungs to the cells and carries carbon dioxide back to the lungs. Each red blood cell contains several hundred molecules of hemoglobin.

hemorrhage: to undergo heavy or uncontrollable bleeding **hemostatic**: an agent that shortens the clotting time of blood **Herceptin®**: the trade name for trastuzumab

hereditary: inherited from one's parents and earlier generations

heredity: the historical distribution of biological characteristics through a group of related individuals via their DNA

heterogeneous (heterogeneity): non-uniform; composed of mixtures of different kinds; in reference to tumors meaning composed of different clones of cells

high dose ketoconazole (HDK): see Nizoral®; An Antiandrogen commonly used as an alternative to Bicalutamide or Flutamide; used with Hydrocortisone

high-intensity focused ultrasound (HIFU): a procedure which utilizes transrectal ultrasound that is highly focused into a small area, creating intense heat which is lethal to prostate cancer tissue. See HIFU Chapter 14 by Rewcastle utilizing Ablatherm and Sonablate 500 treatment technologies

hilum: a shallow depression in one side of a lymph node through which blood vessels pass and efferent lymphatic vessels emerge

histology: the study of the appearance and behavior of tissue, usually carried out under a microscope by a <u>pathologist</u> (who is a physician) or a histologist (who is not necessarily a physician)

histomorphometry: the quantitative measurement and characterization of the microscopic organization and structure of a tissue especially by computer-assisted analysis of images

histone: any of various simple water-soluble <u>proteins</u> that are rich in the basic <u>amino</u> acids lysine and arginine and are complexed with DNA in the <u>nucleosomes</u> of <u>eukaryotic</u> <u>chromatin</u>

histopathologic: tissue changes that affect a part or accompany a disease

HMO: health maintenance organization; an insurance plan in which you choose a primary care physician who must approve referrals to other providers

HMW-uPA: high molecular weight <u>uPA</u>

homeopathy: a system of healing that normally involves remedies being administered in reduced doses.

homeostasis: the ability or tendency of an organism or cell to maintain internal equilibrium by adjusting its physiological processes

homogeneous (homogeneity): uniform; composed of the same element; in reference to a tumor cell population meaning that the cells are of the same clone in contrast to a mixed cell population that would exhibit heterogeneity or be <u>heterogeneous</u>

homologous: corresponding, as in relative position or structure; a homologous <u>tumor</u> is made up of cells resembling those of the tissue in which it is growing

hormone: biologically active chemicals that are responsible for the development of secondary sexual characteristics and other biologic activities

hormone ablation therapy: see **hormone therapy**. **hormone blockade therapy**: see **hormone therapy**. **hormone-naïve**: not having received prior hormone therapy **hormone refractory PC (HRPC) (see <u>AIPC</u>)**: a loosely used term that really should apply to progressive PC in the setting of a <u>testosterone</u> level less than 20 ng/dl and when an <u>ARM</u> has been excluded; the preferred term is AIPC or androgen independent PC.

hormone therapy (HT): the use of <u>hormones</u>, hormone analogs, and certain surgical techniques to treat disease (in this case prostate cancer) either on their own or in combination with other hormones or in combination with other methods of treatment; because prostate cancer is usually dependent on male hormones (ex: <u>testosterone</u>) to grow, hormone blockade or deprivation (also called <u>androgen deprivation therapy</u>) can be an effective means of alleviating symptoms and retarding the development of the disease

hot flash: the sudden sensation of warmth in the face, neck and upper body; a side effect of many forms of <u>hormone</u> <u>therapy</u>

HRPC: see <u>hormone refractory prostate cancer</u>.

HSD (hydroxysteroid dehydrogenase): the <u>enzyme</u> that oxidizes or reduces <u>testosterone</u> to <u>androstenedione</u> or vice versa

hybridization protection assay (HPA): a process that hybridizes the <u>amplicon</u> to singlestranded <u>nucleic acid</u> probes that are labeled with an Acridinium Ester (AE) molecule and then it selects and detects the hybridized probes.

hydrocortisone (HC): a steroid compound synthesized in the <u>adrenal cortex</u> and vital to survival

hydrolyze: undergo hydrolysis; decompose by reacting with water

hydronephrosis: abnormal enlargement of a <u>kidney</u>, may occur secondary to acute <u>ureteral</u> obstruction or chronic kidney disease.

hydroxyapatite: a crystal structure that is a building block for bone; principal bone salt, $Ca_5(PO_4)_3OH$, which provides the compressional strength of vertebrate bone

hydroxyflutamide: the active <u>metabolite</u> of <u>flutamide</u>

hypercalcemia: abnormally high concentrations of calcium in the blood, indicating leeching of calcium from bone (tumors raise serum calcium levels by destroying bone or by releasing PTH or a PTH-like substance, <u>osteoclast</u>-activating factor, <u>prostaglandins</u>, and perhaps, a vitamin D-like sterol). Symptoms of hypercalcemia may include: feeling tired, difficulty thinking clearly, lack of appetite, abdominal pain, frequent urination, increased thirst, constipation, nausea, and vomiting.

hyperechoic: denoting a region in an ultrasound image in which the echoes are stronger than normal or than surrounding structures noting bright areas; the opposite of <u>hypoechoic</u>

hyperintensity: a term used to describe light areas of a scan image due to an increased enhancement of that region

hyperlipidemia, hyperlipemia: an excess of fats (or lipids) in the blood

hyperplasia: enlargement of an organ or tissue because of an increase in the number of cells in that organ or tissue; see also <u>BPH</u>

hypersensitive PSA (ultrasensitive PSA): a laboratory assay for PSA that is more sensitive to detection of low levels of PSA than a standard assay; these assays allow for earlier detection of <u>recurrence</u> and can distinguish an excellent response to <u>ADT</u> from a mediocre response; DPC Immulite® 3rd generation and Tosoh are two examples of hypersensitive PSA assays available

hypertension: arterial disease in which chronic high blood pressure is the primary symptom

hyperthermia: treatment that uses heat; for example heat produced by microwave radiation

hypertrophy: the enlargement or overgrowth of an organ or part due to an increase in size of its constituent cells; compare to <u>hyperplasia</u>; see <u>benign prostatic hyperplasia</u> (BPH)

hypocalcemia: low blood calcium; symptoms may include irritability, muscle spasms or contractions of hands, feet or legs

hypoechoic: A region in an ultrasound image in which the echoes are weaker or fewer than normal or in the surrounding regions showing a darker area; the opposite of <u>hyperechoic</u>

hypofractionated: a radiation treatment that is divided into fewer individual sessions (but correspondingly higher doses of radiation) than usual

hypoglycemia: less than normal level of sugar in the blood

hypointensity: a term used to describe dark areas of a scan image due to a decreased enhancement of that region

hypotension: arterial disease in which chronic low blood pressure is the primary symptom

hypothalamus, (adj.) **hypothalamic**: a portion of the brain which secretes substances that control metabolism by exerting an influence on pituitary gland function.

hypoxia, hypoxic: a deficiency of oxygen reaching the tissues of the body

I

IAD (intermittent androgen deprivation): ADT that discontinues testosterone lowering therapy with the intent to allow the patient to recover from symptoms of ADS as testosterone levels recover to normal; same as IHT or IAS.

IAS: intermittent androgen suppression; same as IAD, IHT

ICTP: carboxy-terminal telopeptide of type 1 collagen (a bone resorption marker like Dpd)

IGF-1: Insulin growth factor 1

IGFBP: Insulin growth factor binding protein; e.g. IGFBP3

IHT: intermittent hormone therapy; see IAD

IL-1(interleukin-1): a cell product involved in the immune response (cytokine) which facilitates osteoblast growth among its many functions; see issue 2 of Insights for a more detailed description with illustrations

IL-1R: Interleukin 1 receptor

IL-6 (interleukin-6): a cytokine that stimulates osteoclast precursors and mature osteoclasts among its many functions; see issue 2 of Insights for a more detailed description with illustrations

imaging: a radiology technique or method allowing a physician to see a graphic representation of something that would not normally be visible

immortalization: the ability of a genetically engineered cell line to reproduce indefinitely

Immulite®: laboratory console manufactured by Diagnostics Products Company (DPC) that evaluates biomarkers such as ultrasensitive PSA

immune reaction: a bodily defense reaction that recognizes an invading substance (an antigen: such as a virus or fungus or bacteria or transplanted organ) and produces antibodies specific against that antigen

immune system: the biological system which protects a person or animal from the effects of foreign materials such as bacteria, viruses, cancer cells, and other things which might make that person or animal sick

immunoassay: a laboratory technique that makes use of the binding between an antigen and its homologous antibody in order to identify and quantify the specific antigen or antibody in a sample

immunoblot: a blot in which a radiolabeled antibody is used as the molecular probe

immunogenic: capable of inducing a strong immune response

immunohistochemistry: of or relating to the application of tissue chemistry and immune reaction methods to analysis of living cells and tissues

immunoperoxidase: stains which are used in the microscopic examination of tissues. These stains are based on antibodies which will bind to specific antigens, usually of protein or glycoprotein origin

immunopositive: a positive result is observed on immunostaining for the target substance

immunoreaction, immunoreactivity: See immune reaction.

immunostaining: the staining of a specific substance by using an antibody against it which is complexed (formed into a complex) with a staining medium

immunotherapy: treatment of disease by inducing, enhancing, or suppressing an immune system response.

implant: a device that is inserted into the body; e.g., a tiny container of radioactive material inserted in or near a tumor (see brachytherapy); also a device inserted in order to replace or substitute for an ability which has been lost; for example, a penile implant is a device which can be surgically inserted into the penis to provide rigidity for intercourse

impotence: the inability to have or to maintain an erection satisfactory for intercourse; also known as ED or *erectile dysfunction*

IMRT (intensity modulated radiation therapy): an approach to radiation therapy allowing the treatment team to specify the tumor target dose and the amount of radiation allowable to the nearby tissues and uses sophisticated computer planning to arrive at acceptable equations; sophisticated hardware is also incorporated into this planning that allows the radiation intensity to be modulated up or down as the delivery system rotates around the patient

incidental: insignificant or irrelevant; for example, incidental prostate cancer (also known as latent prostate cancer) is a form of prostate cancer which is of no clinical significance to the patient in whom it is discovered

incontinence: (urinary incontinence) loss of urinary control; there are various kinds and degrees of incontinence; overflow incontinence is a condition in which the bladder retains urine after voiding; as a consequence, the bladder remains full most of the time, resulting in involuntary seepage of urine from the bladder; stress incontinence is the involuntary discharge of urine when there is increased pressure upon the bladder, as in coughing or straining to lift heavy objects; total incontinence is the inability to voluntarily exercise control over the sphincters of the bladder neck and urethra, resulting in total loss of retentive ability

indication: a reason for doing something or taking some action; also used to mean the approved clinical application of a pharmaceutical

indolent: minimal disease, defined as < 0.5 cc of cancer confined to the prostate with no Gleason grade 4 or 5

induration: an increase in the fibrous elements in tissue, a hardened mass or formation, which if felt during a DRE is worrisome

infiltrate (adj. infiltrative): to penetrate through a porous tissue

inflammation: any form of swelling or pain or irritation

informed consent: permission to proceed given by a patient after being fully informed of the purposes and potential consequences of a medical procedure

in situ: in the natural or usual place

Insights: the newsletter of the Prostate Cancer Research Institute (*PCRI Insights*)

insulin: hormone that helps the body use glucose (sugar) for energy

insulin growth factor1 (IGF-1): a growth factor that stimulates PC cell growth and osteoblast growth

intensity map: representations of energy deposited per unit volume across a treatment volume when the deposition of energy is not delivered in a homogeneous manner

interferon: a body protein that affects antibody production and can modulate (regulate) the immune system

interleukin (IL): any of various compounds of low molecular weight that are produced by T-cells and macrophages and that function especially in regulation of the immune system and cell-mediated immunity

interstitial: within a particular organ; for example, interstitial prostate radiation therapy is radiation therapy applied within the prostate using implanted radioactive pellets or seeds (see also brachytherapy)

intracrinology: the part of endocrinology that focuses on the fact that, in men and women, an important proportion of androgens and estrogens are synthesized locally at their site of action in peripheral target tissues

intraductal: within a duct

intraepithelial: within the layer of cells that forms the surface or lining of an organ

intraglandular prostate cancer: See organ confined disease (OCD).

intraoperative: occurring, carried out, or encountered in the course of surgery

intravascular: within a vessel or vessels

intravenous (IV): into a vein

invasive: requiring an incision or the insertion of an instrument or substance into the body

inverse planning: Treatment planning for radiation therapy in which various aspects of the treatment plan are generated by a computer in order to achieve the dose distribution prescribed by a physician

investigational: a drug or procedure allowed by the FDA for use in clinical trials

in vitro: in an artificial environment e.g. within a Petri dish or test-tube

in vivo: within a living organism

involution: a normal process marked by decreasing size of an organ

ion: atom or molecule that has acquired an electric charge by the loss or gain of one or more electrons

ionize: to dissociate atoms or molecules into electrically charged atoms or radicals

Iressa®: the trade name for gefitinib

isocenter: The center of rotation of a treatment arc/p>

isodose contour: A two or three-dimensional shape that contains the volume receiving a dose greater than or equal to a specified amount

isodose line: A two-dimensional line that circumscribes an area receiving a dose greater than or equal to a specified amount

isoform: One of a set of similar proteins that have the same function but slightly different composition, e.g. free and complexed PSA

isotherm: a line on a chart representing the locations of zones having a particular temperature

isotope: a different form of a chemical element having similar properties

iterations: Repeated series of steps, performed either by the computer or by the user, implemented to develop a treatment plan

IVP (intravenous pyelogram): a procedure that introduces an X-ray absorbing dye into the urinary tract in order to allow the physician a superior image of the tract by taking an x-ray;

K

Kaplan-Meier method: a statistical method that produces a graph showing the percent of a patient population surviving at various intervals of time after the start of the study or treatment

Karnofsky Performance Status: index that allows cancer patients to be classified using a standard way of measuring the ability to perform ordinary tasks. See also: ECOG Performance Status

Kegel exercises: a set of exercises designed to improve the strength of the muscles used in urinating

keratin: any of various sulfur containing fibrous proteins that form the chemical basis of horny epidermal tissues (as hair and nails) and are typically not digested by enzymes of the gastrointestinal tract

ketoconazole: see Nizoral®

kidney: one of a pair of organs whose primary function is to filter the fluids passing through the body

killer cells: white blood cells that attack <u>tumor</u> cells and body cells that have been invaded by foreign substances

kinase: an <u>enzyme</u> that catalyzes the conversion of a pro—enzyme to an active enzyme

kinetics: the study of acceleration, motion or rate of change

L

laparoscopy: a technique that allows the physician to observe internal organs directly through a piece of optical equipment inserted directly into the body through a small surgical incision

laparotomy: an operation in which the <u>abdomen</u> is opened to look for the cause of an undiagnosed illness

latent: 1) insignificant or irrelevant; for example, latent prostate cancer (also known as incidental prostate cancer) is a form of prostate cancer which is of no clinical significance to the patient in whom it is discovered; 2) <u>pathology</u>. in a dormant or hidden stage

LDL cholesterol: low density lipoprotein <u>cholesterol</u>; a lipoprotein of blood plasma that is composed of a moderate proportion of protein with little triglyceride and a high proportion of cholesterol and that is associated with increased probability of developing <u>atherosclerosis</u>

lesions: a localized <u>pathological</u> change in a bodily organ or tissue

leuprolide acetate: a <u>LHRH analog</u>; one trade name is Lupron®

levator: a muscle that raises a structure in the body such as the muscles that support the <u>pelvic organs</u>

Leydig cells: cell population within the <u>testicles</u> that produces <u>testosterone</u>; the other main cell population are the Sertoli cells that make sperm

LH: luteinizing hormone; a pituitary hormone that stimulates the Leydig cells of the testicles to make the male hormone testosterone

LHRH: luteinizing hormone-releasing hormone (also known as GnRH or gonadotrophin releasing hormone; hormone from the hypothalamus that interacts with the LHRH receptor in the pituitary to release LH) see luteinizing hormone releasing hormone

LHRH analogs (or agonists): Synthetic compounds that are chemically similar to Luteinizing Hormone Releasing Hormone (LHRH), but are sufficiently different that they suppress testicular production of testosterone by binding to the LHRH receptor in the pituitary gland and either have no biological activity and therefore competitively inhibit the action of LHRH, or has LHRH activity that exhausts the production of LH by the pituitary; used in the hormonal treatment of advanced prostate cancer and in the adjuvant and neoadjuvant hormonal treatment of earlier stages of prostate cancer; LHRH agonist (mimics natural LHRH but then shuts down LH production after continuous exposure)

LHRH antagonist: an agent that blocks the LHRH receptor by pure antagonism without the initial release of LH seen with LHRH agonists; abarelix (Plenaxis®) is an example

libido: interest in sexual activity; the psychic and emotional energy associated with instinctual biological drives

ligand: An ion, a molecule, a molecular group, a substance or messenger that binds to another chemical entity at a receptor to form a larger complex which is then activated

linear accelerator: A type of high energy X-ray machine that generates radiation fields for external beam radiation therapy. A linear accelerator is typically mounted with a collimator and/or a multileaf collimator in a gantry that revolves vertically around a treatment couch

lipid: fat stored by the body; the two most commonly measured kinds of lipids are triglycerides and cholesterol.

lipomatosis: condition characterized by abnormal localized, or tumor-like, accumulations of fat in the tissues

LNCaP: a line of human prostate cancer cells used in laboratory studies; this cell line is hormonally dependent; See <u>androgen dependent</u>.

lobe: one of the two sides of an organ that clearly has two sides (e.g., the prostate or the brain)

local therapy: treatment that is directed at the prostate and closely surrounding tissue

localized: restricted to a well-defined area

LSESr (LIPO-sterolic extract of *Serenoa repens*): the lipid extracted portion of <u>saw palmetto</u>

lumbar: portion of body between chest and pelvis, often referring to the lower back or spine

lumen: a cavity or channel into any organ or structure of the body

Lupron®: the USA trade or brand name of a leuprolide acetate, a <u>LHRH agonist</u>

luteinizing hormone releasing hormone (LHRH): a <u>hormone</u> responsible for stimulating the production of <u>testosterone</u> in the body by interacting with the LHRH receptor to release <u>LH</u> which in turn stimulates cells in the <u>testicles</u> (<u>Leydig cells</u>) to make testosterone; luteinizing hormone-releasing hormone is also known as GnRH or gonadotrophin-releasing hormone

LUTS: lower <u>urinary</u> tract symptoms; include symptoms of hesitancy in initiating urination, slow urination, dribbling after urination, getting up at night to urinate (<u>nocturia</u>) and frequency of urination; these symptoms are part of the <u>AUA symptom score index</u>

LY294002: a lipid-modifying <u>enzyme</u> that inhibits <u>PI3 kinase</u>

lycopene: A <u>carotenoid</u> responsible for the red color of the tomato, watermelon and pink grapefruit. Recent findings indicate that lycopene may be an important part of the human organism's natural defense mechanism that protects from harmful oxidizing agents

lymph (also lymphatic fluid): the clear fluid in which all of the cells in the body are constantly bathed; carries cells that help fight infection

lymph nodes: the small glands which occur throughout the body and which filter the clear fluid known as lymph or lymphatic fluid; lymph nodes filter out bacteria and other toxins, as well as cancer cells

lymphadenectomy: also known as a pelvic lymph node dissection, this procedure involves the removal and microscopic examination of selected lymph nodes, a common site of metastatic disease with prostate cancer; this procedure can be performed during surgery prior to the removal of the prostate gland, or by means of a small incision a "laparoscopic lymphadenectomy" may be performed, a simple operation requiring only an overnight stay in the hospital

lymphadenopathy: disorder of the lymph nodes or vessels

lymphatic system: the tissue and organs that produce, store and carry cells that fight infection; includes bone marrow, spleen, thymus, lymph nodes, and channels that carry lymph fluid

lymphocele: cystic mass containing lymph from diseased lymphatic channels or following surgical trauma or other injury

lymphocyte: white blood cell

lymphography: radiologic depiction of lymphatic vessels and lymph nodes after use of a contrast material

lytic: of, relating to, or causing a specified kind of decomposition through rupture of cell membranes and loss of cytoplasm

M

M0, M1, Mx: notation of observed metastases, see staging.

MAB (maximal androgen blockade): see CHT, CHB, ADT

macromolecules: a very large molecule, such as a polymer or protein, consisting of many smaller structural units linked together. Also called supermolecule

macrophage: a subset of white blood cells that ingest bacteria, foreign substances, proteins and process them, often presenting them to T cells; one of a kind of <u>antigen</u> presenting cell; see <u>dendritic cells</u>

MAD (maximal androgen deprivation): see <u>ADT</u>, CHB, CHT, TAB, MAB

magnetic resonance: absorption of specific frequencies of radio and microwave radiation by atoms placed in a strong magnetic field

magnetic resonance imaging (MRI): the use of magnetic resonance with atoms in body tissues to produce distinct cross-sectional, and even three-dimensional images of internal organs

malignancy: a growth or tumor composed of cancerous cells

malignant: cancerous; tending to become progressively worse and to result in death; having the invasive and <u>metastatic</u> (spreading) properties of cancer

margin: normally used to mean the "surgical margin", which is the outer edge of the tissue removed during surgery; if the surgical margin shows no sign of cancer ("negative margins"), then the prognosis is better

marker: a diagnostic indication that disease may be present or may develop

MCF-7: human breast cancer cell line

mcg (micrograms): A unit of mass equal to one thousandth (10-3) of a milligram or one millionth (10-6) of a gram

MCP: modified citrus pectin; a substance that is able to interfere with PC growth by preventing cell-cell interaction and adhesiveness by binding to a carbohydrate substance called galectin-3 found on the surface of tumor cells

M-CSF: <u>macrophage</u> colony-stimulating factor

MDR gene: the multi-drug resistance <u>gene</u>; a gene that cells utilize to pump substances such as <u>chemotherapy</u> out of the cell across the cell membrane. The increase in the MDR gene is felt to be a <u>tumor</u> mechanism to overcome the effect of chemotherapy. <u>Nizoral®</u> and <u>tamoxifen</u> decrease MDR activity.

medical oncologist: a physician primarily trained in the use of medicines (rather than surgery) to treat cancer

metabolism, adj. **metabolic**: the organic processes (in a cell or organism) that are necessary for life

metabolite: a substance necessary for or taking part in a particular metabolic (chemical) process in the body

metaphase: Phase of mitosis, or cell division, when the chromosomes align along the center of the cell. Because metaphase chromosomes are highly condensed, scientists use these chromosomes for gene mapping and identifying chromosomal aberrations.

metastasis: (plural **metastases**) a secondary tumor formed as a result of a cancer cell or cells from the primary tumor site (e.g., the prostate) traveling through the body to a new site and then growing there

metastasize: spread of a malignant tumor to other parts of the body

metastatic: having the characteristics of a secondary tumor formed as a result of a cancer cell or cells from the primary tumor site (e.g., the prostate) traveling through the body to a new site and then growing there

metastatic work up: a group of tests, including physical examination, bone scans, X-rays, other imaging studies and blood tests to ascertain whether cancer has metastasized

Metastron®: the brand or trade name of strontium-89, a radioactive isotope used in the treatment of bone pain from metastatic prostate cancer

mg (milligram): a unit of mass equal to one thousandth, **10-3 of** a gram

micromets, micrometastatic cells: microscopic cancer cells in other parts of the body that are similar to those of the original tumor

microtubules: tiny fibers that are basic to DNA structure that assists in the process of cell division

microvessel density: an objective measure of angiogenesis (blood vessel formation)

midgland: the section between the apex and base of the prostate

misstaging: the assignment of an incorrect clinical stage at initial diagnosis because of the difficulty of assessing the available information with accuracy

mitochondria: A spherical or elongated organ in the cytoplasm of nearly all eukaryotic cells, containing genetic material and many enzymes important for cell metabolism, including those responsible for the conversion of food to usable energy

mitosis, mitotic: a process of cell division in which chromosomes separate into two parts, one part of each chromosome is retained in each of two new daughter

mitoxantrone (Novantrone®): a drug used to treat advanced prostate cancer that does not respond to hormones. It is also being studied in the treatment of other cancers. It belongs to the family of drugs called antitumor antibiotics.

MMP-2: matrix metalloprotease-2 (PC cell product involved in angiogenesis)

modality: a therapeutic method or agent, such as surgery, chemotherapy, or electrotherapy, that involves the physical treatment of a disorder

molecular biology: the branch of biology focused on the formation, structure, and function of DNA, RNA and proteins, and their roles in the transmission of genetic information

monoclonal: formed from a single group of identical cells

monotherapy: a treatment that uses one major drug or one major modality of treatment; androgen deprivation therapy using only an LHRH agonist is an example of monotherapy.

morbidity: unhealthy consequences and complications resulting from treatment

morphology, morphologic: a branch of biology that deals with the form and structure of animals and plants

morphometry, morphometric: the quantitative measurement of the form and distribution of parts, especially in living systems

mortality: (1) the quality of being subject to death; (2) the number of deaths in a given time or place or the proportion of deaths to population

motility: the ability to move spontaneously

MRI: see magnetic resonance imaging

MRI/MRSI: the integration of magnetic resonance imaging sequences with magnetic resonance spectroscopic imaging as a sequence.

mRNA: messenger RNA; see RNA.

MRS: magnetic resonance spectroscopy

mucin: the main part of mucus that protects body surfaces from rubbing or wearing down

mucosa: superficial lining cells involving body cavities like the mouth, rectum, bladder; a membrane lining all body passages that communicate with the air, such as the respiratory and alimentary tracts, and having cells and associated glands that secrete mucus

multileaf collimator (MLC): A type of collimator that can define irregularly shaped radiation fields. An MLC has two rows of narrow metal blocks (leaves) that can be independently driven in or out of the radiation beam from opposite sides under computer control

multileaf intensity modulating collimator (MIMIC): A multileaf collimator designed specifically for intensity modulated radiotherapy. The MIMiC treats two slices, each 1 or 2 cm thick with a fan beam of radiation, when the linear accelerator gantry rotates through an arc around the patient. The patient couch is moved to treat adjacent slices if the target is too large to treat with a single arc; see tomotherapy

murine: from or pertaining to mice

mutate, mutation: change in the genetic material (DNA) inside the cell

myalgia: muscle aches, pain or tenderness

N

N0, N1, Nx: notation of lymph nodes metastasis, see <u>staging</u>

nadir: the lowest point

naturopathy: treatment of disease using natural agents and physical manipulation; avoids drugs and surgery

nausea: An unpleasant sensation in the abdomen often leading to vomiting.

NCI: National Cancer Institute

necrosis, adj. **necrotic**: death of cells or tissues through injury or disease

negative: the term used to describe a test result which does not show the presence of the substance or material for which the test was carried out; for example, a negative <u>bone scan</u> would show no sign of bone <u>metastases</u>

negative predictive value: refers to the chance that a negative test result will be correct.

neoadjuvant: The use of a different kind of therapy *before* the use of what is considered a more definitive therapy, e.g. the use of neoadjuvant <u>androgen deprivation therapy</u> (ADT) prior to radiation therapy of PC or the use of neoadjuvant <u>chemotherapy</u> before surgery for breast cancer. Neoadjuvant is contrasted to <u>adjuvant</u>, which relates to the use of another therapy *after* the so-called more definitive therapy, e.g. ADT after RT

neoadjuvant hormone blockade (NHB): use of <u>ADT</u> prior to other therapies such as <u>radiation therapy</u>, surgery or possibly <u>chemotherapy</u> to reduce tumor volume and/or prostate gland volume with the goal to allow these other therapies to work better; also called NHT (Neoadjuvant Hormone Therapy)

neoplasia: the growth of cells under conditions that would tend to prevent the development of normal tissue (e.g., a cancer)

neoplasm, adj. **neoplastic**: new and abnormal growth of tissue, which may be a benign or cancerous tumor

nephrostomy: establishment of an opening for a <u>catheter</u> from the <u>kidney</u> to the exterior of the body.

nerve radicles: small nerve roots that are seen microscopically within specific tissue, like the prostate

nerve sparing: term used to describe a type of <u>prostatectomy</u> in which the surgeon saves the nerves that affect sexual and related functions

Neumega® (oprelvekin): a medication which helps the body produce more <u>platelets</u> in the blood

neuroendocrine: pertaining to the relationships between the nervous and the <u>endocrine</u> systems

neurogenic: originating in the nervous system; compare to <u>psychogenic</u>

neurohormone: any of a group of substances produced by specialized cells (neurosecretory cells) structurally typical of the nervous (rather than of the <u>endocrine</u>) system, but that serve as a link between the two systems

neurologic: meaning it pertains to the nervous system, e.g., a neurologic problem

neurons: nerve cells which make up the central nervous system

neuropathy, adj. **neuropathic**: a disease or an abnormality of the nervous system

neurotoxicity: <u>toxicity</u> to nervous tissue (both brain and peripheral nerves)

neurotransmitter: a chemical that acts as messenger between cells in the brain and nervous system; it transmits impulses across the gap from a neuron to another neuron, a muscle, or a gland.

neurovascular: to both the <u>neurologic</u> and <u>vascular</u> systems or structures

neurovascular bundles: two bundles of nerves between the prostate and the rectum that control erection

neutropenia, neutropenic: a deficiency of neutrophils. A person is considered neutropenic when their white blood cell count drops below 1000.

neutrophil: the principal phagocyte (microbe-eating) cell in the blood. This blood cell is the main cell that combats infections. Often, it is not present in sufficient quantities in patients with acute leukemia or after chemotherapy. A severe deficiency of neutrophils increases the patient's susceptibility to infection.

NHB, NHT: see neoadjuvant hormone blockade (hormone therapy)

NIH: National Institutes of Health

nilutamide (Nilandron®): a non-steroidal antiandrogen

Nizoral®: The brand name of ketoconazole; a medication that blocks testicular and adrenal androgen production while having a direct cytotoxic effect on the PC cell; Nizoral® also is synergistic with certain chemotherapy agents and inhibits the development of the MDR gene

nocturia: the act of needing to getting up at night to urinate. This is usually scored as nocturia x number of times on average patient awakens to urinate. Nocturia x 3, for example, means getting up at night 3 times

nodular: a bump or bumpy tissue

nodule: A growth or lump that may be cancerous or noncancerous.

nomogram: A chart representing numerical relationships

noncoding: In genetics, noncoding DNA describes DNA which does not contain instructions for making proteins (or other cell products such as RNAs)

noninvasive: not requiring any incision or the insertion of an instrument or substance into the body

NSE: neuron-specific enolase; a neuroendocrine marker (see CGA)

N-telopeptides (Ntx): a bone resorption marker

nuclear medicine: branch of medicine dealing with the use of radioactive materials in the diagnosis and treatment of disease

nucleated: formed into a nucleus

nucleic acid: a chemical compound involved in making and storing energy and carrying hereditary characteristics, such as <u>DNA</u>

nucleolus: pl. **nucleoli**: any of the small, dense cell structures made up mostly of RNA (<u>ribonucleic acid</u>)

nucleosomes: the repeating structural units of <u>chromatin</u>, each consisting of approximately 200 base pairs of <u>DNA</u> around a <u>protein</u> core composed of the <u>histones</u>

nucleus: the main controlling body of a living cell

O

oblique: a plane or section not perpendicular to the xyz coordinate system, such as long and short axis views of the heart

occult: detectable only by microscopic examination or chemical analysis, as a minute blood sample

octreotide (Sandostatin®): a synthetic protein that is similar to the naturally-occurring <u>hormone</u> called somatostatin. Octreotide decreases the production of many substances in the body such as insulin and glucagon (involved in regulating blood sugar), growth hormone, and chemicals that affect digestion.

ODC: ornithine decarboxylase; a rate-limiting <u>enzyme</u> in the pathway of mammalian <u>polyamine</u> biosynthesis. Polyamines affect <u>DNA</u>, <u>RNA</u> and <u>protein</u> synthesis. For these reasons, ODC activity is said to be closely associated with <u>tumor</u> promotion. Green tea <u>polyphenols</u> inhibit ODC resulting in a decrease in polyamine synthesis and cell growth.

oncogene: a gene having the potential to cause (or facilitate) a normal cell to become cancerous

oncologist: a physician who specializes in the treatment of various types of cancer

oncology: the branch of medical science dealing with tumors; an oncologist is a specialists in the study of cancerous tumors

oncolytic virus: a virus that causes death of a <u>tumor</u> cell; after the Greek word *onkos* for tumor or mass

opioid: originally, a term denoting synthetic narcotics resembling opiates, but increasingly used to refer to both opiates and synthetic narcotics

orchiectomy (orchidectomy): the surgical removal of the <u>testicles</u>; surgical <u>castration</u>

organ: a group of tissues that work in concert to carry out a specific set of functions (e.g., the heart or the lungs or the prostate)

organ confined disease (OCD): PC that is apparently confined to the prostate <u>clinically</u> or <u>pathologically</u>; not going beyond the confines of the prostatic capsule

organism: any individual living animal or plant

orgasm: the highest point of sexual excitement, characterized by strong feelings of pleasure and marked normally by ejaculation of <u>semen</u> by the male and by vaginal contractions in the female; also called climax

orphan drug: a category created by US <u>FDA</u> for medications used to treat diseases that occur rarely (less than 200,000 cases) or that there is no hope for recovery of development costs, so there is little financial incentive for industry to develop them; orphan drug status gives the manufacturer financial incentives to provide the drug

orthotopic: in the normal or usual position

osseous: consisting of or resembling bone **osteoblast**: cell that forms bone

osteoclast: cell that breaks down bone; osteoclasts are in bone tissue and resorb bone leading to bone loss or <u>osteopenia</u> or <u>osteoporosis</u>

osteoid: uncalcified bone matrix, the product of <u>osteoblasts</u>. Consists mainly of <u>collagen</u>

osteolysis: destruction of bone

osteonecrosis: condition resulting in death of bone tissue

osteopenia: a reduction in the bone density that is more than one standard deviation from the normal bone density; using the T score it is T=-1.0 down to T=-2.4; once the T score is less than 2.4, the patient is defined as having osteoporosis

osteoporosis: a reduction in bone density resulting in a T score of -2.5 or less; a loss of bone due to increased osteoclastic activity leading to bone resorption

overexpress: produce in excess, as does the genetic material of cancer cells

overstaging: the assignment of an overly high clinical stage at initial diagnosis because of the difficulty of assessing the available information with accuracy (e.g., stage T3b as opposed to stage T2b)

oxidant: a substance that causes another substance to combine with oxygen

P

p27: a protein that helps to regulate cell growth and a loss of p27 expression is associated with poor prognosis in prostate cancer

p53: a protein that detects and repairs gene damage, coordinating events that cause the cell to stop its growth and repair the damage. If the damage is too great, p53 becomes the catalyst directing the damaged cell to commit suicide.

paclitaxel (Taxol®): one of the chemotherapy agents called taxanes that block cell division

palliative: designed to relieve a particular problem without necessarily solving it; for example, palliative therapy is given in order to relieve symptoms and improve quality of life, but does not cure the patient

palpable: capable of being felt during a physical examination by an experienced physician; in the case of prostate cancer, this normally refers to some form of abnormality of the prostate which can be felt during a digital rectal examination **palpation**: physical examination in medical diagnosis by pressure of the hand or fingers to the surface of the body especially to determine the condition (as of size or consistency) of an underlying part or organ

pamidronate: a disodium <u>bisphosphonate</u> bone-<u>resorption</u> inhibitor C3H9NNa2O7P2 administered as an intravenous infusion in the treatment of <u>hypercalcemia</u> associated with <u>malignancy</u> called also *pamidronate disodium*

pancreas, pancreatic: A gland situated near the stomach that secretes a digestive fluid into the intestine through one or more ducts and also secretes the <u>hormone</u> insulin

PAP (prostatic acid phosphatase): an <u>enzyme</u> or b<u>iomarker</u> secreted by prostate cells associated with a higher probability of disease outside the prostate when levels are 3.0 or higher; PAP elevations suggest that the disease is not <u>OCD</u> (organ confined disease)

papaverine: a drug which causes blood vessels to expand, thereby increasing blood flow; when papaverine is injected into the penis, it produces an erection by increasing blood flow to the <u>penis</u>; see also <u>phentolamine</u>, "<u>bimix</u>", "<u>trimix</u>"

paracrine: a form of signaling in which the target cell is close to the signal-releasing cell; compare to <u>endocrine</u>.

paramagnetic: a substance in which an induced magnetic field is parallel and proportional to the intensity of the magnetizing field but is much weaker than in ferromagnetic materials

parathormone: a <u>hormone</u> that regulates ion levels in <u>neurons</u> and controls excitability of the nervous system

parathyroid hormone (PTH): one of the principal calcium—regulating <u>hormones</u> in the body

partial response (PR): a 50% or greater decline in parameters that are being used to measure anti-cancer activity; parameters include abnormalities involving physical exam findings, lab and radiologic studies; also see <u>complete</u> <u>response (CR)</u>

partial voluming: the presence of different tissue types (e.g. healthy and malignant) within a <u>spectroscopic</u> volume leading to an averaging of the resulting spectra—a loss of resolution due to excessively large <u>voxels</u>, typically caused by scan slices that are too thick

Partin tables: tables constructed based on results of the <u>PSA</u>, <u>clinical stage</u> and <u>Gleason score</u> involving thousands of men with PC; used to predict the probability that the prostate cancer has spread to the lymph nodes, <u>seminal vesicles</u>, penetrated the <u>capsule</u> or that it remains confined to the prostate; developed by a group of scientists at the Brady Institute for Urology at Johns Hopkins University

pathogen, adj. **pathogenic**: an organism that causes disease in another organism

pathologist: a physician who specializes in the examination of tissues and blood samples to help decide what diseases are present and therefore how they should be treated

pathology, pathological: a science which specializes in the examination of tissues and blood samples to help decide what diseases are present and therefore how they should be treated

PC, PCa: abbreviations for prostate cancer

PC-3: human PC cell line that is <u>androgen independent</u>

PCA3: a specific <u>gene</u> that is profusely expressed in <u>prostate</u> cancer tissue, and not expressed in any other kind of human tissue

PCA3 score: ratio of <u>PCA3</u> to <u>PSA mRNA</u>

PCNA (proliferating cell nuclear antigen): an index of cell division or proliferation

PCRI: The Prostate Cancer Research Institute; a non-profit organization located in Los Angeles whose goal is to educate patients and physicians about PC; telephone number is 310-743-2116; Web site: www.pcri.org

PC SPES: a herbal therapy for PC comprised of 8 herbs that is no longer available

Pd: pyridinoline; a bone <u>resorption</u> marker; a bone <u>collagen</u> breakdown product

PDGF: platelet-derived growth factor; an important factor involved in tumor growth involving <u>angiogenesis</u>

PDQ: physicians data query; a NCI supported database available to physicians, containing current information on standard treatments and ongoing clinical trials

PEENUTS® (Peenuts®): A Complex nutritional formula used to effectively treat non-bacterial prostatitis; Patented (worldwide) and uniquely distributed by Sun Vida

pelvic lymph node dissection: removal of lymph nodes in the area of the pelvis to check for presence of cancer

pelvis, pelvic: that part of the skeleton that joins the lower limbs of the body together

penile: of the penis

penile bulb: the base of the <u>penis</u> that attaches to the <u>perineal</u> membrane

penis: the male organ used in urination and intercourse

peptide: a compound of two or more <u>amino</u> acids where the alpha carboxyl group of one is bound to the alpha amino group of another

percutaneous: through the skin

perfluorocarbon liquid: a colorless and odorless liquid in which all hydrogen atoms have been replaced by fluorine atoms. This liquid is injected within the MEDRAD <u>endorectal</u> <u>coil</u> instead of air to increase image and spectral quality.

perineal: of the perineum; an area of the body between the <u>scrotum</u> and the <u>anus</u>

perineum: the area of the body between the <u>scrotum</u> and the <u>anus</u>; a perineal procedure uses this area as the point of entry into the body

perineural invasion (PNI): PC invading the nerve sheath surrounding the nerves that enter the prostate

peripheral: outside the central region

peripheral neuropathy (PN): any disorder of the nervous system outside the brain and spinal column, such as tingling or numbness in the hands or feet

peripheral zone: the largest portion of the prostate located in the back closest to the rectum

periprostatic: pertaining to the soft tissues immediately adjacent to the prostate

peritoneum, adj. **peritoneal**: the serous membrane that lines the walls of the abdominal cavity and folds inward to enclose the viscera

PET (positron emission tomography) scan: using a radioactive isotope that is taken up by tumor tissue showing that the tumor is functional

PGE-2 (prostaglandin E2): an unfavorable metabolite of arachidonic acid

phagocytosis: the engulfing and ingesting of a substance within a cell; e.g. a macrophage may phagocytize bacteria or other cells

pharmacologic: the characteristics or properties of a drug, especially those that make it medically effective

phase I, II or III clinical trial: see Clinical Trial

phentolamine: given by injection causes blood vessels to expand, thereby increasing blood flow; when injected into the penis, it increases blood flow to the penis, which results in an erection. see also papaverine, "bimix", "trimix"

phenotype, adj. **phenotypic**: the observable physical or biochemical characteristics of an organism or group, as determined by both genetic makeup and environmental influences

phosphodiesterase (PPD) inhibitors: drugs which may help a man achieve an erection

phosphorylation: the addition of phosphate to an organic compound through the action of a phosphorylase or kinase

photon: A unit of energy of a light ray or other form of radiant energy. Most conventional radiation uses photons to deliver ionizing radiation.

physiologic: of or consistent with a living organism's normal functioning

PI3 kinase: an enzyme which influences a wide variety of cellular functions, including cell growth, differentiation and survival, glucose metabolism and cytoskeletal organization

PICP: carboxy-terminal propeptide of type 1 procollagen; a bone formation marker

PIN: prostatic intraepithelial (or intraductal) neoplasia; a pathologically identifiable condition characterized by microscopic changes in the epithelial cells; also known more simply as dysplasia by many physicians; broken down into high-grade PIN or PIN 2 and PIN 3 or low-grade PIN or PIN1. High grade PIN is what is believed to be a precursor to PC

pituitary: a small gland at the base of the brain that supplies hormones that control many body processes including the production of testosterone by the testis

placebo: a form of safe but non-active treatment frequently used as a basis for comparison with pharmaceuticals in research studies

planimetry: the measurement of plane surfaces

planning target volume (PTV): Equivalent to the clinical target volume plus a margin to account for uncertainty in immobilization and localization of the patient anatomy during treatment

plasma: The clear, yellowish fluid portion of blood, lymph, or intramuscular fluid in which cells are suspended. It differs from serum in that it contains fibrin and other soluble clotting elements.

platelet: a particle found in the bloodstream that binds at the site of a wound to begin the blood clotting process; platelets are formed in bone marrow.

plexus: a structure in the form of a network, especially of nerves, blood vessels, or lymphatics

ploidy: a term used to describe the number of sets of chromosomes in a cell; see also diploid and aneuploid

PNI: perineural invasion

polyamine: Any of a group of organic compounds, such as spermine and spermidine, composed of only carbon, nitrogen, and hydrogen and containing two or more amino groups

polymerase chain reaction (PCR): system for in vitro amplification of DNA that involves separating the DNA into its two complementary strands and using DNA enzymes to synthesize two-stranded DNA from each single strand, and repeating the process

polyphenol: Any of a class of aromatic organic compounds comprised of more than one hydroxyl group (-OH) attached directly to a benzene ring

positive: the term used to describe a test result which shows the presence of the substance or material for which the test was carried out; for example, a positive bone scan would show signs of bone metastases

positive margin: the pathologic finding of cancer cells on the outer edge of the tissue removed

positive predictive value: refers to the chance that a positive test result will be correct.

posterior: the rear; for example, the posterior of the prostate is the part of the prostate that faces a man's back

PPO: preferred provider organization—an insurance plan which allows choice of any provider in the network

PR (progesterone receptor): the docking site on a cell that interacts with progestins

preclinical: before a disease becomes recognizable based on direct observation

precursor: a biochemical substance, such as an intermediate compound, from which a more stable or definitive product is formed

prednisone (Orasone® or Deltasone® or Liquid Pred® or Meticorten®): a glucocorticoid steroid used to treat anorexia and cachexia and some cancers. It is similar to a steroid hormone made by the adrenal glands in the body.

priapism: an abnormal, painful erection where the penis remains erect for an extended period of time that is usually not accompanied with sexual desire

procollagen: the soluble precursor of collagen

Procrit®: a recombinant human erythropoietin used to treat anemia

proctitis: inflammation of the rectum; in PC therapy may be associated with radiation therapy

progesterone: a specific steroid hormone used in the treatment of hot flashes in men having suppressions in LH and testosterone; an example of a progestin is Megace® or Depo-Provera®

prognosis: the patient's potential clinical outlook based on the status and probable course of his disease; chance of recovery

progression: continuing growth or regrowth of the cancer

prolactin (PRL): a trophic hormone produced by the pituitary that increases androgen receptors, increases sensitivity to androgens & regulates production & secretion of citrate

proliferative inflammatory atrophy (PIA): chronic inflammatory prostate lesions that may result in prostate cancer

prone: referring to the position of the body when lying face downward

prophylactic, prophylaxis: a drug, procedure or piece of equipment used to prevent disease

Proscar®: brand name of finasteride; a 5 AR inhibitor

prospective: relating to or being a study (as of the incidence of disease) that starts with the present condition of a population of individuals and follows them into the future—compare retrospective

prostaglandin: <u>hormone</u> like substances that stimulate target cells into action; they differ from hormones in that they act locally, near their site of synthesis, and they are metabolized very rapidly; any of various oxygenated unsaturated cyclic fatty acids of animals that have a variety of hormone like actions (as in controlling blood pressure or smooth muscle contraction)

ProstaScint®: a <u>monoclonal antibody</u> test directed against the prostate specific membrane antigen (<u>PSMA</u>); seems to focus on <u>androgen independent</u> <u>tumor</u> tissue which may contain a greater amount of PSMA

prostate: the gland surrounding the <u>urethra</u> and immediately below the <u>bladder</u> in males which provides fluid to nourish and transport <u>sperm</u> during intercourse

prostatectomy: surgical removal of part or all of the prostate gland

prostate specific antigen (PSA): a protein secreted by the <u>epithelial cells</u> of the prostate gland including cancer cells; an elevated level in the blood indicates an abnormal condition of the prostate gland, either <u>benign</u> or <u>malignant</u>; it is used to detect potential problems in the prostate gland and to follow the progress of PC therapy (see <u>screening</u>)

prostate-specific membrane antigen (PSMA): a <u>biomarker</u> of prostate <u>epithelial cell</u> activity that is expressed in the membrane of prostate epithelial cells. PSMA is composed of a short 19 <u>amino</u> acid intra-cellular domain, a 24 amino acid transmembrane domain and a 707 amino acid extra-cellular domain. PSMA <u>antigen</u> is radiologically identified (imaged) using a <u>monoclonal</u> <u>antibody</u> attached to a radioactive Indium 111 isotope (ProstaScint scan) to allow visualization of PSMA antigen-containing tissue found within lymph nodes and/or prostate gland.

prostatic acid phosphatase (PAP): an <u>enzyme</u> or <u>biomarker</u> secreted by prostate cells associated with a higher probability of disease outside the prostate when levels are 3.0 or higher; PAP elevations suggest that the disease is not OCD (organ confined disease)

prostatism: a symptom resulting from compression or obstruction of the <u>urethra</u>, due most commonly to <u>hyperplasia</u> of the prostate; results in urinary difficulties and, occasionally, <u>urinary</u> retention

prostatitis: infection or inflammation of the prostate gland treatable by medication, nutritionals like Peenuts® and/or manipulation; (<u>BPH</u> is a more permanent laying down of fibrous and connective tissue caused when the prostate tries to contain a relatively silent chronic lower-grade infection, often requiring a <u>TURP</u> to relieve the symptoms)

prosthesis: a manufactured device used to replace a normal body part or function

protease: any <u>enzyme</u> that catalyzes the splitting of <u>proteins</u> into smaller <u>peptide</u> fractions and <u>amino</u> acids by a process known as proteolysis

protease inhibitor: a substance that inhibits the action of a <u>protease</u>

protein: any of a group of complex organic macromolecules that contain carbon, hydrogen, oxygen, nitrogen, and usually sulfur and are composed of one or more chains of <u>amino</u> acids. Proteins are fundamental components of all living cells and include many substances, such as <u>enzymes</u>, <u>hormones</u>, and <u>antibodies</u>, that are necessary for the proper functioning of an organism. They are essential in the diet of animals for the growth and repair of tissue and can be obtained from foods such as meat, fish, eggs, milk, and legumes

protocol: a precise set of methods by which a treatment or research study is to be carried out

proton beam radiation therapy: a form of RT that uses the proton, a positively charged nuclear particle, to deliver ionizing radiation. The proton can be programmed to stop at a particular depth within tissue for the delivery of its radiation payload

proton pump inhibitors (PPI): drugs that reduce gastric acidity by inhibiting the proton pump within the gastric lining cells; examples of PPI include Prilosec® and Nexium®

proximal: a part of the body that is nearer to the point of reference, compare to <u>distal</u>

PSA: see <u>prostate-specific antigen</u>; the 'barometer of prostate disease'

PSA density (PSAD): The amount of <u>PSA</u> per unit volume of the prostate gland; the quotient of PSA divided by gland volume; a reflection of tumor density within the prostate

PSA doubling time (PSADT): the calculation of the time it takes for the <u>PSA</u> value to double based on at least three values separated by at least three months each; before diagnosis, a PSADT of less than 10 years may be an indication of the presence of PC

PSA failure: the <u>ASTRO</u> definition of <u>PSA</u> failure as being three consecutive increases in PSA level following treatment.rising <u>PSA</u> as seen in 3 consecutive determinations; also called biochemical relapse-free survival (bRFS)

PSAII: See % Free PSA

PSA slope: the rate of rise in the <u>PSA</u> level normally expressed as ng/mL per month

PSA velocity (PSAV): the calculation of the rate of increase in <u>PSA</u> levels in succeeding PSA tests; before diagnosis, a PSAV of 0.75 ng/ml/year (or higher) may be an indication of the presence of PC

PSM: prostate specific membrane; a membrane that surrounds the protoplasm (cytoplasm) of prostate cells

PSMA: <u>prostate specific membrane antigen</u>

psychogenic: produced or caused by psychological or mental factors rather than organic factors; compare to <u>neurogenic</u>

PTEN: a <u>gene</u> acts as a <u>tumor</u> suppressor gene by deactivating <u>Akt</u> and rendering prostate cancer cells more susceptible to suicide

PTHrP: Parathyroid hormone-related protein; a protein involved in <u>osteoblast</u> stimulation; a product also of the PC cell elaborated by <u>neuroendocrine</u> cells that make <u>CGA</u> (chromogranin A)

Pub Med: a Web site which allows access to thousands of published medical studies. It is a service of the National Institute of Health and can be found at www.pubmed.com

pubic arch: the arch formed by the inferior rami of the pubic bones

pulmonary embolism: a blood clot in a lungs, causing a severe impairment of respiratory function

Pyrilinks-D (Dpd): a urine test that quantitates bone resorption; the second voided urine specimen is ideal to use; other markers of bone resorption are ICTP and N-telopeptide

pyrophosphate: a salt or ester of pyrophosphoric acid

Q

qCT: quantitative CT bone densitometry; an alternate way to evaluate bone density besides the DEXA scan; qCT is not falsely elevated due to calcium deposits in blood vessels or due to degenerative joint disease

quality of life (QOL): an evaluation of health status relative to the patient's age, expectations and physical and mental capabilities

PSA mRNA: messenger RNA which replicates the DNA code of the PSA protein

PSA nadir (PSAN): the lowest value the PSA reaches during or after a particular treatment; a progressive rise after a PSA nadir has been reached usually indicates biologic activity of PC

PSA relapse-free survival: survival of the PC patient that relates to no evidence of biochemical relapse based on the presence of prostate specific antigen

R

RAD: A unit of absorbed radiation dose, **100 rads = 1 joule/kg = 1 Gray**

radiation cystitis: inflammation of the bladder lining due to the ionizing effects of radiation therapy

radiation oncologist: a physician who has received special training regarding the treatment of cancers with different types of radiation

radiation proctitis: inflammation of the rectal mucosa lining due to the ionizing effects of radiation therapy

radiation therapy (RT): the use of X-rays and other forms of radiation to destroy malignant cells and tissue

radical: (in a surgical sense) directed at the cause of a disease; thus, radical prostatectomy is the surgical removal of the prostate with the intent to cure the problem believed to be caused by or within the prostate

radical prostatectomy (RP): an operation to remove the entire prostate gland and seminal vesicles

radio sensitivity: the degree to which a type of cancer responds to radiation therapy

radiobiology adj. **radiobiological**: the study of the effects of radiation on living organisms

radiography: producing an image by radiation other than visible light, e.g., x-rays of one's teeth is done by radiography.

radioimmunometric: a measurement using radioimmunology, a system for testing antigen antibody reactions using radioactive labelling of antigen or antibody to detect the extent of the reaction

radioisotope: a type of atom (or a chemical which is made with a type of atom) that emits radioactivity

radiolabeled, radiolabel: an antibody that has been joined with a radioactive substance

radiology: the branch of medicine that deals with radioactive substances for diagnosing and treating disease

radionuclide: an unstable form of a chemical element that radioactively decays, resulting in the emission of nuclear radiation

radiopharmaceutical: a drug containing a radioactive substance that is used in the diagnosis and treatment of cancer and in pain management of bone metastases. Also called a radioactive drug.

radiotherapy: see radiation therapy

ramus, pl. rami: the arch formed by the inferior rami of the pubic bones

randomized: the process of assigning patients to different forms of treatment in a research study in a random manner

rapamycin, also called sirolimus (Rapamune®): a peptide drug used to help prevent the body from rejecting organ and bone marrow transplants. It is also has been shown to block one of the survival pathways under Akt control

rb: a protein which plays an important role in sensing whether appropriate growth factors and nutrients are present to allow for cell growth and division; loss of Rb fosters the evolution of hormone-resistant disease and may impair the response to radiation therapy

receptor: a docking site which interacts with a ligand; receptors may be on the cell membrane or within the cell cytoplasm or nucleus; estrogen receptors and androgen receptors are examples; all cells have multiple receptors

rectal exam: see digital rectal examination

rectoprostatic: the area between the prostate and its neighboring rectal wall

rectum adj. **rectal**: the final part of the intestines that ends at the anus

recurrence: the reappearance of disease; this can be manifested clinically as findings on the physical examination (e.g. DRE) or as a laboratory recurrence only (e.g. rise in PSA)

refractory: resistant to therapy; e.g., hormone refractory prostate cancer is resistant to forms of treatment involving hormone manipulation

regression: reduction in the size of a single tumor or reduction in the number and/or size of several tumors

remission: the real or apparent disappearance of some or all or the signs and symptoms of cancer; the period (temporary or permanent) during which a disease remains under control, without progressing; even complete remission does not necessarily indicate cure

renal: pertaining to the kidneys

resection: surgical removal

resectoscope: instrument inserted through the <u>urethra</u> and used by a <u>urologist</u> to cut out tissue (usually from the prostate) while the physician can actually see precisely where he is cutting

resistance: (in a medical sense) a patient's ability to fight off a disease as a result of the effectiveness of the patient's immune system

resorption: loss of bone through increased breakdown via <u>osteoclasts</u> or other mechanism causing a reduction in bone mass

response: a decrease in disease that occurs because of treatment; divided into complete response (remission) or partial response (remission)

retention: difficulty in initiation of urination or the inability to completely empty the <u>bladder</u>

reticuloendothelial: the widely diffused bodily system constituting all <u>phagocytic</u> cells except certain white blood cells

retinoid: derivatives of vitamin A used clinically in the treatment of severe acne and psoriasis; under investigation for treating cancer

rectoprostatic: the area between the prostate and its neighboring <u>rectal</u> wall

retropubic prostatectomy: surgical removal of the prostate through an incision in the <u>abdomen</u> above the pubic bones

retrospective: relating to a study (as of a disease) that starts with the present condition of a population of individuals and collects data about their past history to explain their present condition—compare to <u>prospective</u>

ribosome: A minute round particle composed of <u>RNA</u> and protein that is found in the <u>cytoplasm</u> of living cells and serves as the site of assembly for polypeptides encoded by messenger RNA

risk: the chance or probability that a particular event will or will not happen

risk factor: that which causes an individual or group of individuals to have an increased risk of a condition or disease

RNA (ribonucleic acid): found mostly in the cytoplasm of cells is important in the synthesis of proteins. It is a chain made up of subunits called nucleotides. Messenger RNA (mRNA) replicates the DNA code for a protein and moves to organelles (specialized cell structures) called ribosomes, which are themselves composed of protein and a type of RNA called ribosomal RNA (rRNA). At the ribosomes, transfer RNA (tRNA) assembles amino acids to form the protein specified by the messenger RNA.

robotic prostatectomy: a new minimally invasive type of surgery that features telemanipulation devices allowing the performance of complex surgical tasks with dexterity and minimal fatigue due to their ergonomic design. They also provide expanded degree of movements, tremor filtering, and 3-D stereoscopic visualization.

RP: see radical prostatectomy

RT-PCR: reverse transcriptase polymerase chain reaction; a technique which allows a physician to search for tiny quantities of a protein, such as PSA, in the blood or other body fluids and tissues; see RT-PCR PSA

RT-PCR PSA: reverse transcriptase-polymerase chain reaction; a blood test that detects micrometastatic cells circulating in the blood stream; may be useful as a screening tool to help avoid unnecessary invasive treatments (RP, RT, etc.) on patients with metastasized PC

Rx: standard abbreviation for medication prescribed

S

sagittal: a plane, slice or section of the body cutting from front to back through the sagittal suture of the skull, and continued down through the body in the same direction, dividing it into two parts

sagittal localizer: an anatomic image which is acquired quickly to provide information about how to select high resolution images of the organ of interest—specifically, the first imaging sequence acquired for a prostate MRI/MRSI exam to determine the proper placement of the endorectal coil and prescribe other images acquired during the exam

salvage: a procedure intended to "rescue" a patient following the failure of a prior treatment; for example, a salvage prostatectomy would be the surgical removal of the prostate after the failure of prior radiation therapy or cryosurgery

Sandostatin®: trade name for octreotide

SARM (selective androgen receptor modulator): a drug that selectively inhibits androgen receptors of a specific tissue(s) while allowing the normal interaction of the androgen with androgen receptors at other sites (see SERM)

saturation biopsy: a systematic biopsy using 3-D mapping to obtain thorough coverage of a half or the full prostate involving as many as 30-80 samples, depending on gland volume

saw palmetto: The dwarf palm plant indigenous to Florida that is the source of Serenoa repens and its lipid extract (lipido-sterol extract of *Serenoa repens* or LSESr) that is sometimes used for treating BPH; Shown to be ineffective in reducing voiding symptoms or PSA in a study sponsored by the NIH

SCF: stem cell factor

sclerotic: [tissue] hardened by causes like inflammation, mineral accumulation, etc.

screening: evaluating populations of people to diagnose disease early

scrotum: the pouch of skin containing a man's testicles

secondary to: derived from or consequent to a primary event or thing

secretion: 1. the process of secreting (releasing) a substance, especially one that is not a waste, from the blood or cells; 2. a substance, such as saliva, mucus, tears, bile, or a hormone, that is secreted

seed, seeding: brachytherapy; the implantation of radioactive seeds or pellets (may also be called "capsules") which emit low energy radiation in order to kill surrounding tissue, e.g., the prostate, including prostate cancer cells. Also known as "seed implantation" or "SI"

selenium: a relatively rare nonmetallic element found in food in small quantities that has some effect in prevention of prostate cancer

semen: the whitish, opaque fluid emitted by a male at ejaculation

seminal: related to the semen; for example, the seminal vesicles are structures at the base of the bladder and connected to the prostate that provide nutrients for the semen

seminal vesicles (SV): glandular structures located above and behind the prostate that secrete and store seminal fluid; the seminal vesicles connect with the ejaculatory ducts; the seminal fluid contains nutrients for the sperm that improves their viability and mobility

seminal vesicle invasion or **involvement (SVI)**: prostate cancer cells are found in the seminal vesicle(s)

senescence: the state of being old the process of becoming old

sensitivity: the probability that a diagnostic test can correctly identify the presence of a particular disease assuming the proper conduct of the test; specifically, the number of true positive results divided by the sum of the true positive results and the false negative results; see specificity

sequential androgen blockade (SAB): a variation of ADT involving a two-medication (anti-androgen plus a 5 alpha reductase inhibitor) approach intended to stop PC growth using androgen deprivation focused at the level of the tumor cell, while at the same time maintaining normal serum testosterone levels so that the sexual function will hopefully be preserved

Serenoa repens: the dwarf palm and source of the active herb used in saw palmetto preparations such as permixon and found in Peenuts®. Serenoa blocks various pathways in testosterone metabolism such as the conversion of testosterone to androstenedione as well as the conversion of testosterone to DHT; albeit controversial. By itself, Serenoa repens has been used in the treatment of LUTS.

SERM (selective estrogen receptor modulator): a drug that selectively blocks one estrogen receptor but allows the other receptors at specific sites to function normally with estrogen; raloxifene or toremifene is an example of a SERM—it blocks the ER in the breast and uterine tissue but allows the ER in bone tissue to be operative

seroma: a mass or swelling caused by the localized accumulation of serum within a tissue or organ

serotonin: neurotransmitter that relays impulses between nerve cells (neurons) in the central nervous system. Serotonin is involved in mood and behavior, physical coordination, appetite, body temperature, and sleep.

serous: of, relating to, producing, or resembling serum; especially : having a thin watery constitution

serum: any clear, watery fluid such as the pale yellow liquid that separates from the clot in the coagulation of blood

sex hormone binding globulin (SHBG): a protein that binds testosterone to make it unavailable for function; SHBG production is increased by estrogens such as DES. SHBG binds to DHT four times more avidly than to testosterone.

sextant: having six parts; thus, a sextant biopsy is a biopsy that takes six samples

SGOT: **serum glutamic-oxaloacetic transaminase**; a liver cell enzyme; elevation of SGOT is seen as an effect of liver cell injury by drugs, alcohol and viruses. Supplements such as silymarin, alpha lipoic acid and curcumin may protect and repair the liver cell and help reduce elevations of SGOT.

SGPT: **serum glutamic pyruvic transaminase**; a liver cell enzyme; elevation of SGOT is seen as an effect of liver cell injury by drugs, alcohol and viruses

SI: **seed implantation**; insertion of radioactive seeds, usually iodine 125 or palladium 103 into the prostate tissue to destroy prostate cancer (PC); see brachytherapy

side effect: a reaction to a medication or treatment (most commonly used to mean an unnecessary or undesirable effect)

sign: physical changes which can be observed as a consequence of an illness or disease

signal excitation: the excitation of signals using a strong magnetic field and radio frequency (RF) pulses to produce resonances or peaks due to water or other chemicals (metabolites) within tissue

sildenafil: the active ingredient of Viagra®, which may help to produce erections

sinusoidal: any of the venous cavities through which blood passes in various glands and organs, such as the adrenal gland and the liver

skeletal-related events: include bone fracture, spinal cord compression or the need for radiation or surgery for the treatment of bone metastasis

small cell PC: an aggressive variant of prostate cancer with a tendency to metastasize early due to rapidly dividing cells

sonogram, sonographic: an image of a structure that is produced by ultrasonography

spatial-resolution: a term that refers to the number of pixels utilized in construction of a digital image—images having higher spatial resolution have a greater number of pixels

specificity: the probability that a diagnostic test can correctly identify the absence of a particular disease assuming the proper conduct of the test; specifically, the number of true negative results divided by the sum of the true negative results and the false positive results;

a method that detects 95% of true PC cases is highly sensitive, but if it also falsely indicates that 40% of those who do not have PC do have PC then its specificity is only 60%; see sensitivity.

SPECT:(singlephotonemissioncomputedtomography)—Tomography using emissions from radionuclides and a computer algorithm to reconstruct the image. SPECT allows visualization of the body in slices from recalculated planar views of the patient.

spectroscopy: the science of measuring the emission and absorption of different wavelengths (spectra) of visible and non-visible light; a sequence noted in MRIS or MRSI scans

sperm: a male reproductive cell

spermidine: A polyamine compound, C7H19N3, found in ribosomes and living tissues and having various metabolic functions. It was originally isolated from semen

spermine: A crystalline polyamine compound, C10H26N4, present in ribosomes and found widely in living tissues along with spermidine. It was originally isolated from semen

sphincter: a muscle which surrounds, and by its contraction tends to close, a natural opening; as, the sphincter of the bladder

SPIO (spios): Small particles of Iron Oxide used to identify lymph node disease activity

stage: a term used to define the size and physical extent of a cancer

staging: the process of determining extent of disease in a specific patient in light of all available information; it is used to help determine appropriate therapy; there are two staging methods: the Whitmore-Jewett staging classification (1956) and the more detailed TNM (tumor, (lymph) nodes, metastases) classification (1992) of the American Joint Committee on Cancer and the International Union Against Cancer. Staging should be subcategorized as clinical staging and pathologic staging. Clinical stage is based on the digital rectal exam findings. Pathologic stage usually relates to what is found at the time of surgery. The TNM system is now most commonly used.

—TNM stages:

T Primary Tumor

TX: Primary tumor cannot be assessed

T0: No evidence of primary tumor

T1: Clinically inapparent tumor not palpable or visible by imaging

T1a: Tumor incidental <u>histologic</u> finding in > 5% of tissue resected via TURP

T1b: Tumor incidental histologic finding > 5% of tissue resected via TURP

T1c: Tumor identified by needle <u>biopsy</u> (e.g., because of elevated PSA)

T2: Tumor palpable but confined within the prostate

T2a: Tumor involves half of a lobe or less

T2b: Tumor involves more than half a lobe, but not both lobes

T2c: Tumor involves both lobes

T3: Tumor extends through the prostatic capsule

T3a: Unilateral extracapsular extension

T3b: Bilateral extracapsular extension

T3c: Tumor invades the <u>seminal vesicle</u>(s)

T4: Tumor is fixed or invades adjacent structures other than the seminal vesicles

T4a: Tumor invades any of bladder neck, external <u>sphincter</u> or <u>rectum</u>

T4b: Tumor invades levator muscles and/or is fixed to the <u>pelvic</u> wall

N Regional Lymph Nodes

NX: Regional lymph nodes cannot be assessed

N0: No regional lymph nodes metastasis

N1: Metastasis in a single lymph node, 2 cm or less in greatest dimension

N2: Metastasis in a single lymph node, more than 2 cm but not more than 5cm in greatest dimension; or multiple lymph node metastases, none more than 5 cm in greatest dimension

N3: Metastasis in a lymph node more than 5 cm in greatest dimension

M Distant Metastases

MX: Presence of distant metastasis cannot be assessed

M0: No distant metastasis

M1: Distant metastasis

M1a: Nonregional lymph node(s) M1b: Bone(s)

M1c: Other site(s)

-—**Whitmore-Jewett Stages**:

stage A is clinically undetectable <u>tumor</u> confined to the gland and is an incidental finding at prostate surgery.

A1: well-<u>differentiated</u> with focal involvement

A2: moderately or poorly differentiated or involves multiple foci in the gland

stage B is tumor confined to the prostate gland. B0: non-<u>palpable</u>, PSA-detected

B1: single nodule in one lobe of the prostate B2: more extensive involvement of one lobe or involvement of both lobes

stage C is a tumor clinically localized to the periprostatic area but extending through the prostatic <u>capsule</u>; seminal vesicles may be involved.

C1: <u>clinical extracapsular extension</u>

C2: extracapsular tumor producing bladder outlet or ureteral obstruction

stage D is <u>metastatic</u> disease.

D0: clinically localized disease (prostate only) but persistently elevated enzymatic serum acid phosphatase

D1: regional lymph nodes only

D2: distant lymph nodes, metastases to bone or visceral organs

D3: D2 prostate cancer patients who relapse after adequate endocrine therapy

stem cell: cell that has the ability to divide for indefinite periods in culture and to give rise to specialized cells; the ultimate stem cell might be a fertilized egg capable of producing the entire organism

stenosis: abnormal narrowing of a bodily canal or passageway

stent: a tube used by a surgeon to drain fluids

step-section histopathology: the sectioning of diseased tissues into ordered slices used for microscopic analysis

stepper: a motor (especially an electric motor) that moves or rotates in small discrete steps

steroid: any one of the hormones made in the outer layer of the adrenal glands (adrenal cortex)

stratified: In an analysis of data, a particular clinical or pathologic feature(s) is used as the basis for comparison, e.g. clinical stage, pathologic stage, PSA, Gleason score

stress incontinence: passing a small amount of urine when coughing, lifting, etc.

stricture: scarring as a result of a procedure or an injury that constricts the flow of a fluid; for example, a urethral stricture would restrict the flow of urine through the urethra

stroma: the supporting tissue of an organ

stromal BPH: a non-cancerous cause of prostate enlargement (BPH) within the connective tissue framework of the prostate

strontium-89: an injectable radioactive product that is used to relieve bone pain in some patients with prostate cancer that no longer responds to hormones or appropriate forms of chemotherapy

subcapsular: under the capsule; for example, a subcapsular orchiectomy is a form of castration in which the contents of each testicle is removed but the testicular capsules are then closed and remain in the scrotum

subcutaneous: located, found, or placed just beneath the skin

SUO: Society of Urologic Oncology

superficial : pertaining to or situated near the surface, especially relating to the skin

suprapubic: above the pubic bone; a suprapubic tube is placed into the <u>bladder</u> by puncturing the skin and soft tissue above the pubic bone

surgical margins: the outer edge of the tissue removed during surgery

suture: surgical stitching used in the closure of a cut or incision

SVI: see <u>seminal vesicle invasion</u>.

symptom: a feeling, sensation or experience associated with or resulting from a physical or mental disorder and noticeable by the patient

symptomatic: having symptoms, evidence of disease

synergistic: assists or adds to the activity of another substance, such as a drug

systematic biopsy: sampling of various sectors of the <u>prostate</u> under <u>ultrasound</u> guidance

systemic: throughout the whole body; affecting the entire body

Sx: an abbreviation for symptoms

T

T-cell: An immune-system cell that orchestrates an immune response to infected or <u>malignant</u> cells, sometimes by direct contact with the abnormal cells; T-cells are lymphocytes that develop in the <u>thymus</u> and circulate in the blood and lymphatic system; see <u>dendritic cell</u>.

T-score: a comparison of an individual's bone mass with the average bone mass of a young adult; a negative indicates a loss of bone density; see <u>osteopenia</u> and <u>osteoporosis</u>

T1a, T1b, T1c, T2a, T2b, T2c, T3a, T3b, T3c, T4: see <u>staging</u>

tamoxifen: the generic name for Nolvadex®; an anti—<u>estrogen</u> that works by blocking the <u>estrogen receptor</u> (ER) on the cell.

target capture: (genetics) a process that isolates the target nucleic acid from clinical specimens and purifies the nucleic acid for amplification

taxanes: anticancer drugs that inhibit cancer cell growth by stopping cell division. Includes paclitaxel and docetaxel.

Taxol®: the trade name for paclitaxel

Taxotere®: trade or brand name for docetaxel, a chemotherapy agent

TCAP: targeted cryoablation of the prostate

telemanipulation: the direct human control of a robotic manipulator, where the operator and the manipulator are at different locations

tesla: unit of measurement to describe magnetic field strength

testicle, adj. **testicular**: see testis

testis, pl. **testes**: one of two male reproductive glands located inside the scrotum that are the primary sources of the male hormone testosterone

testosterone (T): the male hormone or androgen which comprises most of the androgens in a man's body; chiefly produced by the testicles but also is derived from adrenal androgen precursors such as DHEA and androstenedione. T is highly important to a man's sexual interest or libido and his ability to achieve erection. T plays a key role in virtually every tissue in the human body e.g. brain, bone, blood formation, skin, nails, muscle.

testosterone inactivating pharmaceuticals (TIP): also known as androgen deprivation therapy (ADT) or hormone therapy.

tetraploid: having two times the normal amount of DNA or chromosomal material

TGF-b (transforming growth factor beta): a bone-derived growth factor that stimulates the PC cell and osteoblast, among many other functions

thalidomide: a drug that belongs to the family of drugs called angiogenesis inhibitors. It prevents the growth of new blood vessels into a solid tumor.

therapeutic: the treatment of disease or disability

therapeutic index: an index based on the ratio of <u>tumor</u> control probability (TCP) to normal tissue complication probability (NTCP) used in radiation therapy to assess the likelihood of effective treatment vs. the likelihood damage to surrounding tissues

therapy: the treatment of disease or disability

thermocouple: a thermoelectric device used to measure temperatures accurately

thermoluminescent dosimeter: A device that registers the radiation dose (energy per unit mass) indicated by changes in color induced by temperature change. A device that directly measures absorbed dose

thoracic: pertaining to or affecting the chest.

thrombocytopenia: a blood disorder in which there are not enough platelets. Platelets are cells in the blood that help blood to clot.

thromboembolism, thromboembolic: the blocking of a blood vessel by a blood clot dislodged from its site of origin

thrombosis: the formation or presence of a thrombus (a clot of coagulated blood attached at the site of its formation) in a blood vessel

thymus: a small glandular organ that is situated behind the top of the sternum (breastbone), consisting mainly of lymphatic tissue and serving as the site of <u>T cell</u> differentiation. The thymus increases gradually in size and activity until puberty, becoming <u>atrophic</u> thereafter

tibial: of or pertaining to a tibia (the larger bone of the lower leg)

tissue vascularity: the state at which a tissue circulates an adequate flow of liquid components such as blood and nutrients within its <u>vessels</u>

TNF-alpha: tumor necrosis factor alpha; a protein produced by <u>macrophages</u> in the presence of an <u>endotoxin</u> and shown experimentally to be capable of attacking and destroying cancerous <u>tumors</u>

TNM (tumor, nodes, metastases): see staging

tomography: a procedure where internal body images at a predetermined plane are recorded by means of the tomograph, a computer-driven device that builds the image from multiple X-ray measurements; tomography is used in CAT scan and PET scan

tomotherapy: Rotational radiotherapy delivery using an intensity-modulated fan beam. Intensity-modulated delivery is achieved by moving multiple collimator vanes into and out of the fan beam. The length of time that a leaf spends out of the beam is proportional to the intensity of radiation allowed through that particular portion of the beam

total PSA: the total of free PSA plus bound PSA

toxicity: the degree to which something is poisonous

transcription: (genetics) the synthesis of mRNA from a DNA template

transcription mediated amplification (TMA): a process that uses two enzymes, Reverse Transcriptase and RNA Polymerase, to produce billions of copies of RNA amplified target from the purified target nucleic acid

transducer: a substance or device that converts input energy of one form into another

transition zone: area of the prostate closest to the urethra which has features that distinguish it from the much larger peripheral zone

translation: (genetics) the process by which the mRNAcode is converted to a sequence of amino acids (a protein)

translational research: a sharing of information between laboratory research and patient care, often referred to as "from bench to bedside"

transperineal: through the perineum **transrectal**: through the rectum **transurethral**: through the urethra **transurethral resection (TUR)**: see TURP.

transverse: acting, lying, or being across : set crosswise

trastuzumab (Herceptin®): a type of monoclonal antibody which blocks the effects of the growth factor protein HER2, which transmits growth signals to cancer cells

treatment (Tx): administration of remedies to a patient for a disease

trimix, tri-mix: a mixture of papaverine, phentolamine and prostaglandin E-1 that is injected into the penis to cause an erection.

trophic: the starting of cell reproduction and enlargement by nurturing and causing growth

tropism: the movement of an organism in response to an external source of stimulus

true pelvis, true pelvic cavity: the lower more contracted part of the pelvic cavity

TRUS (transrectal ultrasound): a method that uses echoes of ultrasound waves (far beyond the hearing range) to image the prostate by inserting an ultrasound probe into the rectum; commonly used to visualize and guide prostate biopsy procedures

TRUSP: see TRUS

tumor: an excessive growth of cells caused by uncontrolled and disorderly cell replacement; an abnormal tissue growth that can be either benign or malignant; see benign, malignant

tumorigenesis, tumorigenic: the formation of tumors or tendency to form tumors

TURP (transurethral resection of the prostate): a surgical procedure to remove tissue obstructing the urethra; the technique involves the insertion of an instrument called a resectoscope into the penile urethra, and is intended to relieve obstruction of urine flow due to enlargement of the prostate

Tx: an abbreviation for treatment

tyrosine kinase: an enzyme involved in communication within cells, or signaling pathways

U

ultrasound (US): sound waves at a particular frequency (far beyond the hearing range) whose echoes bouncing off tissue can be used to image internal organs

understaging: the assignment of an overly low clinical stage at initial diagnosis because of the difficulty of assessing the available information with accuracy (e.g., stage T2b as opposed to stage T3b)

undetectable PSA (UDPSA): defined in our research as a PSA of <0.05 using a hypersensitive assay

unit: a blood-banking term for a pint of blood or plasma but can be used to quantitate other blood products such as platelets

uPA (urokinase-like plasminogen activator): a protease or digestive enzyme that is made by the PC cell, stimulates PC cell and osteoblast growth, and is involved with invasion and metastasis

uPM3 urine test: a new molecular test for detecting prostate cancer cells based on PCA3, a specific gene that is profusely expressed in prostate cancer tissue. Patients who receive the uPM3(TM) undergo a thorough digital rectal prostate examination by a urologist which causes cells from the patient's prostate to be shed into the urine.

up-regulation: the process of increasing the response to a stimulus

uptake: the absorption by a tissue of a substance, such as a nutrient, and its permanent or temporary retention

urea: the main nitrogen part of urine made from protein breakdown

uremia: the presence of excessive amounts of urea and other waste products in the blood, as occurs in kidney

ureter: an anatomical tube that drains urine from one of the two kidneys to the bladder

urethra: the tube that drains urine from the bladder through the prostate and out through the penis

urge incontinence: the need to urinate which is sudden and uncontrollable

urinary system: the group of organs and their interconnections that permits excess, filtered fluids to exit the body, including (in the male) the <u>kidneys</u>, the <u>ureters</u>, the <u>bladder</u>, the <u>urethra</u> and the <u>penis</u>

urinate: to discharge urine, a fluid produced by the <u>kidneys</u>

urodynamics: The mechanical laws of fluid dynamics as they apply to urine transport

urologist: a doctor trained first as a surgeon who specializes in disorders of the <u>genitourinary system</u>

uropathy: a disorder involving the <u>urinary</u> tract

UTI (urinary tract infection): an infection identifiable by the presence of bacteria (or theoretically viruses) in the urine; may be associated with fever or a burning sensation on urination

V

vacuum erection device (VED): a device that creates an erection with vacuum; it is usually a hard, plastic device placed over the <u>penis</u>; a vacuum is then created by a pump, bringing blood into the penis

vas deferens: tube through which <u>sperm</u> travel from the <u>testes</u> to the prostate prior to ejaculation

vascular: relating to a blood vessel

vasectomy: operation to make a man sterile by cutting the *vas deferens*, thus preventing passage of <u>sperm</u> from the <u>testes</u> to the prostate

vasoconstrictor: relating to a process, condition or substance that causes a narrowing of an opening of a blood vessel

vasodilator: a drug which cause blood vessels to expand, thereby increasing blood flow; vasodilators are used in Viagra® and other drugs (e.g., <u>trimix</u>) to cause erections

vasomotor: causing or regulating dilation or constriction of the blood vessels

VEGF (vascular endothelial growth factor): a substance known to stimulate blood vessel growth or <u>angiogenesis</u> and hence stimulate <u>tumor</u> growth

Veil of Aphrodite: a superficial membrane on the surface of the prostate critical for preservation of neurovascular bundle **venous**: of, relating to, or contained in the veins: e.g. *venous circulation*

vesicle: a small sac containing a biologically important fluid

vessel: a tube in which a body fluid circulates

vinblastine (trade name Velban®): periwinkle plant derivative used as an <u>antineoplastic</u> drug that disrupts cell division

visceral: relating to the internal organs of the body cavity

virus: ultramicroscopic infectious agent that replicates itself only within cells of living hosts; many are <u>pathogenic</u>; a piece of nucleic acid (<u>DNA</u> or RNA) wrapped in a thin coat of <u>protein</u>

voxels: three-dimensional pixels (volumes) which display spectral data that consist of a series of peaks at distinct frequencies for different chemicals (<u>metabolites</u>) within tissue.

W

watchful waiting (WW): active observation and regular monitoring of a patient without actual treatment; also called active objectified surveillance

WBC: white blood cell count; cells that are important to combating infection as well as being part of the immune system; comprised of granulocytes (neutrophils), lymphocytes and monocytes

WBC/HPF: white blood cells counted per high powered field during a microscopic evaluation

WHITMORE-JEWETT staging: see <u>staging</u>

wortmannin: a lipid-modifying <u>enzyme</u> that inhibits <u>PI3 kinase</u>

X

X-ray: a type of high energy radiation that can be used at low levels to make images of the internal structures of the body and at high levels for <u>radiation therapy</u>

xenograft: a graft of tissue taken from a donor of one species and grafted into a recipient of another species

Z

Zoladex®: trade or brand name for goserelin acetate, an <u>LHRH agonist</u>

<u>Special thanks is given to PCRI in recognition of the work they did to provide us with an excellent glossary of terminology relevant to this book while enhancing an improved understanding for the topic of prostate related disease!</u>

REFERENCES

Chapter 1

"Inflammation and Prostate Cancer" by S. Vasto, et al.: Future Oncology, 2008 Vol. 4, No. 5 pp. 637-45)

Greenlee RT, Harmon MB, Murray T et. al: Cancer Statistics, 2001. Journal Clinical Cancer, Vol. 51, 15-36, 2001American Cancer Society: Cancer Facts and Figures 2004. Atlanta, Georgia: American Cancer Society, Page 16-7, 2004

Chan JM, Jou RM, and Carroll PR.: The Relative Impact and Future Burden of Prostate Cancer (4th International Conference). Journal of Urology (supplement), Vol. 172, S13-S17, 2004

Fowler FJ, McNaughton-Collins M, Albertsen MS, et. al: Comparison of Recommendations by Urologists and Radiation Oncologists for Treatment of Clinically Localized Prostate Cancer. JAMA Vol. 283, No. 24, 3217-22, 2000

Tefilli MV, Gheiler EL, Tiguert R, etal. Should Gleason Score 7 Prostate Cancer Be Considered a Unique Grade Category? Urology, Vol. 53, 372-377, 1999

Lamb DJ and Zhang L: Challenges in Prostate Cancer Research: Animal Models for Nutritional Studies of Cehmoprevention and Disease Progression. Journal of Nutrition, Vol. 135 (12 Supplement), 3009S-3015S, 2005

Wolk A.: Diet, Lifestyle and Risk of Prostate Cancer. Acta Oncologica, Vol. 44, No. 3, 277-81, 2005

Walker M, Aronson KJ, King W, et. al: Dietary Patterns and Risk of Prostate Cancer in Ontario, Canada. International Journal of Cancer, Vol. 116, No. 4, 592-8, 2005

McCann SE, Ambrosone CB, Moysich KB, et. al: Intakes of Selected Nutrients, Foods, and Phytochemicals and Prostate Cancer Risk in Western New York: Nutrition and Cancer, Vol. 53, No. 1, 33-41, 2005

Cohen JH, Kristal AR and Stanford JL: Fruit and Vegetable Intake and Prostate Cancer Risk. Journal of the National Cancer Institute, Vol. 92, No. 1, 61-8, 2000

Michaud DS, Augustsson K, Rimm EB, et. al: A Prospective Study on Intake of Animal Products and Risk of Prostate Cancer. Cancer Causes and Control, Vol. 12, No. 6, 557-67, 2001

Cross AJ, Peters U, Kirsh VA, et. al: A Prospective Study of Meat and Meat Mutagens and Prostate Cancer Risk. Cancer Research, Vol. 65, No. 24, 11779-84, 2005

Mayer J: Prospective Studies of Dairy Product and Calcium Intakes and Prostate Cancer Risk: A Metaanalysis. Journal of the National Cancer Institute, Vol. 97, No. 23, 1768-77, 2005

Xu J, Thornburg T, et. al: Serum Levels of Phytanic Acid Are Associated With Prostate Cancer Risk. Prostate, Vol. 63, No. 3, 209-14, 2005

Dagnelio PC, Schuurman AG, Goldbohm RA and Van den Brandt PA: Diet, Anthropomorphic Measures and Prostate Cancer Risk: A Review of Prospective Cohort and Intervention Studies. British Journal of Urology International, Vol. 93, No. 8, 1139-50, 2004

Giovannucci E, Rimm EB, Colditz GA, et. al: A Prospective Study of Dietary Fat and Risk of Prostate Cancer. Journal of the National Cancer Institute, Vol. 85, No. 19, 1571-9, 1993

Mydlo, JH: The impact of Obesity in Urology. Urologic Clinics of North America, Vol. 31, No. 2, 275-8, 2004

Trichopoulou A, Lagiou P, Kuper H, and Trichopoulos D: Cancer and Mediterranean Dietary Traditions. Cancer, Epidemiology, Biomarkers and Prevention, Vol. 9, No. 9, 869-73, 2000

Chapter 2

Dixon C. Diagnosis and Treatment of Chronic Prostatitis. The Clinician's New Paradigm, Abbott Labs & Thomas R. Beam, Jr; Memorial Institute for CME, 1998.

Moon TD. Questionnaire Survey of Urologists and Primary Care Physicians' Diagnostic and Treatment Practices for Prostatitis: Urology 50:543-547, 1997. McNaughton-Collins M., Barry MJ: Epidemiology of Chronic Prostatitis, Current Opinion Urology 8:33-27, 1998.

Schapert SM: National Ambulatory Care Survey: 1991 Summary, National Center for Health Statistics. Vital Health Stat 13:1-84, 1994.

McNaughton-Collins M., Stafford RJ, Oleary MF ET.AL: How Common is Prostatitis? A National Survey of Physician Visits. Jurol.: 159:1224-1228, 1998.

Wheeler RE: Pilot Data: The Effectiveness of Antibiotics and an All Natural Formula on Prostatitis, Abstract, 1998.

Wenninger K, Heiman Jr, Rothman 1. ET AL: Sickness Impact of Chronic Non-Bacterial Prostatitis and its Correlates; J Urol.: 155: 965968, 1996.

Alexander RB, Trissel D: Chronic Prostatitis: Results of an Internet Survey; Urology 48:568-574, 1996

Wheeler RE.: The Incidence of Chronic Prostatitis in 235 Consecutive Adult Men with Voiding Symptoms, Abstract, 1999.

Nickel JC etal; Diagnosis and Treatment of Prostatitis in Canada Urology 52: 792-802, 1998

Kohnen PW, Drach GW: Patterns of inflammation in prostatic hyperplasia: A histologic and bacteriologic study. JUrol 121: 755-60, 1979.

Nelson WG, DeMarzo AM, DeWeese TL, etal. The Role of Inflammation in the Pathogenesis of prostate cancer. JUrol. Vol. 172, S6-S12, 2004.

Schaeffer AJ, Wendel EF, Dunn JK. etal. Prevalence and Significance of prostate inflammation. JUrol.125: 215, 1981.

Anderson RU, Weller C: Prostatic Secretion Leukocyte Studies in Non-bacterial Prostatitis. JUrol. 121: 292, 1979.

American Cancer Society: Cancer Facts & Figures, 2004. Atlanta, Ga. American Cancer Society, Page 16-17, 2004.

Knoops K, deGrout L, Kromhout D, etal. Mediterranean Diet, Lifestyle Factors, and 10-year Mortality in Elderly European Men and Women (The Hale Project). JAMA: Vol. 292, No.12, 1433-39, 2004.

Coley CM, Barry MJ, Mulley AG. Clinical Guideline: Part III, Screening for Prostate Cancer. AnnIntMed. 126: 480-84, 1997.

Rose DP, Connelly JM: Effects of Fatty Acids and Eicosanoid Synthesis Inhibitors on the Growth of Two Human Prostate Cancer Cell Lines. Prostate Vol. 18, 243-254, 1991

Chapter 3

Greenlee RT, Harmon MB, Murray T et. al: Cancer Statistics, 2001. Journal Clinical Cancer, Vol. 51, 15-36, 2001American Cancer Society: Cancer Facts and Figures 2004. Atlanta, Georgia: American Cancer Society, Page 16-7, 2004

Chan JM, Jou RM, and Carroll PR.: The Relative Impact and Future Burden of Prostate Cancer (4th International Conference). Journal of Urology (supplement), Vol. 172, S13-S17, 2004

Fowler FJ, McNaughton-Collins M, Albertsen MS, et. al: Comparison of Recommendations by Urologists and Radiation Oncologists for Treatment of Clinically Localized Prostate Cancer. JAMA Vol. 283, No. 24, 3217-22, 2000

Tefilli MV, Gheiler EL, Tiguert R, etal. Should Gleason Score 7 Prostate Cancer Be Considered a Unique Grade Category? Urology, Vol. 53, 372-377, 1999

Lamb DJ and Zhang L: Challenges in Prostate Cancer Research: Animal Models for Nutritional Studies of Cehmoprevention and Disease

Progression. Journal of Nutrition, Vol. 135 (12 Supplement), 3009S-3015S, 2005

Wolk A.: Diet, Lifestyle and Risk of Prostate Cancer. Acta Oncologica, Vol. 44, No. 3, 277-81, 2005

Walker M, Aronson KJ, King W, et. al: Dietary Patterns and Risk of Prostate Cancer in Ontario, Canada. International Journal of Cancer, Vol. 116, No. 4, 592-8, 2005

McCann SE, Ambrosone CB, Moysich KB, et. al: Intakes of Selected Nutrients, Foods, and Phytochemicals and Prostate Cancer Risk in Western New York: Nutrition and Cancer, Vol. 53, No. 1, 33-41, 2005

Cohen JH, Kristal AR and Stanford JL: Fruit and Vegetable Intake and Prostate Cancer Risk. Journal of the National Cancer Institute, Vol. 92, No. 1, 61-8, 2000

Michaud DS, Augustsson K, Rimm EB, et. al: A Prospective Study on Intake of Animal Products and Risk of Prostate Cancer. Cancer Causes and Control, Vol. 12, No. 6, 557-67, 2001

Cross AJ, Peters U, Kirsh VA, et. al: A Prospective Study of Meat and Meat Mutagens and Prostate Cancer Risk. Cancer Research, Vol. 65, No. 24, 11779-84, 2005

Mayer J: Prospective Studies of Dairy Product and Calcium Intakes and Prostate Cancer Risk: A Metaanalysis. Journal of the National Cancer Institute, Vol. 97, No. 23, 1768-77, 2005

Xu J, Thornburg T, et. al: Serum Levels of Phytanic Acid Are Associated With Prostate Cancer Risk. Prostate, Vol. 63, No. 3, 209-14, 2005

Dagnelio PC, Schuurman AG, Goldbohm RA and Van den Brandt PA: Diet, Anthropomorphic Measures and Prostate Cancer Risk: A Review of Prospective Cohort and Intervention Studies. British Journal of Urology International, Vol. 93, No. 8, 1139-50, 2004

Giovannucci E, Rimm EB, Colditz GA, et. al: A Prospective Study of Dietary Fat and Risk of Prostate Cancer. Journal of the National Cancer Institute, Vol. 85, No. 19, 1571-9, 1993

Mydlo, JH: The impact of Obesity in Urology. Urologic Clinics of North America, Vol. 31, No. 2, 275-8, 2004

Trichopoulou A, Lagiou P, Kuper H, and Trichopoulos D: Cancer and Mediterranean Dietary Traditions. Cancer, Epidemiology, Biomarkers and Prevention, Vol. 9, No. 9, 869-73, 2000

Chapter 4

Greenlee RT, Harmon MB, Murray T et. al: Cancer Statistics, 2001. Journal Clinical Cancer, Vol. 51, 15-36, 2001American Cancer Society: Cancer Facts and Figures 2004. Atlanta, Georgia: American Cancer Society, Page 16-7, 2004

Chan JM, Jou RM, and Carroll PR.: The Relative Impact and Future Burden of Prostate Cancer (4th International Conference). Journal of Urology (supplement), Vol. 172, S13-S17, 2004

Fowler FJ, McNaughton-Collins M, Albertsen MS, et. al: Comparison of Recommendations by Urologists and Radiation Oncologists for Treatment of Clinically Localized Prostate Cancer. JAMA Vol. 283, No. 24, 3217-22, 2000

Tefilli MV, Gheiler EL, Tiguert R, etal. Should Gleason Score 7 Prostate Cancer Be Considered a Unique Grade Category? Urology, Vol. 53, 372-377, 1999

Lamb DJ and Zhang L: Challenges in Prostate Cancer Research: Animal Models for Nutritional Studies of Cehmoprevention and Disease Progression. Journal of Nutrition, Vol. 135 (12 Supplement), 3009S-3015S, 2005

Wolk A.: Diet, Lifestyle and Risk of Prostate Cancer. Acta Oncologica, Vol. 44, No. 3, 277-81, 2005

Walker M, Aronson KJ, King W, et. al: Dietary Patterns and Risk of Prostate Cancer in Ontario, Canada. International Journal of Cancer, Vol. 116, No. 4, 592-8, 2005

McCann SE, Ambrosone CB, Moysich KB, et. al: Intakes of Selected Nutrients, Foods, and Phytochemicals and Prostate Cancer Risk in Western New York: Nutrition and Cancer, Vol. 53, No. 1, 33-41, 2005

Cohen JH, Kristal AR and Stanford JL: Fruit and Vegetable Intake and Prostate Cancer Risk. Journal of the National Cancer Institute, Vol. 92, No. 1, 61-8, 2000

Michaud DS, Augustsson K, Rimm EB, et. al: A Prospective Study on Intake of Animal Products and Risk of Prostate Cancer. Cancer Causes and Control, Vol. 12, No. 6, 557-67, 2001

Cross AJ, Peters U, Kirsh VA, et. al: A Prospective Study of Meat and Meat Mutagens and Prostate Cancer Risk. Cancer Research, Vol. 65, No. 24, 11779-84, 2005

Mayer J: Prospective Studies of Dairy Product and Calcium Intakes and Prostate Cancer Risk: A Metaanalysis. Journal of the National Cancer Institute, Vol. 97, No. 23, 1768-77, 2005

Xu J, Thornburg T, et. al: Serum Levels of Phytanic Acid Are Associated With Prostate Cancer Risk. Prostate, Vol. 63, No. 3, 209-14, 2005

Dagnelio PC, Schuurman AG, Goldbohm RA and Van den Brandt PA: Diet, Anthropomorphic Measures and Prostate Cancer Risk: A Review of Prospective Cohort and Intervention Studies. British Journal of Urology International, Vol. 93, No. 8, 1139-50, 2004

Giovannucci E, Rimm EB, Colditz GA, et. al: A Prospective Study of Dietary Fat and Risk of Prostate Cancer. Journal of the National Cancer Institute, Vol. 85, No. 19, 1571-9, 1993

Mydlo, JH: The impact of Obesity in Urology. Urologic Clinics of North America, Vol. 31, No. 2, 275-8, 2004

Trichopoulou A, Lagiou P, Kuper H, and Trichopoulos D: Cancer and Mediterranean Dietary Traditions. Cancer, Epidemiology, Biomarkers and Prevention, Vol. 9, No. 9, 869-73, 2000

Chapter 5

Greenlee RT, Harmon MB, Murray T et. al: Cancer Statistics, 2001. Journal Clinical Cancer, Vol. 51, 15-36, 2001American Cancer

Society: Cancer Facts and Figures 2004. Atlanta, Georgia: American Cancer Society, Page 16-7, 2004

Chan JM, Jou RM, and Carroll PR.: The Relative Impact and Future Burden of Prostate Cancer (4th International Conference). Journal of Urology (supplement), Vol. 172, S13-S17, 2004

Fowler FJ, McNaughton-Collins M, Albertsen MS, et. al: Comparison of Recommendations by Urologists and Radiation Oncologists for Treatment of Clinically Localized Prostate Cancer. JAMA Vol. 283, No. 24, 3217-22, 2000

Tefilli MV, Gheiler EL, Tiguert R, etal. Should Gleason Score 7 Prostate Cancer Be Considered a Unique Grade Category? Urology, Vol. 53, 372-377, 1999

Lamb DJ and Zhang L: Challenges in Prostate Cancer Research: Animal Models for Nutritional Studies of Cehmoprevention and Disease Progression. Journal of Nutrition, Vol. 135 (12 Supplement), 3009S-3015S, 2005

Wolk A.: Diet, Lifestyle and Risk of Prostate Cancer. Acta Oncologica, Vol. 44, No. 3, 277-81, 2005

Walker M, Aronson KJ, King W, et. al: Dietary Patterns and Risk of Prostate Cancer in Ontario, Canada. International Journal of Cancer, Vol. 116, No. 4, 592-8, 2005

McCann SE, Ambrosone CB, Moysich KB, et. al: Intakes of Selected Nutrients, Foods, and Phytochemicals and Prostate Cancer Risk in Western New York: Nutrition and Cancer, Vol. 53, No. 1, 33-41, 2005

Cohen JH, Kristal AR and Stanford JL: Fruit and Vegetable Intake and Prostate Cancer Risk. Journal of the National Cancer Institute, Vol. 92, No. 1, 61-8, 2000

Michaud DS, Augustsson K, Rimm EB, et. al: A Prospective Study on Intake of Animal Products and Risk of Prostate Cancer. Cancer Causes and Control, Vol. 12, No. 6, 557-67, 2001

Cross AJ, Peters U, Kirsh VA, et. al: A Prospective Study of Meat and Meat Mutagens and Prostate Cancer Risk. Cancer Research, Vol. 65, No. 24, 11779-84, 2005

Mayer J: Prospective Studies of Dairy Product and Calcium Intakes and Prostate Cancer Risk: A Metaanalysis. Journal of the National Cancer Institute, Vol. 97, No. 23, 1768-77, 2005

Xu J, Thornburg T, et. al: Serum Levels of Phytanic Acid Are Associated With Prostate Cancer Risk. Prostate, Vol. 63, No. 3, 209-14, 2005

Dagnelio PC, Schuurman AG, Goldbohm RA and Van den Brandt PA: Diet, Anthropomorphic Measures and Prostate Cancer Risk: A Review of Prospective Cohort and Intervention Studies. British Journal of Urology International, Vol. 93, No. 8, 1139-50, 2004

Giovannucci E, Rimm EB, Colditz GA, et. al: A Prospective Study of Dietary Fat and Risk of Prostate Cancer. Journal of the National Cancer Institute, Vol. 85, No. 19, 1571-9, 1993

Mydlo, JH: The impact of Obesity in Urology. Urologic Clinics of North America, Vol. 31, No. 2, 275-8, 2004

Trichopoulou A, Lagiou P, Kuper H, and Trichopoulos D: Cancer and Mediterranean Dietary Traditions. Cancer, Epidemiology, Biomarkers and Prevention, Vol. 9, No. 9, 869-73, 2000

Chapter 6

Koppie, T.M., Grady, B.P., Shinohara, K.: Rectal wall recurrence of prostatic adenocarcinoma. Journal of Urology, Vol. 168, 2120, November 2002

Moul, J.W., Bauer, J.J., Srivastava, S., colon, E., Ho, C.K., Sesterhenn, I.A. et. Al: Perineal seeding of prostate cancer as the only evidence of clinical recurrence 14 years after needle biopsy and radical prostatectomy: molecular correlation. Urology, 51: 158, 1998

Haddad, F.S. and Somsin, A.A.: Seeding and perineal implantation of prostatic cancer in the track of the biopsy needle: three case reports and a review of the literature, Journal Surgical Oncology, 35: 184, 1987

Bastacky, S.S., Walsh, P.C. and Epstein, J.I.: Needle biopsy associated tumor tracking of adenocarcinoma of the prostate. Journal of Urology, 145: 1003, 1991

Chapter 7

Gaylis, F.F., Lin, D.W., Ignatoff, J.M., Amling, C.L., et. al: Prostate cancer in men using testosterone supplementation. J Urol, 174: 534-538, 2005

Chan, J.M., Gann P.H., Giovannucci, E.L.: Role of diet in prostate cancer development and progression. J Clin Oncol, 23: 81, 42-60, 2005

Coussens, L.M., Werb, Z.: Inflammation and cancer. Nature, 420: 860-867, 2002

Margolis, S., Carter, H.B., Prostate disorders. The Johns Hopkins White Paper. Baltimore: Johns Hopkins, P 28, 2002

Nelson, W.G., DeMarzo, A.M., DeWeese, T.L., et. al: The role of inflammation in the pathogenesis of prostate cancer. J Urol, 172: S6-S12, 2004

American Association of Clinical Endocrinologists. Medical guidelines for clinical practice for the evaluation and treatment of hypogonadism in adult male patients. Endocr Pract, 8: 440-456, 2002

Ornish, D., Weidner, D, Fair, W.R., et. al: Intensive lifestyle changes may affect the progression of prostate cancer. J Urol, 174: 1065-1070, 2005

Mulligan, T., Frick, M.F., Zuraw, Q.C., et. al: Prevalence of hypogonadism in males aged at least 45 years: the HIM study. Int J Clin Pract, 60 (7): 762-769, 2006

Morales A, Heaton J.W.P., Carson C.C.; Andropause: A misnomer for a true clinical entity, Journal of Urology, 163: 705, 2000.

Loughlin, K.R., Richie, J.P.: Prostate cancer after exogenous testosterone treatment for impotence. J Urol, 157: 1845, 1997

Curran, M.J., Birhrle, W.: Dramatic rise in prostate specific antigen after androgen replacement in a hypogonadal man with occult adenocarcinoma of the prostate. Urology, 53: 423, 1999

Morentaler, A., Bruning, C.O., DeWolf, W.C.: Occult prostate cancer in men with low serum testosterone levels. JAMA, 275: 1904, 1996

Rhoden, E.L., Morgentaler, A.: Risks of testosterone replacement therapy and recommendations for monitoring. N Engl J Med, 350: 482, 2004

Bhasin, S., Singh, A.B., Mac, R.P., et. al: Managing the risks of prostate disease during testosterone replacement therapy in older men: recommendations for a standardized monitoring plan. J Androl, 24: 299, 2003

Livermore, C.T., Blazer, D.G.: Testosterone and aging: Clinical research directions. Institute of Medicine of the National Academies Press, 2004

Bhasin, S., Buckwalter, J.G.: Testosterone supplementation in older men: a rational idea whose time has not come yet. J Androl, 22: 718, 2001

Chapter 8

Gaylis, F.F., Lin, D.W., Ignatoff, J.M., Amling, C.L., et. al: Prostate cancer in men using testosterone supplementation. J Urol, 174: 534-538, 2005

Wheeler, R.E., Is it necessary to cure prostate cancer when it is possible? (understanding the role of prostate inflammation resolution to prostate cancer evolution). J Clin Interventions in Aging, 2 (1): 153-161, 2007

Chan, J.M., Gann P.H., Giovannucci, E.L.: Role of diet in prostate cancer development and progression. J Clin Oncol, 23: 81, 42-60, 2005

Coussens, L.M., Werb, Z.: Inflammation and cancer. Nature, 420: 860-867, 2002

Margolis, S., Carter, H.B., Prostate disorders. The Johns Hopkins White Paper. Baltimore: Johns Hopkins, P 28, 2002

Nelson, W.G., DeMarzo, A.M., DeWeese, T.L., et. al: The role of inflammation in the pathogenesis of prostate cancer. J Urol, 172: S6-S12, 2004

American Association of Clinical Endocrinologists. Medical guidelines for clinical practice for the evaluation and treatment of hypogonadism in adult male patients. Endocr Pract, 8: 440-456, 2002

Ornish, D., Weidner, D, Fair, W.R., et. al: Intensive lifestyle changes may affect the progression of prostate cancer. J Urol, 174: 1065-1070, 2005

Mulligan, T., Frick, M.F., Zuraw, Q.C., et. al: Prevalence of hypogonadism in males aged at least 45 years: the HIM study. Int J Clin Pract, 60 (7): 762-769, 2006

Loughlin, K.R., Richie, J.P.: Prostate cancer after exogenous testosterone treatment for impotence. J Urol, 157: 1845, 1997

Curran, M.J., Birhrle, W.: Dramatic rise in prostate specific antigen after androgen replacement in a hypogonadal man with occult adenocarcinoma of the prostate. Urology, 53: 423, 1999

Morgenthaler, A., Bruning, C.O., DeWolf, W.C.: Occult prostate cancer in men with low serum testosterone levels. JAMA, 275: 1904, 1996

Rhoden, E.L., Morgentaler, A.: Risks of testosterone replacement therapy and recommendations for monitoring. N Engl J Med, 350: 482, 2004

Bhasin, S., Singh, A.B., Mac, R.P., et. al: Managing the risks of prostate disease during testosterone replacement therapy in older men: recommendations for a standardized monitoring plan. J Androl, 24: 299, 2003

Livermore, C.T., Blazer, D.G.: Testosterone and aging: Clinical research directions. Institute of Medicine of the National Academies Press, 2004

Bhasin, S., Buckwalter, J.G.: Testosterone supplementation in older men: a rational idea whose time has not come yet. J Androl, 22: 718, 2001

Chapter 12

Jemal A, Siegel R, Ward E, et al. Cancer statistics, 2006. *CA Cancer J Clin.* Mar-Apr 2006;56(2):106-130.

Bostwick DG. Prospective origins of prostate carcinoma. Prostatic intraepithelial neoplasia and atypical adenomatous hyperplasia. *Cancer.* Jul 15 1996;78(2):330-336.

McNeal JE, Bostwick DG. Intraductal dysplasia: a premalignant lesion of the prostate. *Hum Pathol.* Jan 1986;17(1):64-71.

Bostwick DG, Brawer MK. Prostatic intra-epithelial neoplasia and early invasion in prostate cancer. *Cancer.* Feb 15 1987;59(4):788 794.

Ramos CG, Carvahal GF, et al. The effect of high-grade prostatic intraepithelial neoplasia on serum total and percentage of free prostate specific antigen levels. *J Urol.* Nov 1999; 162(5): 1587-1590.

Abbas F, Hochberg D, Civantos F, et al. Incidental prostatic adenocarcinoma in patients undergoing radical cystoprostatectomy for bladder cancer. *Eur Urol.* 1996;30(3):322-326.

Taneja SS, Smith MR, Dalton JT, et al. Toremifene—a promising therapy for the prevention of prostate cancer and complications of androgen deprivation therapy. *Expert Opin Investig Drugs.* Mar 2006;15(3):293-305.

Steiner MS, Pound CR. Phase IIA clinical trial to test the efficacy and safety of Toremifene in men with high-grade prostatic intraepithelial neoplasia. *Clin Prostate Cancer.* Jun 2003;2(1):24-31.

Alberts SR, Novotny PJ, Sloan JA, et al. Flutamide in Men with Prostatic Intraepithelial Neoplasia: A Randomized, Placebo Controlled Chemoprevention Trial. *Am J Ther.* July/August 2006;13(4):291-297.

Iczkowski KA, MacLennan GT, Bostwick DG. Atypical small acinar proliferation suspicious for malignancy in prostate needle biopsies: clinical significance in 33 cases. *Am J Surg Pathol.* 1997;21(12):1489-1495.

Iczkowski KA Current prostate biopsy interpretation: criteria for cancer asap, high-grade prostatic intraepithelial neoplasia, and use of immunostains. Arch Pathol Lab Med. 2006 Jun;130(6):835-43.

Brausi M, Castagnetti G, Dotti A, et al. Immediate radical prostatectomy in patients with atypical small acinar proliferation. Over treatment? *J Urol.* Sep 2004;172(3):906-908; discussion 908 909.

Cheng L, Koch MO, Juliar BE, et al. The combined percentage of Gleason patterns 4 and 5 is the best predictor of cancer progression after radical prostatectomy. J Clin Oncol 23:2911-2917, 2005.

Augustin H, Eggert T, Wenske S, et al. Comparison of accuracy between the Partin tables of 1997 and 2001 to predict final pathological stage in clinically localized prostate cancer. *J Urol.* Jan 2004;171(1):177-181.

Bostwick DG, Grignon DJ, Hammond ME, et al. Prognostic factors in prostate cancer. College of American Pathologists Consensus Statement 1999. *Arch Pathol Lab Med.* Jul 2000;124(7):995-1000.

Montironi R, Mazzuccheli R, Scarpelli M, et al. Gleason grading of prostate cancer in needle biopsies or radical prostatectomy specimens: contemporary approach, current clinical significance and sources of pathology discrepancies. *BJU Int.* Jun 2005;95(8):1146 1152.

Lopez-Beltran A, Mikuz G, Luque RJ, et al. Current practice of Gleason grading of prostate carcinoma. *Virchows Arch.* Nov 23 2005:1-8.

Oyama T, Allsbrook WC, Jr., Kurokawa K, et al. A comparison of interobserver reproducibility of Gleason grading of prostatic carcinoma in Japan and the United States. *Arch Pathol Lab Med.* Aug 2005;129(8):1004-1010.

Thompson CA. Finasteride may prevent prostate cancer. Am J Health Syst Pharm. 2003 Aug 1;60(15):1511.

Jacobsen SJ, Roberts RO. Re: Effect of nonsteroidal anti inflammatory agents and finasteride on prostate cancer risk. *J Urol.* May 2003;169(5):1798-1799.

Brawley OW. Hormonal prevention of prostate cancer. *Urol Oncol.* Jan-Feb 2003;21(1):67-72.

Lowe FC, McConnell JD, Hudson PB, et al. Long-term 6-year experience with finasteride in patients with benign prostatic hyperplasia. *Urology.* Apr 2003;61(4):791-796.

Vaughan D, Imperato-McGinley J, McConnell J, et al. Long-term (7 to 8-year) experience with finasteride in men with benign prostatic hyperplasia. *Urology.* Dec 2002;60(6):1040-1044.

Grignon DJ, Bostwick DG, Civantos F, et al. Pathologic handling and reporting of prostate tissue specimens in patients receiving neoadjuvant hormonal therapy: report of the Pathology Committee. *Mol Urol.* 1999; 3: 193—198.

Vailancourt L, Têtu B, Fradet Y, et al. Effect of neoadjuvant endocrine therapy (combined androgen blockade) on normal prostate and prostatic carcinoma. A randomized study. *Am J Surg Pathol.* Jan 1996;20(1):86-93.

Montironi R, Schulman CC. Pathological changes in prostate lesions after androgen manipulation. *J Clin Pathol.* Jan 1998;51(1):5-12.

Goldstein NS, Begin LR, Grody WW, et al. Minimal or no cancer in radical prostatectomy specimens. Report of 13 cases of the "vanishing cancer phenomenon". *Am J Surg Pathol.* Sep 1995;19(9):1002-1009.

Thompson IM, Coltman CA, Jr., Crowley J. Chemoprevention of prostate cancer: the Prostate Cancer Prevention Trial. *Prostate.* Nov 1 1997;33(3):217-221.

Thompson IM, Goodman PJ, Tangen CM, et al. The influence of finasteride on the development of prostate cancer. *N Engl J Med.* Jul 17 2003;349(3):215-224.

Andriole GL, Roehrborn C, Schulman C, et al. Effect of dutasteride on the detection of prostate cancer in men with benign prostatic hyperplasia. Urology. 2004 Sep;64(3):537-41; discussion 542-3.

Cheng L, Sebo TJ, Slezak J, et al. Predictors of survival for prostate carcinoma patients treated with salvage radical prostatectomy after radiation therapy. *Cancer.* Nov 15 1998;83(10):2164-2171.

Goldstein NS, Martinez A, Vicini F, et al. The histology of radiation therapy effect on prostate adenocarcinoma as assessed by needle biopsy after brachytherapy boost. Correlation with biochemical failure. *Am J Clin Pathol.* Dec 1998;110(6):765-775.

Burke HB, Qian J, Fitch W. PCA3: The Next Generation Molecular Test for Prostate Cancer. Submitted.

Ornstein DK, Tyson DR. Proteomics for the identification of new prostate cancer biomarkers. *Urol Oncol.* May-Jun 2006;24(3):231-236.

Chapter 13

Greenlee RT, Harmon MB, Murray T et. al: Cancer Statistics, 2001. Journal Clinical Cancer, Vol. 51, 15-36, 2001American Cancer Society: Cancer Facts and Figures 2004. Atlanta, Georgia: American Cancer Society, Page 16-7, 2004

Chan JM, Jou RM, and Carroll PR.: The Relative Impact and Future Burden of Prostate Cancer (4th International Conference). Journal of Urology (supplement), Vol. 172, S13-S17, 2004

Fowler FJ, McNaughton-Collins M, Albertsen MS, et. al: Comparison of Recommendations by Urologists and Radiation Oncologists for Treatment of Clinically Localized Prostate Cancer. JAMA Vol. 283, No. 24, 3217-22, 2000

Tefilli MV, Gheiler EL, Tiguert R, etal. Should Gleason Score 7 Prostate Cancer Be Considered a Unique Grade Category? Urology, Vol. 53, 372-377, 1999

Lamb DJ and Zhang L: Challenges in Prostate Cancer Research: Animal Models for Nutritional Studies of Cehmoprevention and Disease Progression. Journal of Nutrition, Vol. 135 (12 Supplement), 3009S-3015S, 2005

Wolk A.: Diet, Lifestyle and Risk of Prostate Cancer. Acta Oncologica, Vol. 44, No. 3, 277-81, 2005

Walker M, Aronson KJ, King W, et. al: Dietary Patterns and Risk of Prostate Cancer in Ontario, Canada. International Journal of Cancer, Vol. 116, No. 4, 592-8, 2005

McCann SE, Ambrosone CB, Moysich KB, et. al: Intakes of Selected Nutrients, Foods, and Phytochemicals and Prostate Cancer Risk in Western New York: Nutrition and Cancer, Vol. 53, No. 1, 33-41, 2005

Cohen JH, Kristal AR and Stanford JL: Fruit and Vegetable Intake and Prostate Cancer Risk. Journal of the National Cancer Institute, Vol. 92, No. 1, 61-8, 2000

Michaud DS, Augustsson K, Rimm EB, et. al: A Prospective Study on Intake of Animal Products and Risk of Prostate Cancer. Cancer Causes and Control, Vol. 12, No. 6, 557-67, 2001

Cross AJ, Peters U, Kirsh VA, et. al: A Prospective Study of Meat and Meat Mutagens and Prostate Cancer Risk. Cancer Research, Vol. 65, No. 24, 11779-84, 2005

Mayer J: Prospective Studies of Dairy Product and Calcium Intakes and Prostate Cancer Risk: A Metaanalysis. Journal of the National Cancer Institute, Vol. 97, No. 23, 1768-77, 2005

Xu J, Thornburg T, et. al: Serum Levels of Phytanic Acid Are Associated With Prostate Cancer Risk. Prostate, Vol. 63, No. 3, 209-14, 2005

Dagnelio PC, Schuurman AG, Goldbohm RA and Van den Brandt PA: Diet, Anthropomorphic Measures and Prostate Cancer Risk: A Review of Prospective Cohort and Intervention Studies. British Journal of Urology International, Vol. 93, No. 8, 1139-50, 2004

Giovannucci E, Rimm EB, Colditz GA, et. al: A Prospective Study of Dietary Fat and Risk of Prostate Cancer. Journal of the National Cancer Institute, Vol. 85, No. 19, 1571-9, 1993

Mydlo, JH: The impact of Obesity in Urology. Urologic Clinics of North America, Vol. 31, No. 2, 275-8, 2004

Trichopoulou A, Lagiou P, Kuper H, and Trichopoulos D: Cancer and Mediterranean Dietary Traditions. Cancer, Epidemiology, Biomarkers and Prevention, Vol. 9, No. 9, 869-73, 2000

Chapter 14

Blana A, Walter B, Rogenhofer S, Wieland WF, High-intensity focused ultrasound for the treatment of localized prostate cancer: 5-year experience Urology. 2004 Feb.; 63(2):297-300.

Chaussy C, Thüroff S. Results and side effects of high-intensity focused ultrasound in localized prostate cancer. J Endourol. 2001; 15:437-440.

Gelet A, Chapelon JY, Bouvier R, et al. Transrectal high-intensity focused ultrasound for the treatment of localized prostate cancer: Factors influencing the outcome. Eur Urol. 2001; 40:124-129.

Poissonnier L, gelet A, Chapelon JY, Bouvier R, Rouviere O, Pangaud C, Lyonnet

D, Dubernard JM. Results of transrectal-focused ultrasound for the treatment of localized prostate cancer (120 patients with PSA < or + 10ng/ml. Prog Urol. 2003 Feb.; 13(1):60-72.

Thüroff S, Chaussy C, Vallancien G, et al. High-intensity focused ultrasound and localized prostate cancer: Efficacy results from the European Multicentric study. J Endourol. 2003; 17:673-677.

Uchida T, Sanghvi NT, Gardner TA, et al. Transrectal high-intensity focused ultrasound for treatment of patients with stage T1b-2N0M0 localized prostate cancer: A preliminary report. Urology. 2002; 59:394-399.

Uchida T, Ohkusa H, Nagata Y, Hyodo T, Satoh T, Irie A. Treatment of localize Rewcastle, John, Ph.D.; Department of Radiology, University of Calgary, Alberta, Canada; (rewcastle@shaw.ca)

APPENDIX—1

ProCap Trial—A Prostate Cancer Prevention Trial

(Does Inflammation reduction Decrease Prostate Cancer risk?)

Date of Proposal: January 10, 2011

Format: Randomized, Double blind, Placebo Controlled, Age-Matched and PSA Matched

Trial Accrual: 500-1000 patients without evidence of prostate cancer will be randomly divided between the placebo and the active formula while being performed at multiple Veterans Administration Clinic States in Florida (actual number of entrants will depend upon a statistical analysis associated with the projected outcome that the study is powered to measure)

Trial Entry: Men aged 40-69 years old (three decades represented)

Trial Qualification:
- No evidence of prostate cancer based on digital rectal exam
- PSA must be ≥ 1 ng/ml, but ≤ 4 ng/ml to avoid a qualifying negative biopsy
- Men with a PSA of 4 ng/ml—9.9 ng/ml will also qualify if there is a preceding biopsy that validates a lack of cancer
- IPSS-Index (international Prostate Symptom Score Index)

Trial Variables:
1. Prostate-specific antigen (PSA) using Quest Diagnostics
2. Digital rectal exam
3. International Prostate Symptom Score Index (IPSS)
4. Biopsy specimens will be interpreted by pathologists who routinely evaluate biopsy specimens at the VA; **Second opinions will be sent to Bostwick laboratories under the auspices of David Bostwick, M.D.**

Frequency of Office Visits: Every six months (Evaluate and record all variables)

Study Trial Endpoint: Prostate cancer diagnosis

Length of study trial: 3-5 years is the anticipated time frame to reach statistical significance, albeit, 3 years is very realistic

Study Guideline: In the event that men evaluated note a change in PSA (velocity change) or digital rectal findings that support suspicion for prostate cancer, a prostate biopsy will be performed following a complete consented disclosure. In the event the biopsy is negative, the patient will be returned to the previously assigned treatment arm while a diagnosis of prostate cancer will prompt immediate termination options with subsequent implementation. The entirety of the study tenets represented will be usual and customary to the protocols normally practiced by urologists in a community setting.

Funding: Private resources are requested, albeit, this offering presents an opportunity to "Create a legacy" through a foundation donation or business opportunity

Premise: Prostate disease is the number one health risk that an adult male will face with 90 men dying daily from this menacing disease while a new case of prostate cancer is diagnosed every three minutes, according to the American Cancer Society. Based upon scientific data, it is believed that a worldwide patented prostate nutritional formula (Peenuts®) will provide a major health care benefit. Specifically, Peenuts® is expected to decrease the pool of prostate biopsy candidates based on eradication of prostatitis as a sentinel disease that many experts believe is associated with the evolution of prostate cancer, according to the American Association of Cancer Research, AACR. Improvement in prostatitis will be noted by a reduction in PSA (prostate-specific antigen), a surrogate marker for prostatitis. Therefore, it's believed that a reduction in prostatitis (a non-bacterial inflammatory condition) will lead to a decrease in the diagnosis of prostate cancer. To reiterate, the expectation is noted for the health care system to benefit through a reduction in unnecessary prostate biopsies associated with a reduction in PSA, improved patient health anticipated with improvement in voiding abilities, a reduction or resolution of signs and symptoms associated with inflammation as well as an ultimate decrease in the incidence of prostate cancer (validated by study design).

Background Data: Prostate disease is the number one health risk that men face associated with prostate enlargement (Benign Prostatic Hyperplasia, BPH), prostatitis (a non-bacterial inflammation of the prostate in greater than 95 percent of cases) and/or prostate cancer. All diseases of the prostate are epidemic individually and collectively. Fifty percent of 50-year-old men have evidence of BPH, while the signs and symptoms are the number one reason that men visit the doctor, according to McNaughton-Collins. Voiding symptoms common to BPH are also common to prostatitis. In a clinical trial presented at the National Institute of Health in 1999, 235 consecutive men with any level of voiding symptoms were evaluated clinically for prostatitis. Prostatitis was noted to be present in 81 percent of men less than 50 years old (n = 83) while 88 percent of men 50 years old or older (n= 152) were noted with the disease, according to the NIH Presentation, by Dr. Wheeler in 1999.

PSA (prostate-specific antigen) represents the most dominant male health disease marker associated with BPH, prostatitis, and prostate cancer. Data from Johns Hopkins, associated with the Baltimore Longitudinal Study, notes that men aged 40-60 years with a PSA reading of greater than 0.6-0.7 ng/ml have a three-four fold increased risk for prostate cancer within their subsequent 20 years. In a separate study, Gann and Hennekens noted a five to nine times increased risk for the evolution of an aggressive cancer within the subsequent 10 years when the PSA was identified between 2-4 ng/ml. It is further noted that 30 percent of 30-year-old men have prostate cancer, adding an inordinate amount of financial stress to an already beleaguered health care system, according to the Detroit Autopsy Study. While the search for novel, cost effective prostate cancer diagnostic and treatment models continues, the cost of needless prostate biopsies, based on the PSA blood test primarily, costs the United States health care system in excess of 2.2 billion dollars yearly. The most significant portion of these costs would likely be eliminated by the resolution of prostatitis with the subsequent decrease in PSA. Prostatitis is the number one reason that PSA rises and arguably the prime culprit in why men are asked to undergo a prostate biopsy. Minimizing the impact of prostatitis would promote a quantum shift in health care expenditure to the cost savings side as the majority of the 70-80 percent of the negative biopsies could be avoided. Additionally, as prostatitis is resolved, annoying symptoms that prompt men to visit the doctor may also be eliminated.

A proposed prostate cancer prevention trial (**the ProCap Trial**) comparing a patented, synergistic blend of natural ingredients for the prostate versus a placebo in a randomized, double blind, age-matched study is expected to alter the landscape of disease understanding. Peenuts®, a prostate nutritional formula was chosen for study consideration based on its worldwide *patent status* and effectiveness in reduction of signs and symptoms associated with prostatitis reported through clinical evaluation referencing the recently published research study, entitled, **"*Is it necessary to cure prostate cancer when it is possible?*"** Peenuts®, a synergistic blend of vitamins, minerals, herbs and amino acids is associated with anti-inflammatories, immune boosters, antioxidants and beta sitosterols. Peenuts® has been validated previously to reduce voiding symptoms in a randomized, placebo controlled, double blind study. The study findings were statistically significant. Reasons for enhanced academic excitement is furthered by the published results of the prospective study mentioned above, evaluating the benefit of the Peenuts® formula with diet in men with known prostate cancer. At an average of 38.5 months, prostate cancer is suppressed in 87 percent of the study participants. This is a sentinel finding as it demonstrates that man can now safely live with prostate cancer similarly to living with rheumatoid arthritis, diabetes or hypertension. The overall effect on the health care budget could be monumental as 50-60 percent of men with prostate cancer have cancer characteristics (Gleason Score) similar to the men studied in this prospective trial.

The ability of nutritional ingredients to have an impact in the evolution of prostate cancer is well chronicled in the literature through the Alpha-tocopherol, Beta-carotene (ATBC-Finnish Study) and through the work of Larry Clark, Ph.D. at the University of Arizona who evaluated the benefit of Selenium on prostate cancer. Specifically, Vitamin E (50 IU) daily was noted to decrease the incidence of prostate cancer by 34 percent while Selenium (200 mcg) was noted to decrease the incidence of prostate cancer by 66 percent, respectively. Notwithstanding the premature termination of an NCI (National Cancer Institute) study intended to evaluate the benefit of the aforementioned Selenium and Vitamin E in prostate cancer prevention, the Peenuts® formula works by reducing inflammation in the prostate. This data has enabled patents to be issued internationally in recognition of formula excellence.

To state further, it is felt that based on the fact that Peenuts® formula can suppress and/or stabilize all cases of prostate cancer in the prospective study, it may be possible for this formula to prevent prostate cancer. The mechanism of action with the Peenuts® formula is believed to be associated with the resolution of non-bacterial prostatitis through a decrease in cellular oxidative stress. Beyond an expected decrease in anxiety as the PSA decreases, inflammation is decreased as noted by a comparative analysis of the expressed prostatic secretion with a predictable decrease in white blood cells as well as an improvement in voiding symptoms; the expected number of doctor visits is expected to drop.

While the health care budget is strained due in part to the diagnosis and treatment of prostate cancer, the ability to prevent prostate cancer gives men and improved opportunity to extend their quality of life while saving the health care system hundreds of millions of dollars, if not, billions. Beyond the expected prevention of prostate cancer (the ultimate goal of the study), the number of biopsies requested is expected to drop precipitously with an anticipated decrease in PSA level with the Peenuts® formula when compared to placebo. Presently, in excess of 2.2 billion dollars are spent yearly on prostate biopsy with the majority of procedures performed based on an elevation of PSA only. Despite our best efforts, only 20-30 percent of biopsies yield a cancer, suggesting our current model for biopsy consideration qualifies men excessively and inappropriately. None of this is surprising when it is noted that PSA elevation is more commonly associated with inflammation than prostate cancer.

A paradigm shift to an improved health care model for men has been proposed. This study is about . . . more than altering a disease course . . . it is about altering or eliminating the number one health risk for every adult male while ensuring a healthy, more productive society. The only remaining challenge is to locate the financial commitment to fund the study. Finding a person(s) or organization to embrace this noble project remains difficult despite an anticipated outcome that promises to tame an epidemic and foster wellness for all men.

Ronald E. Wheeler, M.D.
Medical Director of the Diagnostic Center for Disease™

NOTES:

APPENDIX—2

Incidence of initial local therapy among men with lower-risk prostate cancer in the United States

Miller DC, Gruber SB, Hollenbeck BK, Montie JE, Wei JT
Department of Urology, University of Michigan, Ann Arbor,
MI, USA

BACKGROUND: THE FREQUENTLY indolent nature of early-stage prostate cancer in older men and in men with low—or moderate-grade tumors and the demonstration that the survival benefits of radical prostatectomy are primarily among men younger than 65 years have led to **concerns about prostate cancer overtreatment**. METHODS: Using data from 13 Surveillance, Epidemiology and End Results registries, we performed a retrospective cohort study of 71,602 men who were diagnosed with localized or regional prostate cancer between 2000 and 2002. We quantified the incidence of initial curative therapy (i.e., surgery or radiation therapy) among men with lower-risk cancers as defined by their limited likelihood of either dying from expectantly managed prostate cancer or achieving a survival benefit from local therapy. Stratified analyses and multinomial logistic regression models were used to quantify the absolute and relative rates of curative therapy among men in various age-grade strata. All statistical tests were two-sided. RESULTS: We identified 24,405 men with lower-risk prostate cancers and complete data for the first course of treatment. Initial curative therapy was undertaken in 13,537 of these men (55 percent); 81 percent of treated men received radiation therapy. The likelihood of curative therapy, relative to expectant management, varied statistically significantly among lower-management and is appropriate for all lower-risk cancers. 2,564 men (10 percent) of this population-based sample were over treated with radical prostatectomy and 10,973 (45 percent) with radiation therapy. CONCLUSIONS: This data quantifies a target population for whom greater use of expectant approaches may reduce overtreatment and improve the quality of localized prostate cancer care.

APPENDIX—3

New European Study Confirms Effectiveness of PSA Test

~Prostate cancer deaths cut by up to 31 percent and unnecessary biopsies by 33 percent~

NEW DATA FROM the European Randomized Study of Screening for Prostate Cancer (ERSPC) shows the PSA test reduces prostate cancer deaths by as much as 31 percent.

ERSPC also announced yesterday a new research study showing biopsies could be reduced by as much as 33 percent. This is based on physicians adhering to a PSA test cut-off level of 3 ng/ml. Other factors that must be taken into account include: the patient's age, prostate size, digital rectal exam and ultrasound test results.

"This new ERSPC research provides scientifically-based data to show that taking the PSA test can save your life," said ZERO's CEO Skip Lockwood. "The PSA test is as important to men as a mammogram is to women. Everyone has the right to know if they have cancer."

The new ERSPC findings, shown online in the January 2010 issue of *European Urology*, should provide a better guide to assist doctors in providing an appropriate level of care for their patients, Lockwood said.

"The PSA test is not to blame—it's what the physician decides to do following the PSA test," he said. "Some doctors are too quick to pull the trigger by providing additional medical care such as biopsies that prove to be unnecessary."

"We all know that over-diagnosis is a common trait of mammograms, PSA tests and other health care screening tools, and it should be emphasized that **the real issue is over-treatment of prostate cancer, resulting from the over zealously performed biopsies on far too many men as noted by ERSPC."**

ERSPC is the world's largest randomized screening trail on prostate cancer, consisting of more than 162,000 men in seven European countries who were followed over a 17-year period. Preliminary ERSPC findings earlier this year (*New England Journal of Medicine*, March 2009) noted that PSA testing produced a 20 percent reduction in prostate cancer deaths.

This latest ERSPC analysis, which scrubs out data contamination issues and concentrates only on men who were actually PSA tests, shows up to a 31 percent reduction in prostate cancer deaths.

Contamination issues, such as non-participants; being counted or control group members inadvertently receiving the PSA test, make it difficult to measure effectiveness. Contamination is one of the reasons why a smaller prostate cancer screening study—known as the Prostate, Lung, Colorectal and Ovarian (PLCO) study—has failed to show any reduction in prostate cancer deaths.

Dr. Wheeler's Commentary:

In a couple of words . . . I concur!!!!

NOTES:

APPENDIX—4

Dr. Wheeler's Commentary to US Preventive Services Task Force (USPSTF)

~Article regarding PSA Testing for Older Men~

THE POLICY STATEMENT by the U.S. Preventive Services Task Force (USPSTF) to stop PSA testing in men age 75 or older recently published is counter-intuitive to health and sends the wrong message. Men who commonly live into their late 80s or 90s should be encouraged to obtain accurate laboratory tests to allow the best personal health decisions to be made. It is not immortality that we seek to protect but rather quality of life and peace of mind as we age. It is for this reason that the debate whether or not to perform PSA testing must stop. **The question should not be whether to get a PSA but rather what to do with the PSA number once obtained.** I do not disagree with the USPSTF commentary that suggests with sufficient certainty that "The risk of being harmed exceeded potential benefits starting at age 75. I believe these concerns are understated for men of all ages. Ultimately, the PSA conundrum centers on an overly aggressively interpretation and application of PSA by family physicians and urologists alike, resulting in unnecessary biopsies. An egregious misappropriation of medical common sense can be demonstrated by one of my recent case reviews, featuring an 81-year-old gentleman who was scheduled for a radical prostatectomy despite a Gleason score of 10 and a PSA value of 29. **Not only do prediction tables address the unlikely scenario of organ confinement, a successful outcome cannot be achieved in this patient.** Using data from Dr. Michael Barry at Harvard, assuming success in removal of the prostate in this individual, a week or two more of life is all that would be achieved. Clearly, the benefit does not outweigh the risk in this individual, while inviting criticism to a profession that should know better.

On the other hand, to ignore PSA would be comparable to regarding blood pressure, pulse, temperature and cholesterol levels as meaningless. Obviously, this makes no sense. PSA is a well-known and accepted prostate disease marker. Rather than react to an elevated PSA with a biopsy, it would be far more prudent to treat non-bacterial Prostatitis ("prostate inflammation"); the number one reason PSA elevates. In this regard, PSA serves as a "barometer of prostate health," rather than a clarion for the coming of prostate cancer. The inability to lower PSA with conservative measures better suggests biopsy, if at all, as a secondary response.

In a recent Pilot study, the failure to decrease the PSA to less than 4 ng/ml in 12 months, with a nutritional Prostatitis formula (Peenuts®) resulted in 90 percent of these men ultimately being diagnosed with prostate cancer, as confirmed with biopsy. In other words, the majority of men who responded to this nutritional approach with a lower PSA were spared a needless and intrusive biopsy. **This allows us to do for a disease what is required and nothing more.** Implementation of such a protocol would be economically favorable and be a quantum leap above the usual 20-30 percent yield for cancer, when biopsies are randomly performed as a primary response to an elevated PSA. This logical strategy would save the health care system hundreds of millions of dollars over time.

Beyond what has been stated, it is important to note that disease starts early. In this regard, an educated older generation should become better qualified to teach younger men the value of prostate health. Memorial Sloan-Kettering and the Detroit Autopsy Study have shown that 30 percent of 30-year-old men have prostate cancer, generally unrecognized until later in life. It is, therefore, our obligation as professionals to delay the onset of disease, if not prevent it, whenever possible. Efforts to reverse the progression of prostate disease with a strategy of addressing Prostatitis, plus lifestyle changes, promises to have a positive impact for present and future generations to come. **Let's not "throw out the baby with the bath water" and minimize the importance of PSA testing to the number one health risk men face.**

References:

Barry MJ, PSA screening for prostate cancer: The current controversy—a viewpoint. Annals of Oncology, 9: 1279-1282, 1998

APPENDIX—5

Adult Urology

Change in Prostate-Specific Antigen Following Androgen Stimulation is an Independent Predictor of Prostate Cancer Diagnosis

Robert S. Svatek, Michael J. Shulman, Elie A. Benaim, Thomas E. Rogers and Vitaly Margulis
Departments of Urology and Pathology (TER), Dallas Veterans Administration Hospital, University of Texas Southwestern Medical Center at Dallas, Dallas, Texas

Purpose

We tested the hypothesis that a single exogenous androgen injection in men with low prostate-specific antigen would provoke a differential specific antigen response that would correlate with the presence and volume of cancer at biopsy.

Materials and Methods

Following institutional review board approval, 40 men with prostate-specific antigen between 2.5 and 4 ng/ml were given one intramuscular injection of 400 mg testosterone cypionate at the start of the study. Prostate specific antigen and early morning serum testosterone were measured at baseline, 48 hours, and weeks one, two and four. All men underwent 12-core transrectal ultrasound guided biopsy at week four.

Results

Of the 40 men, 18 (45 percent) were diagnosed with prostate cancer. The mean change in prostate specific antigen from baseline to four weeks was 3.1 to 3.4 ng/ml (9.7 percent) in men found to have benign findings on biopsy compared to a mean increase of 2.9 to 3.8 ng/ml (29 percent) in those with prostate cancer (p = 0.006). **The change in prostate-specific antigen following androgen stimulation was significantly associated with the percent of involved with cancer and it was an independent predictor of cancer diagnosis on univariate and multivariate analysis.**

Conclusions

An increase in prostate-specific antigen following androgen stimulation in men with prostate specific antigen between 2.5 and 4 ng/ml was highly predictive of the subsequent diagnosis of prostate cancer and it correlated with disease volume. If these findings are corroborated, prostate-specific antigen provocation may become an important strategy to identify men at risk for harboring prostate cancer and minimize the number undergoing unnecessary biopsies.

Dr. Wheeler's Commentary:

I have always maintained that Testosterone supplementation or replacement therapy associated with a rising PSA is pathognomonic for the diagnosis of prostate cancer. This study does nothing to alter that opinion!

Key Words: prostate; prostate-specific antigen; androgen; prostatic neoplasms; biopsy

Abbreviations: PSA, prostate specific antigen

APPENDIX—6

Men's Health is in Chaos

"Failure to establish health among men is driven by a lack of vision, a lack of intellectual curiosity, a lack of common sense, and greed"

HARVEY S IS a 67-year-old African-American male who like so many other males is concerned about prostate cancer. While his risk for prostate cancer was enhanced based on race, he also had a family history of prostate cancer in an uncle and an elevated PSA. Since 2004, Harvey has had five negative prostate biopsy sessions prompted by PSA values that have ranged from 8.5 to 18.89 ng/ml. Despite every effort made by the urology staff at the Veteran's Administration Facility to find cancer, none of the needle cores ever produced a cancer. Based on the frustration and futility of trying to find a cancer and the perceived health risk to the patient of not finding an occult disease that may end his life prematurely, the treating urologist suggested to the patient that it was time to try a new diagnostic technology being utilized in Sarasota, Fla. at the Diagnostic Center for Disease™ (DCD). The DCD uses a 3.0 Tesla Magnetic Resonance Imaging scanner that predictably locates prostate cancer when present. Historically for more than 20 years, radiologists had not been able to achieve sufficient success with a scanner that had half the imaging resolution (a 1.5 T Magnet) of the aforementioned

3 T magnet, thereby precluding urologists the opportunity to embrace diagnostic imaging as a complement to "blind biopsies." While a 20-30 percent yield for prostate cancer is not something to be proud of, urologists have been dependent on this ancient and inexact art form for more than 50 years. Based on the fact that men have not demanded more, doctors have not been obliged to provide more to an apathetic, yet unwitting population. The modus operandi has been the status quo. What had been passed from one generation to another was that if prostate cancer was to be diagnosed, random biopsies represented the "gold standard" or standard of care. **Who has the right to declare a 20-30 percent yield for prostate cancer as a "gold standard, much less a standard of care?"**

Following the advice of his trusted physician, Harvey made an appointment for the 3 T MRI scan at the DCD. Based on concern that a prostate cancer was growing, consistent with a PSA value in excess of 18, the patient was put on an anti-androgen to suppress what was suspected to be an occult cancer. **The PSA responded to the anti-androgen by decreasing to less than 2 consistent with a marked suppression of the disease, giving our team a chance to evaluate the entirety of the prostate without the added anxiety of a cancerous process out of control.** The scan showed regions of interest bilaterally while the most dominant region of interest was evident on the left side of the prostate in the mid-base portion of the peripheral zone. Despite an offer to the VA doctor to target the area in question with another set of biopsy needles, the patient was directed to go to the Diagnostic Center for Disease™ for a targeted biopsy based on their collective expertise in merging MRI image findings with ultrasound. While sepsis prevention measures were put in place with a course of antibiotics and needle tracking was precluded with an anti-androgen, six targeted biopsies were performed. The biopsy specimens were sent to Bostwick Laboratories for an independent analysis. Biopsies targeted to the region(s) of interest discovered the presence of prostate cancer in the left mid-prostate and the left mid-base of the prostate corresponding to the exact location of the cancer identified on the 3 T MRI scan.

In a 2 billion dollar a year industry, more than a million men like Harvey are told during a 12-month span they need a biopsy secondary to a rising or elevated PSA blood test. Unlike other diseased organs where imaging is always the first test performed before a biopsy is recommended, urologists have become complacent and overly secure in their ability to preferentially place invasive needles blindly into an organ without any real accountability. **It is unconscionable to allow physicians to continue to perform and perpetuate an art form practiced by their forefathers with minimal outside objection or criticism when the risks to the patient are so significant.** While it is beyond the scope of this article to discuss the perils of biopsy including the potential spread of cancer cells beyond the capsule, we must generate an academic enthusiasm and curiosity within the specialty of urology that will allow all urologists to appreciate why blind random biopsies can never be a standard with which to be proud.

In another, equally profound case, **Phil M**, a 67-year-old gentleman from Cincinnati, Ohio came to the DCD with a PSA value of 7.5 ng/ml. All totaled, four previous negative biopsies were performed over a six-year span with the highest PSA value being 10.5 in 2002. The standard operating procedure of the Department of Urology at the University of Cincinnati Medical School is and forever shall be; **"random biopsies will be performed routinely when we suspect the presence of prostate cancer based on an elevated PSA. Imaging of the prostate does not have a place in the diagnosis of prostate cancer."** This was the statement from the Chairman of Urology at the University of Cincinnati Medical School. From my urologic perspective, this language represents arrogant and egregious rhetoric. This level of bravado is inconsistent with a practice pattern that routinely shows an inability to make a diagnosis with blind biopsies. In this case, the 3 T MRI scan isolated the cancer on the left side in the mid-prostate. Fortunately for the Urology Chairman in question, a knowledgeable radiologist was available to assist and isolate the prostate lesion for him based on the previously performed scan at the Diagnostic Center for Disease™. The subsequent targeted biopsy guided by MRI imaging revealed a Gleason score of 6, enabling this patient to finally make appropriate, albeit delayed, arrangements regarding treatment.

In yet another case of futility, **Tom C**, a 62-year-old gentleman from Florida was trying to qualify for a study whereby a new and exciting prostate cancer treatment procedure called high-intensity focused ultrasound (HIFU) would be made available to him at no charge once a current biopsy (less than 2 months old) reconfirmed the presence of prostate cancer. Historically, cancer had been detected by his urologist three years prior on the left and right sides using the random biopsy technique. In an effort to accommodate his patient, a 12 core biopsy session was carried out absent any interest in viewing a 3 T MRI scan that had confirmed the presence of cancer with organ confinement only six months earlier. **Ironically, the result of the 12 core random biopsy performed by the original Urologist failed to identify the cancer he had originally diagnosed previously. The weakness in our diagnostic abilities becomes blatantly obvious for all to see as we can now appreciate the predicted epitome of futility and lack of skill set associated with a blind biopsy.** To compound this embarrassment, the inability to confirm cancer prevents the patient from entering a clinical trial in an attempt to cure his cancer. In this case his only option is a saturation biopsy (upwards of 30-40 additional cores or more) or an image-guided biopsy at the DCD.

How long will society tolerate this type of behavior? How many men need to be exposed to this guessing game before a conscientious effort is made to study the benefit of imaging versus random biopsies in earnest? How long do we need to continue to spend billions of dollars per year on an obsolete diagnostic exercise that requires little to no skill? Haven't we already proven the futility of the blind biopsy procedure based on a paltry 20-30 percent yield of cancer with random biopsies? I can't be the only physician who sees the lack of medical common sense in random biopsies. There is a reason we image first and foremost at the DCD. When the location of a lesion is identified consistent with disease, then and only then, is there a predictable opportunity to hit the target. **Institutions of higher learning like Memorial Sloan-Kettering, the Medical School at Cincinnati and organizations like the American Urology Association must bear some responsibility in the gamesmanship of trying to protect the turf of urologists.** Due to a lack of vision and/or intellectual curiosity; urologists will continue to routinely miss upwards of 35-50 percent of prostate cancers using traditionally rooted blind biopsies; due in part to a reluctance to understand and accept 3 T MRI scanning with or without Spectroscopy scanning as the next greatest diagnostic test. Furthermore, **acceptance of defined obsolescence as represented by a blind biopsy prompts a more extensive and equally traumatic diagnostic process of fiscal and ethical consequence.** This is troubling data for any public health model and an issue of significant social and professional concern to say the least. Combined with Dr. Michael Karin's startling research at the University of California at San Diego that notes prostate biopsies actually increase the likelihood of metastasis while stimulating the growth of prostate cancer through mutation of up-regulated inflammatory cells, patients will be asked to pay the ultimate price of professional ignorance and the status quo.

APPENDIX—7

Patient questionnaire response: Prostate Biopsy Exposed

First & Last Name Chieko Higuchi
City Mililani
State HI

"My husband just had a prostate biopsy done in the doctor's office which resulted in him having an E Coli infection. The E Coli bacterium was resistant to the Cipro (an antibiotic, also known as Ciprofloxacin) that he took before the biopsy. On top of that, my husband has diabetes and the E Coli made his blood sugar go sky high (almost 300) and sky rocketed his blood pressure, putting him into a semi-conscious state requiring admission to the hospital with a high fever and chills. His blood cultures were positive for E Coli to no one's surprise. Please let urologists in the State of Hawaii know of your MRI procedure in an effort to prevent another male from getting what my husband contracted. He was in the hospital for more than 10 days trying to rid himself of the E Coli blood infection."

Dr. Wheeler's Commentary: What happened to this man is all too common with prostate biopsies, while in my opinion underreported! A recent medical article cited the prostate biopsy procedure associated with an increasing risk of antibiotic resistant sepsis. **In layman's terms, the antibiotic no longer works versus the common bowel bacteria in question.** Doctors collectively are concerned for the future of prostate biopsy because of the increasing tendency for bacterial resistance. To be sure, this patient could have died as did a Neurosurgeon from London, England who came to Johns Hopkins in the summer of 2010 to have a biopsy performed associated with an elevated PSA. In the case at John's Hopkins, biopsies were carried out and the patient became septic (high fever, chills and rigors) and died! Imaging with MRI and treatment without a biopsy would have allowed this patient an improved opportunity for success, while avoiding death. While I don't know whether the patient truly had prostate cancer or not; he only had a 20-30% chance for cancer based on a PSA value of less than 10.0. In this case, the patient paid the ultimate price with his life; trying to live another day without the threat of cancer. All I can hope is that we have learned something from both cases discussed above. Unfortunately, in a 2 Billion dollar per year business, I do not think we have. **All patients must fully understand that imaging (with MRI) will one day be the 'standard of care' and standard of excellence for the diagnosis of prostate cancer.**

APPENDIX—8

From: MarkSchoenberg in a letter to Dr. Wheeler (unedited)
markschoenberg@internationalhifu.com
Date: Wed, Mar 23, 2011 6:56 p.m.

Dr. Wheeler,

The following is a notice to you and your staff that the selection criteria, as determined by the Medical Review Committee of International HIFU, LLC (the Company), for patients who are to be treated for prostate cancer using **Sonablate 500 devices** (Sonablate HIFU) **owned by the Company** must have written evidence or certification that **(1)** the patient received a prostate biopsy during the 12 months prior to the treatment date and **(2)** that biopsy demonstrated histologically confirmed prostate malignancy. **The diagnosis of prostate cancer by imaging alone will no longer constitute adequate preoperative evaluation for a patient to undergo Sonablate HIFU; and patients diagnosed on the basis of modalities other than biopsy will not be scheduled to receive Sonablate HIFU after May 1, 2011.**

Please let me know if you or your staff has questions regarding these criteria.

Regards,
Mark Schoenberg, MD
Chief Medical Officer
USHIFU
801 E. Morehead St.
Suite 202

Charlotte, NC 28202
Primary: 386-748-0497
Secondary: 443-928-8093

Dr. Wheeler's commentary:
You may ask yourself why I put a Policy letter from
International HIFU into this book. The reason this letter is
included is because patients need to understand the politics
taking place behind the scenes and how the decisions made by
invested parties could affect your future with a diseased prostate.
To state preferentially, International HIFU is a manufacturer
of a device called the Sonablate 500. This is a technology that
produces High Intensity Focused Ultrasound energy utilized
for BPH (benign prostatic hyperplasia) and prostate cancer
currently; outside of the USA. HIFU technology is utilized
commonly and currently in the USA to treat Uterine Fibroids in
women; a benign or non-malignant condition! **International
HIFU's Medical Director, Mark Schoenberg, M.D stated that
all patients undergoing treatment with the Sonablate 500
technology had to have a biopsy proven cancer, prior to
treatment. He may have a best practice pattern or scenario
for the technology's use, but should have no authority
to dictate to treating Urologists across the USA on how to
utilize this therapy when performed outside this country
or inside this country once FDA approved.** It is the treating
physician who must decide how this therapy should be utilized;
no one else! Dr. Schoenberg's comments appear to be coming
from the 'bully pulpit' whereby he is trying to influence doctors
preferentially to his way of thinking! From my perspective, this
is very odd, irregular and unacceptable behavior! Moreover,
Dr. Schoenberg has no professional experience with the HIFU
technology from which to draw his conclusion, relevant to a
prostate biopsy or imaging! Dr. Schoenberg, as Medical Director

of the company, has effectively influenced many unwitting and inexperienced physicians to his point of view. By making his **proclamation; that as of May 1, 2011 all men who undergo the HIFU procedure had to have a biopsy proving prostate cancer,** Dr. Schoenberg has ignored the fact that HIFU is utilized for benign disease in women and approved in the USA by the FDA for this purpose. Additionally, Dr. Schoenberg is trying to influence treating physicians to obtain biopsies when he knows full well; there is a risk to the patient for spreading cancer cells through the process of **'needle tracking', associated with the biopsy.** This statement is referenced in the **Journal of Urology, November 2002** principally and other resources available to Dr. Schoenberg! Because of his intellectual posturing, he is also unceremoniously dismissing the diagnostic ability of physician clinical judgment to make the diagnosis of prostate cancer while negating the abilities of imaging through MRI with or without Spectroscopy to make this call.

To be sure, **Dr. Schoenberg should not have the authority to tell any doctor how to treat prostate cancer; regardless of the technology used! Patients who choose to be treated with the Sonablate 500 Technology after May 1, 2011 have been forced and/or coerced mentally by treating physicians, and Dr. Schoenberg's dictum, to accept whatever the fate that 'needle tracking' will bring to them years after the biopsy and a subsequent HIFU procedure.**

It should be noted that prior to May 1, 2011; International HIFU's position on biopsy was not in place, articulated in print and/or enforced. This allowed treating physician's prior to May 1, 2011 to decide with their patients what represented the best diagnostic and treatment strategy. **By insisting now, that doctors performing the Sonablate 500 HIFU procedure must qualify their patients (by biopsy) ignores the safety issues of biopsy, which in effect enhances patient risk in**

the diagnostic and treatment processes. To be sure, there is a reason that 40-60% of men fail to be cured by 7-10 years! 'Needle tracking' commonly associated with a biopsy is at the top of the list of potential causative procedures.

Rather than accept what Dr. Schoenberg has said without discussion or hesitation, patients need to know there is an alternative to the Sonablate 500 HIFU model. The alternative HIFU procedure is **Ablatherm®**, the more venerable and studied procedure, manufactured and trademarked by EDAP, the world leader in HIFU technology, based on the total successful procedures performed. **To learn more, interested men are encouraged to understand the perils of the biopsy issue as well as the advantages of imaging to cancer recognition. Additionally, men are encouraged to contact our office to discuss the needle tracking issue with our advocacy staff as well as the advantages of the patient friendly and totally robotic Ablatherm® technology. Using this approach, patients will have the opportunity to avoid a biopsy with a high likelihood for cure without the need to bear the scars of ignorance and persuasion.**

The Literature speaks volumes regarding the value of MRSI or MRIS to the Diagnostic Evaluation

In September, 2011 an important question was raised in an online Urology News posting by *Medscape*[i]. Author Greg Freiherr examined the implications of using a powerful noninvasive diagnostic imaging technique called proton MR spectroscopy, or MRS, to distinguish cancerous tissue from healthy tissue. **This topic is of interest within the prostate cancer community, as some patients believe that the MRS replaces the more invasive prostate needle biopsy.** Essentially, Freiherr confronted this issue, asking if an imaging tool can both identify cancerous cells and adequately characterize them.

The author points out that certain types of cancer manifest unique "fingerprints" or biochemical signatures. The cancer cells have cellular metabolites that show up in MRS images as "spectral peaks" that can be compared to the way nearby healthy tissues show up. With the proper technology, this type of analysis adds less than 15 minutes to a standard MRI (Magnetic Resonance Imaging) exam.

MRS is promising in diagnosing prostate cancer, which has a "distinct signature of reduced citrate and elevated choline," writes Freiherr. In fact, an 8-center clinical trial correlated MRS images with tissue from surgically removed prostates, validating that the MRS images had correctly distinguished between cancerous and noncancerous tissues[1]

Dr. Wheeler's Commentary: Maybe Dr. Schoenberg should review this article also! We the people with the disease can only hope so! Jurgen Futterer and others have correlated biopsies statistically to imaging, thereby, validating the diagnostic protocol scientifically.

APPENDIX—9

Unintended Deception—
Observations by Dr. Wheeler

THE PROSTATE CANCER Symposium sponsored by the American Society of Clinical Oncology (ASCO) in 2006 presented data that showed a survival advantage for men who underwent definitive treatment for prostate cancer when compared to men in a "Watchful Waiting" group. The research presented by Dr. Wong from Fox Chase Cancer Center in Philadelphia was intended to show that men with prostate cancer who underwent definitive surgery or radiation had a survival advantage when compared to men who were minimizing their disease anxiety through watchful waiting. **This study made national news despite the inherent bias associated with patient selection.** Heretofore, men who ignore the disease treatment usually do so based on their overall health. If we examine the facts, a group of men too old or too sick or both with prostate cancer or other disease(s) were spared definitive therapy because they were too old or too sick or both to endure definitive therapy or it was obvious there would be little to no benefit relevant to their life expectancy. While the observations from the Fox Chase research were not consistent with a fair analysis of scientifically relevant data, to state the outcomes as beneficial is misleading, if not fraudulent. Their analysis hardly seems like an observation worthy of reporting to local colleagues, much less, a national audience of healthcare providers at a major Prostate Cancer Symposium, sponsored by ASCO. That stated, there is nothing news worthy as the better candidates by virtue of a better health status received definitive treatment while the more infirmed were watched. The observational data noted that most men aged 65 years or older received radiation while a smaller percentage received either surgery or watchful waiting. My question . . . why is this news? **Notwithstanding the lack of scientific rigor, wouldn't we expect a definitive treatment to outperform doing nothing?** Since when does anyone get excited from data that should be obvious to most of us? The truth is, there are studies that debate the survival advantages and therefore the comparison can be made, albeit, not scientifically. **The analysis by Dr. Wong and colleagues is observational only and should not have been presented to the news media as the observations mean little.** Men who read about this study are now questioning whether they are doing the right thing by being conservative when a three-year difference in the time of death is factored into the debate. In this case, the observational study merely muddies the water and heightens the anxiety and confusion regarding what to do when prostate cancer is encountered in an older population. If men were minimally randomized, the outcomes would have meant something. Additional data that would have improved the analysis of the outcome data would be to match the patients for age, disease co-morbidity, PSA (prostate-specific antigen), Gleason Score and stage of disease. Before the Radiation Oncologists and Surgeons get too excited by the small margin of victory versus doing nothing in a meaningless biased observational exercise, I would propose that men in this age group consider a program of Chronic Disease Management (CDM) versus radiation or surgery. CDM is a strategy of active surveillance that treats patients with diet, nutrition, exercise, stress reduction and education while protecting quality of life issues. Patients in this group will receive a protocol that is proactive including the use of diet, nutrition and/or intermittent hormonal manipulation dictated by PSA rise and disease status. Not surprisingly, many patients in this age range can suppress or stabilize their disease with diet and nutrition only. This was presented at this meeting as well but received no press coverage. When compared to radiation or surgery, CDM patients maintain potency and urinary continence associated with validation of disease stabilization as judged by PSA reduction or lack of elevation. I trust my friends at Fox Chase or any institution around this great country of ours should consider my challenge. The results will truly be newsworthy as men will be shown to live at least as long if not longer with Chronic Disease Management while avoiding the inherent side effect profile common to radiation or surgery.

APPENDIX—10

Endorectal MRI found valuable prior to salvage RP

NEW YORK—ENDORECTAL MAGNETIC resonance imaging can be used prior to salvage prostatectomy to identify tumor sites and show extracapsular extension and seminal vesicle invasion with "reasonable accuracy," say investigators from Memorial Sloan-Kettering Cancer Center.

However, interobserver variability and limited sensitivity to predict seminal vesicle invasion, both of which were observed in the Sloan-Kettering study, are reasons to proceed with caution, according to one urologist.

The study consisted of 45 consecutive patients who underwent salvage radical prostatectomy at Sloan-Kettering over a period of almost six years. Patients, who ranged in age from 43 to 76 years, all had failed radiation treatments and underwent endorectal MRI before surgery.

"In clinical practice, it has been generally accepted that MRI was of limited use in these patients," said study co-author Oguz Akin, MD, assistant professor of radiology.

Indeed, previous research had shown that irradiated tissue was difficult to image in this manner.

In this current study, published in *Radiology* (2006), primary radiation treatments among the 45 patients had included external beam radiation therapy, brachytherapy, and combined therapy. Seventeen of the patients also received chemotherapy or hormonal therapy before salvage prostatectomy.

Patients had to be otherwise healthy, with a life-expectancy of at least 10 years, along with having a locally-confined, biopsy-determined recurrence of cancer and no evidence of metastasis.

Two radiologists at Memorial Sloan-Kettering independently read MR images for tumor localization and determination of local stage. Their individual interpretations were then compared with pathologic findings from surgical specimens, and inter-rater variability was estimated with the kappa statistic.

Areas under the receiver operating characteristic curve (AUCs) were used to determine the accuracy of endorectal MRI in tumor detection and determination of extracapsular extension and seminal vesicle invasion AUCs—all with 95 percent confidence interval—were:

* Tumor detection: Reader 1, **0.75**; Reader 2, **0.61**
* Prediction of extracapsular extension: Reader 1, **0.87**; Reader 2, **0.72**
* Prediction of seminal vesicle invasion: Reader 1, **0.76**; Reader 2, **0.70**

Dr. Akin said that endorectal MRIs are now commonly used with these patients at Sloan-Kettering.

"Training in prostate cancer MR imaging and experience is necessary for accurate evaluation," he said.

Raj Pruthi, MD, director of urologic oncology at the University of North Carolina, Chapel Hill, expressed concern over the potential for significant variability among those reading MR images.

"This is a study performed by a group with tremendous experience and expertise in prostate MRI," Dr. Pruthi said. "One concern is that the application of endorectal MRI before salvage radical prostatectomy is subject to significant interobserver variability, as reported by the authors even when performed within the same institution by such a highly skilled group.

"The concern is that such variability in interpretation is likely to be even more substantial when this technique is compared between different institutions and by different radiologists with varying experience."

Dr. Pruthi had also hoped that endorectal MRI could aid in surgical planning by, for example, predicting seminal vesicle invasion.

"Unfortunately, the sensitivity to predict invasion was limited to this study: only 38 percent to 62 percent," he said.

Dr. Wheeler's Commentary:

Dr. Pruthi accurately points out the variability in interpretation from doctor to doctor of MRI results. The most important factor in assessment of the prostate is the experience of the radiologist. In my opinion, doctors who review prostate MRI images must review dozens of cases with clinical and pathologic feedback before they can qualify to review a scan accurately. Courses are available at major teaching institutions like UCSF and Sloan-Kettering for doctors with interest in the topic. There are significant sequences to the diagnosis that must be performed in association with minimally 2 mm slices. **Prostate MRI interpretation requires a unique skill set that takes years of experience to develop associated with a steady state high volume of cases and oversight from the true industry experts!**

APPENDIX—11

Robotic High-intensity Focused Ultrasound for Prostate Cancer: What Have We Learned in 15 Years of Clinical Use?

Christian G. Chaussy & Stefan F. Thüroff
Springer Science+Business Media, LLC 2011

ABSTRACT HIGH-INTENSITY FOCUSED ultrasound (HIFU) is an emerging, noninvasive, local treatment of prostate cancer with 15 years of clinical experience, during which about 30,000 HIFU treatments have been performed worldwide. In this paper we review relevant publications regarding the means by which new and old prostate cancer technologies are evaluated, the outcomes of HIFU by Ablatherm (EDAP TMS, Lyon, France), and the evolution currently underway regarding how prostate cancer is diagnosed and treated. We show the potential of HIFU utilized as a local therapy for men with any stage of prostate cancer and how this additional therapeutic option can fit within the future armamentarium of a sequential multimodality therapeutic concept.

Keywords—High-intensity focused ultrasound. HIFU. Prostate cancer. Localized prostate cancer. Advanced prostatic cancer.

Focal therapy. Immune response. Transurethral resection of the prostate. TURP. Combination therapy

Introduction

Currently, on average, men live almost 4 years longer and prostate cancer is diagnosed 10 years earlier compared to 25 years ago [1, 2].This means that the therapeutic necessity is more than double the time than it was then. None of the classical therapies is effective enough to cover this time frame as a monotherapy without a significant risk of aggressive recurrence during these years. Therefore, new concepts of multimodal and sequential therapies have to be introduced to cover the time effectively to maintain the patient's quality of life (QOL). One of these new therapeutic modalities may be the treatment of prostate cancer with high-intensity focused ultrasound (HIFU).

This review evaluates what we have learned in 15 years of clinical development by focusing on significant and relevant publications that have appeared in the past few years. The focus also covers ongoing clinical research and development in all possible indications and tumor stages of prostate cancer.

During the past 15 years, over 30,000 prostate HIFU treatments have been performed, mainly in Europe, but also throughout the world, including the United States (under an investigational device–exemption protocol, approved by the US Food and Drug Administration). In 2010, two transrectal HIFU devices are on the market (Ablatherm [EDAPTMS, Lyon, France] and Sonablate [Misonix, Inc., Farmingdale, NY]), differing significantly in technology, installed units, number of treatments performed, scientific evaluation, and publications. Data received by one device cannot be pooled with the other. The authors' personal experiences and data are based on the Ablatherm technology.

Method

HIFU is a single-session therapy in spinal anesthesia with a duration of 2 to 3 hours. It is accomplished by placing a probe that contains a curved piezoelectric crystal and a transrectal ultrasound (TRUS) scanner into the rectum. This probe collects emitted ultrasound beams at a focal point. The applicators' intrarectal position is controlled and corrected automatically on time according to a treatment plan, ensuring highest intraoperative precision of the applied ultrasound.

Physically, HIFU tissue ablation occurs via two modes of action: thermal and mechanical. The thermal effect is a temperature increase as the ultrasound energy is absorbed into the tissue and converted into heat. The resulting temperature increase and the geometry within this increase depend on the shape and size of the crystal, the amount of energy (ultrasound frequency and intensity) focused on the point, the applicators' movement algorithm, power settings, and the thermal capacity of the tissue itself. When sufficient temperature increase occurs ($> 80°C$) over a sufficient duration of time (> 4 seconds), irreversible tissue damage through coagulative necrosis results. Mechanically, a negative pressure imparted on the tissue by the ultrasound wave causes bubbles to form inside the cells, which increase in size to the point at which resonance is achieved. Sudden collapse of these bubbles results in a very high pressure (20,000–30,000 bars), which damages cells. The primary single lesions are small (1.7×19–26 mm), are applied side by-side, and produce reproducible volumes of sharply demarcated ablation. During the clinical procedure, due to the steep temperature gradient between the tissue in the focus, the surrounding tissue-sensitive adjacent structures, namely the rectum, external sphincter, and the neurovascular bundles, are not compromised [3, 4].

High-intensity Focused Ultrasound in Localized Prostate Cancer

Diagnosis of prostate cancer was based on the histopathological examination of biopsies in cases of suspicious prostate specific antigen (PSA), digital rectal examination, magnetic resonance imaging, or transrectal ultrasound (TRUS) or unexpected findings in resected tissue after open adenomectomy, holmium, or transurethral resection. The group of "localized prostate cancers" contains three subgroups of patients: primary localized, incidental, and mono-focal prostate cancer.

Primary Localized Prostate Cancer

Several reports of HIFU as a primary treatment of localized prostate cancer have emerged (Table 1). Blana et al. [12] reported multicenter results from 140 patients (T1-2, PSA < 15 ng/mL, Gleason ≤7) treated in Germany and France with HIFU and followed for a minimum of 5 years. The negative biopsy rate was 86.4% and the biochemical disease–free rates were 77% at 5 years and 69% at 7 years. Blana et al. [13•] also reported an 8-year experience of 163 patients in Germany (T1-2, N0M0, PSA ≤20 ng/mL, Gleason ≤7) followed for 4.8±1.2 years and observed a 5-year biochemical survival rate of 75%. More recently, Crouzet et al. [14] reported a multicenter analysis consisting of 803 patients from six French centers followed for 42 ±33 months. They observed 5—and 7-year biochemical survivals according to the Phoenix definition of 83% and 75%, respectively, for the low-risk group and 72% and 63%, respectively, for the intermediate-risk group. The negative biopsy rate for the low—and intermediate-risk groups were 84.9% and 73.5%, respectively. **They also observed 8-year overall, metastasis-free, and cancer specific survivals of 89%, 97%, and 99%, respectively.** Comparing to radiation therapy outcomes, Crouzet et al. [14] concluded that primary

HIFU outcomes are at least equivalent to radiation therapy. This is a very reasonable conclusion. It also is reasonable to extend this conclusion to the outcomes of radical prostatectomy as well when one considers the 2008 report of 5277 men who underwent prostate cancer treatment in the United States and were tracked in the CaPSURE (Cancer of the Prostate Strategic Urological Research Endeavor) database [15]. Recurrence occurred in 587 of the 935 men (63%) who underwent external-beam radiation therapy (XRT) at a mean time of 38 months after treatment. Of the 4342 men who underwent prostatectomy, 1590 (30%) failed at a mean of 34 months.

Incidental Prostate Cancer

Histological examination shows prostate cancer in up to 8% of patients who undergo adenomectomy/holmium-laser enucleation or transurethral resection of the prostate (TURP) because of symptomatic benign prostatic hyperplasia. Consequently, these patients need a therapeutic approach for their prostate cancer. We offered these patients HIFU as a local therapy and analyzed efficacy and side effects since 2000 [16].

Overall, 65 patients with incidental prostate cancer at an age of 70 years (57–87 y) have been treated. Initial PSA was 4.9 ng/mL (1–32 ng/mL) and prostate volume was 39 mL (16–130 mL), and 20 g (1–95 g) had been resected. Histology showed 5% (5%–50%) positive chips and a Gleason of 5 (3–9). Patients were treated completely with transrectal HIFU (robotic Ablatherm-integrated imaging) in spinal anesthesia in a single session. In follow-up, PSA nadir of 0.07 ng/mL (0–3.67 ng/mL) was measured after 1.8 months (0.7–5.9 mo), including 62% with PSA less than 0.1 ng/mL and 81% with PSA less than 0.5 ng/mL. A median PSA of 0.13 ng/mL (0–8.3 ng/mL) equivalent to a median PSA velocity of 0.01 ng/mL/y was found after a mean follow-up of 48 months (3–110 mo). Intra-operative and postoperative side effects were minimal (Clavien classification: < 15% I–III). **Long-term follow-up showed 45% of secondary obstructions caused by necrotic tissue or bladder neck stenosis.** Other long-term side effects were mild: intermediate grade I urinary stress incontinence was found in 11% (no Grade II or III stress incontinence), and UTI in 14%. There was no cancer-specific mortality. The PSA nadir of 0.07 ng/mL and the PSA velocity of 0.01 ng/mL/year indicate that HIFU can be used as a curative therapy for patients with incidental prostate cancer. These results show that the psychological burden of these patients, who are confronted either with untreated cancer disease in cases of "wait and see" or with fear of side effects in cases of radical surgery or radiation, can be avoided by this noninvasive therapy.

Focal High-intensity Focused Ultrasound

The overtreatment of prostate cancer is recognized and the need for less-aggressive minimally sufficient treatments is paramount [17, 18]. Focal therapy for prostate cancer is in the same vein as the progress that has been made for the treatment of breast cancer, where lumpectomy is suggested as a first-line treatment of patients with lesions of limited size. In the same way, for moderate-sized kidney cancers (less than 40 mm), it actually has been shown that conservative treatment (lumpectomy or partial nephrectomy) is as effective as extensive nephrectomy in terms of oncology while preserving a maximum of renal functioning. For superficial TCC bladder cancer, focal resection has been a "gold standard" for decades.

Therefore, it seems logical to propose a strategy of this type to a patient who has a monofocal prostatic tumor with a good prognosis. The objective is to propose a partial treatment that is limited to the tumor and a safety margin for the patient with noninvasive, monofocal, localized prostate cancer. This type of

Table 1 High-intensity focused ultrasound: efficacy summary

Study	Patients, n	Pretreatment PSA, ng/mL	Gleason score	Stage	Median follow-up, mo	Negative biopsy rate, %	Biochemical survival	Retreatment rate,%
Chaussy and Thueroff [5]	184	12	–	T1–2 Nx	–	80	NR	26.1
Gelet et al. [6]	102	8.38 (mean)	54% 2–6; 46% 7–10	T1–2	19	75	66% at 5 years (ASTRO)	78.4
Poissonnier et al. [7]	120	5.67 (mean) 100%<10	64% 2–6; 36% 7–10	T1–2	27	86	76.9% at 5 years (ASTRO)	1.4 Tx per patient
Thüroff et al. [8]	402	10.9 (mean)	13.2% 2–4; 77.5% 5–7; 9.3% 8–10	T1–2	13	87.2	NR	36.7
Blana et al. [9]	146	7.6 (mean)	5±1.2	T1–2 N0M0	22	93.4	84% at 22 months (PSA <1.0)	18.7
Ficarra et al. [10]	30	18 (median)	17% 7; 33% 8; 37% 9; 13% 10	30% T2b; 70% T3; 70% T3	6	77	90% at 1 year (PSA >0.3)	0
Poissonnier et al. [11]	227	7.0 (mean)	67% 2–6; 33% 7	T1–2	20.5	86	NR	42.7
Blana et al. [12]	140	7.0 (mean)	5.2±1.4	T1–2 N0M0	76.8[a]	96.4	77% at 5 years (Phoenix)	29.3
Blana et al. [13•]	163	5 (median)	7.9±3.7	T1–2 N0M0	57.6[a]	92.7	75% at 5 years (Phoenix)	20.8

[a] Mean

ASTRO American Society for Therapeutic Radiology and Oncology, *NR* not reported; *Nx* lymph nodes not tested; *PSA* prostate-specific antigen, *Tx* T grading unknown treatment should enable treatment to be "totaled up" in the event of failure or recurrence. Thus, the object is twofold: preserve normal sphincter function, sexual performance, and fertility on one hand, and on the other, treat the disease with sufficient efficacy. This would achieve the same morbidity goal of active surveillance but lower the psychological burden resulting from the definitive treatment of the known disease for the patient [19, 20].

The primary idea of carrying out a focal treatment goes back to Onik et al. [21•], who were the first to use cryoablation to offer patients "a prostate lumpectomy." This concept paper was followed by the first outcomes of focal cryoablation in 2007 [22–24] and a report of focal ablation with HIFU [25]. Bahn et al. [22] followed 31 men treated with hemi-spherical cryoablation using stage as the primary

Table 1 High-intensity focused ultrasound: efficacy summary Study Patients (n), Pretreatment PSA, ng/mL, Gleason score Stage Median follow-up (months), Negative biopsy rate, % Biochemical survival, Retreatment rate (%)

ASTRO American Society for Therapeutic Radiology and Oncology, NR not reported; Nx lymph nodes not tested, PSA prostate-specific antigen, Tx T grading unknown selection criteria (26.6% of men had a Gleason of 7 and 9.7% had a PSA >10 ng/mL). With a median follow-up of 70 months, 92.8% of men had a stable PSA (American Society for Therapeutic Radiology and Oncology [ASTRO] definition) and 96% had negative biopsies. In the Ellis et al. [24] series, 60 patients were selected for hemi-spherical cryoablation via a 12-core biopsy. The average follow-up was 15 months and the biological progression-free survival rate was 80.4%, the incontinence rate was 3.6%, and erectile function was preserved in 70.6% of patients. It should be noted that 33% of patients included in this series were of intermediate risk or higher. In the Onik et al. [23] series (55 patients with a follow-up of more than 1 year), a stable PSA was obtained in 95% of the patients and sexual function was preserved in 86% of the patients. **Not all patients in these two series were reevaluated by biopsy after the focal treatment and, under these conditions, the rate of negative biopsies is therefore subject to caution (100% in the Onik et al. [23] series and 77% in the Ellis et al. [24] series).**

In the Muto et al. [25] article, 29 patients underwent focal HIFU with a biochemical progression-free survival rate at 2 years of 83.3% for patients at low risk (TA-T2A, and Gleason 6 and PSA <10 ng/mL) and of 53.6% for patients at intermediate risk (T2B or Gleason 7 or PSA > 10). The rate of negative biopsies was 76.5% at 12 months in 17 patients who were re-biopsied. It should be noted that the focal treatment in this series consisted of treating the entire peripheral zone of the two prostate lobes and the transitional area of the diseased lobe (in the end, only the transitional area of the lobe presumed to be healthy was saved). **Focal therapy for prostate cancer is a noninvasive answer to the question of overtreatment.** Studies in the United States, France, and Germany are on the way.

Side Effects after Primary High-intensity Focused Ultrasound in Localized Prostate Cancer

The most common observed side effects of HIFU for prostate cancer include prolonged voiding dysfunction and retention caused by edema, necrosis, or bladder outlet obstruction. **To reduce the time of urinary diversion and the postoperative morbidity (sludging, obstruction, infection), studies were undertaken to observe the effect of a combination therapy (HIFU and TURP).** In 30 patients with localized prostate cancer, a one-stage (a single Anesthetic—general or spinal) combination therapy with TURP and HIFU was performed. The mean treatment duration was 2 hours and 48 min. The transurethral catheter time was 2 days and the mean hospitalization period was 3 days. After 6 months, control biopsies were negative in 80% of patients, and the median PSA was 0.9 ng/mL. The mean Post-treatment International Prostate Symptom Score was 6.7, compared with a pre-treatment score of 7.5. Potency was preserved in 73% of patients who had reported no erectile dysfunction before treatment [26].

The beneficial effect of a combination of TURP and HIFU was demonstrated in a series of 271 patients with prostate cancer and an initial median PSA less than 15 ng/ mL. Of these 271 patients, 96 received HIFU monotherapy, while 175 were treated with combination therapy. The mean resection weight was 15.7 g (2–110 g; median: 12.5 g). In 51.6% of the patients, carcinoma was found in the resection material. The mean follow-up time in the monotherapy group was 18.7±12.1 months, and was 10.9±6.2 months for the combination-therapy group. The histological results in both groups were similar after treatment, with negative biopsies in 87.7% versus 81.6%. The median PSA nadir was 0.0 ng/mL in both groups. **The monotherapy group required a suprapubic catheter for 40 days, while in the combination group, it was removed after 7 days.** The benefits of a combination therapy have been demonstrated with this study [27•].

The rate of adverse events among patients with primary therapy is low (Table 2). Grade I stress incontinence was observed in 4% to 6% of patients, grade II in up to 2%, and secondary infra-vesical obstruction in 5% to 10%. Severe incontinence (grade III) and rectourethral fistulae are rare (< 1%). Preservation of erectile function is directly dependent on the position of the primary lesion in relation to the neurovascular bundle. Although sparing the contralateral side for neurovascular preservation can improve potency, this results in a higher retreatment rate [29–32].

Results from a prospective QOL study from Japan recently have been reported [33]. They evaluated QOL impact using standard questionnaires, including the Functional Assessment of Cancer Therapy-Prostate and the Sexual Health Inventory for Men administered to 326 men before HIFU and then at follow-up months 6, 12, and 24. Their primary conclusion was that functional and QOL outcomes after HIFU for localized prostate cancer are better than those after other treatment modalities. Based on these results, HIFU as therapy for localized prostate cancer has definitively emerged from the experimental stage, and is, since 2000, in the investigational stage for this indication. **(Editorial comment: Radical Prostatectomy remains in the investigational stage to this day)**

Salvage High-intensity Focused Ultrasound Therapy after Failed Primary Therapy

HIFU can be used as local salvage therapy after almost any previous primary prostate cancer therapy: for patients with recurrent cancer after external radiation, after low–dose rate and high–dose rate brachytherapy, after cryoablation or biochemically progressing PSA, after failed primary HIFU, and after combined pretreatments, including radical prostatectomy. This is due to the poor treatment options for recurrent disease. **According to CaPSURE data, 63% of the patients who underwent radiation therapy had disease recurrence.** The salvage therapy employed for this population almost always was androgen deprivation, which was applied in 93.5%. Definitive local therapy was employed only in 3.9% (salvage radical prostatectomy: 0.9% and cryoablation: 3.0%). It has been well recognized that salvage radical prostatectomy and cryoablation are more theoretical options with high morbidity rates. The cause of this may be due to the complexity of the procedure, the high

Table 2 Summary of morbidity results following high-intensity focused ultrasound

Study	Patients, n	INC,%	ED,%	FIS,%	S&S,%	PR,%	UTI,%	CA, d	Pain,%
Blana et al. [9]	146	5.8	57.2	0.7	11.7	NR	4.1	SP: 12.7	1.4
Thüroff et al. [8]	402	GI 10.6; GII 2.5; GIII 1.5	13	1.2	3.6	8.6	13.8	F: 5 SP: 34	NR
Gelet et al. [6]	102	GI 8.8; GII 9.8; GIII 3.9	61	1	17	5	NR	9.1	2
Chaussy et al. [27•][a]	96	GI 9.1; GII 4.6; GIII 1.7	40	NR	27.1	NR	47.9	SP: 45.1	NR
Chaussy et al. [27•][b]	175	GI 4.6; GII 2.3	31.8	NR	8	NR	11.4	SP: 13.7	NR
Ficarra et al. [10]	30	7	NR	0	10	13	16	SP: 12	NR
Lee et al. [28]	58	GI 16	NR	0	NR	3.4	NR	SP: 15	NR
Poissonnier et al. [11]	227	GI 9.0; GII 3.0; GIII 1.0	39	0	12	9	2	7	3
Blana et al. [12]	140	GI 5.0; GII 0.7	43.2	0	13.6	–	7.1	NR	5.7
Blana et al. [13•]	163	GI 6.1; GII 1.8	44.7	0	24.5	–	7.8	NR	3.7

[a] No TURP. [b] TURP

CA postoperative catheter duration, *ED* erectile dysfunction, *F* Foley catheter, *FIS* fistula, *GI* incontinence grade I (loss of urine under heavy exercise requiring 0–1 pad/d), *GII* incontinence grade II (loss of urine under light exercise requiring > 1 pad/d), *GIII* incontinence grade III (loss of urine under any exercise requiring >2 pads/day). *INC* incontinence, *NR* not reported, *PR* postoperative retention, *SP* suprapubic catheter, *S&S* stricture and stenosis, *TURP* transurethral resection of the prostate, *UTI* urinary tract infection rates of side effects, and/or the procedure costs. Two significant publications regarding salvage HIFU recently appeared.

Murat et al. [34] updated the Lyon series of patients and reported outcomes of 167 men who underwent salvage HIFU, observing a 73% negative-biopsy rate and a 5-year overall survival rate of 84%. Surprisingly, they did not present a biochemical disease–free survival rate. **No rectal complications were observed, but the urinary incontinence rate was 49.5%, which is similar to rates reported in salvage radical prostatectomy series.** Berge et al. [35] reported early results from a prospective study of salvage HIFU and observed a biochemical failure rate of 39.1%. Significantly, the urinary incontinence rate was much lower in their cohort than in the Lyon group, with 17.3% developing either grade II or grade III incontinence. One patient developed a rectourethral fistula.

Salvage HIFU remains an attractive treatment option for those men who have had a recurrence after radiation therapy, although the postoperative course does have an associated higher morbidity due to the alterations of the tissue after radiation therapy. **It is a curative option that should be discussed with any patient who is thought to have a localized recurrence after radiation therapy.**

High-intensity Focused Ultrasound in Locally Advanced (T3-4) or Non-metastatic Hormone-resistant Prostate Cancer

Although not yet published as full manuscripts, a few important abstracts regarding the use of HIFU for the treatment of more aggressive disease were presented in 2010 and need to be mentioned because the results are compelling and encouraging. Most HIFU outcome reports are limited to T1-2 or radiation failures. The first report of T3-4 disease came recently, with 113 patients followed for a median of 4.6 years [36]. The median PSA velocity of this cohort was 0.19 ng/mL/y and the cancer-specific survival was 96.4%. A series of 55 men with PSA progression during their definitive hormonal ablation with a local biopsy-proven tumor recurrence were reported [37]. With a mean follow-up of 21 months, the prostate-specific survival was 87.3%. This is impressive and encouraging because this is a group of patients with a very poor prognosis and a short median survival.

Immune Induction: More than Just a High-intensity Focused Ultrasound "Side Effect"?

Recent progress has been made in developing an effective immune strategy for treating prostate cancer.

Table 2 Summary of morbidity results following high-intensity focused ultrasound Study Patients (n) Incontinence %, Erectile Dysfunction %, Fistula %, S&S%, PR %, UTI %, CA d, Pain % CA postoperative catheter duration, ED erectile dysfunction, F Foley catheter, FIS fistula, GI incontinence grade I (loss of urine under heavy exercise requiring 0–1 pad/d), GII incontinence grade II (loss of urine under light exercise requiring >1 pad/d), GIII incontinence grade III (loss of urine under any exercise requiring >2 pads/day), INC incontinence, NR not reported, PR postoperative retention, SP suprapubic catheter, S&S stricture and stenosis, TURP transurethral resection of the prostate, UTI urinary tract infection A number of immunotherapy regimens are being studied, including immunomodulatory cytokines/effectors, peptide and cellular immunization, viral vaccines, dendritic cell vaccines, and antibody therapies. Immunomodulatory agents, such as granulocyte-macrophage colony-stimulating factor, Flt3 ligand, and interleukin 2, have been used to stimulate the immune system to generate an antitumor response against prostate cancer.

Several recent studies have looked at the potential of HIFU to initiate an immune response. Wu et al. [38•] examined the effect of HIFU on systemic antitumor immunity, particularly T lymphocyte-mediated immunity in patients with cancer.

The same group investigated whether the tumor antigens expressed on breast cancer cells may be preserved after HIFU treatment [39]. Primary lesions in 23 patients with biopsy-proven breast cancer were treated with HIFU, then submitted to modified radical mastectomy. Breast cancer specimens then were stained for a variety of cellular molecules, including tumor antigens and heat-shock protein 70. A number of tumor antigens were identified and these could provide a potential antigen source to stimulate antitumor immune response.

It has been suggested that endogenous signals from HIFU-damaged tumor cells may trigger the activation of dendritic cells, and that this may play a critical role in a HIFU-elicited antitumor immune response [40].

Status of tumor-infiltrating lymphocytes (TILs) after HIFU ablation of human breast cancer has been investigated [41]. Results show that TILs infiltrated along the margins of the ablated region in all HIFU-treated neoplasms, and the numbers of tumor-infiltrating CD3, CD4, CD8, CD4/CD8, B lymphocytes, and NK cells was increased significantly with HIFU treatment. The number of FasL (+), granzyme (+), and perforin (+) TILs was significantly greater in the HIFU group than in the control group.

The "Randomized Trial" Pipe Dream

One of the biggest lessons of 2010 is that it still appears to be impossible to objectively compare two definitive local therapies for localized prostate cancer.

Donnelly et al. [42] made the best attempt in the past 25 years to accrue patients to a cryoablation versus XRT (radiation) trial in Calgary, but it still fell short of the accrual target. This is the most recent in a string of randomized clinical trials that fall short of their accrual target. Importantly, it is noted that the Calgary trial was done in Canada in the early 2000s, when the treatment options were not as extensive or as confusing as they are today. The two standard options at that time were prostatectomy and XRT. Those not interested in or not indicated for prostatectomy would have only one option: XRT. If they wished to have cryoablation, they could do so only by entering the trial. If they were not randomized to the cryoablation arm, they would get the treatment they would have had anyway. Today, with so many options, this environment is essentially impossible to recreate. Another randomized clinical trial comparing different definitive local therapies is not underway nor on the horizon. As such, it should finally be admitted that accruing patients to a randomized trial comparing two different definitive therapies for localized prostate cancer is a pipe dream.

It is important to distinguish between two phases of development and evaluation of a technology. "Experimental" indicates that the effect of the treatment in terms of both morbidity and efficacy is essentially unknown. An "investigational" procedure is one for which the efficacy and morbidity have been established, but the long-term (> 10 years) durability remains to be established. Prostate cancer, being a slowly progressing disease in most cases, necessitates its treatments to be followed for a very long time (> 15 years) to completely determine efficacy.

In fact, the foundation procedures for management of localized prostate cancer have become "standards," not due to rigorous research that long ago, but more due to the simple fact that they have been the longest practiced treatments. The only successful randomized trial comparing prostatectomy to active surveillance; however, it is not a comparison of two definitive treatment options, and only yielded meaningful results in 2008 [43]. This is more than 100 years after Young [44] first defined the radical prostatectomy in 1905. Demanding that a new treatment be vetted via a randomized clinical trial is not feasible while demanding one . . . simply is blocking innovation and ignoring reality. Today, everyone wants to be treated with the newest technology, and at the same time, on a highest possible evidence level. This is a dilemma that cannot be solved by a randomized trial. **(Editorial comment: the utilization of HIFU cannot be associated with a 'double standard', therefore, I submit to the medical world; a diseased prostate as witnessed by an elevated PSA has met the threshold for prostate treatment with HIFU when compared to the use of HIFU for uterine fibroids in women. A Uterine fibroid is a benign (non-malignant) condition. No one can argue this point successfully)**

Conclusions

Since 2000, HIFU by Ablatherm is a non-experimental therapy under long-term investigation for primary treatment of localized prostate cancer as well as salvage therapy after radiation failure. It appears to have a high potential to treat on either side of this spectrum in focal and in incidental prostate cancer as well as adjuvant in T3/T4 disease or in non-metastatic hormone-resistant prostate cancer. The versatility of HIFU appears to be unique in the treatment of the entire spectrum of prostate cancer, which is a multifaceted increasing and long-lasting disease. HIFU does not substitute or is not competitive to only one classical therapy, but its indications overlap in a certain range with all therapies.

As an additional localized one-session tumor debulking therapy option with low perioperative morbidity, HIFU is feasible for patients at any age and health status. HIFU helps to delay the need for surgery, radiation, or hormonal ablation at a point in a patients' life when they (the patients) are truly looking to avoid caustic treatment measures. An eventual HIFU-provoked induction of the immune response as supportive therapeutic effect is under investigation.

Acknowledgements The authors thank Mrs. Regina Nanieva, Dr. Tina Chaussy, and Dr. John Rewcastle for their invaluable help. Disclosures: No potential conflicts of interest relevant to this article were reported.

References:
Papers of particular interest, published recently, have been highlighted as: • Of importance

1. Marberger M. Prostate cancer 2008. Challenges in diagnostic and management. Europ Urol. 2009;8 Suppl 3:1989-96.
2. van Leeuwen PJ, Connolly D, Tammela TL, et al. Balancing the harms and benefits of early detection of prostate cancer. Cancer. 2010;116:4857–65.
3. Chaussy C, Thueroff S. The use of high-intensity focused ultrasound in prostate cancer. In: Ukimura O, Gill IS, editors. Contemporary Interventional Ultrasonography in Urology, Chapter7. London: Springer; 2009. p. 63–73.
4. Chaussy C, Thueroff S, Rebillard X, et al. Technology insight: high-intensity focused ultrasound for urologic cancers. Nat Clin Pract Urol. 2005;2(4):191–8.
5. Chaussy C, Thueroff S. Results and side effects of high-intensity focused ultrasound in localized prostate cancer. J Endourol. 2001;15:437–40.
6. Gelet A, Chapelon JY, Bouvier R, et al. Transrectal high intensity focused ultrasound for the treatment of localized prostate cancer: factors influencing the outcome. Eur Urol. 2001;40:124–9.
7. Poissonnier L, Gelet A, Chapelon JY, et al. Results of transrectal focused ultrasound for the treatment of localized prostate

cancer (120 patients with PSA < or +10 ng/ml). Prog Urol. 2003;13:60–72.

8. Thüroff S, Chaussy C, Vallencien G, et al. High-intensity focused ultrasound and localized prostate cancer: efficacy results from the European multicentric study. J Endourol. 2003;17:673–7.

9. Blana A, Walter B, Rogenhofer S, et al. High intensity focused ultrasound for the treatment of localized prostate cancer. Urology. 2004;63(2):297–300.

10. Ficarra V, Antoniolli SZ, Novara G, et al. Short-term outcome after high-intensity focused ultrasound in the treatment of patients with high-risk prostate cancer. BJU Int. 2006;98:1193-8.

11. Poissonnier L, Chapelon JY, Rouvière O, et al. Control of prostate cancer by transrectal HIFU in 227 patients. Eur Urol. 2007;51:381–7.

12. Blana A, Murat FJ, Walter B, et al. First analysis of the long-term results with transrectal HIFU in patients with localized prostate cancer. Eur Urol. 2008;53(6):1194–201.

13. • Blana A, Brown SC, Chaussy C, et al. High-intensity focused ultrasound for prostate cancer: comparative definitions of biochemical failure. Int BJU. 2009;104 (8):1058–62. This article provides the outcome from a large registry of HIFU patients, which showed good 5-year results in low—and medium-risk patients.

14. Crouzet S, Rebillard X, Chevallier D, et al. Multicentric oncologic outcomes of high-intensity focused ultrasound for localized prostate cancer in 803 patients. Eur Urol. 2010;58:559–66.

15. Agarwal PK, Sadetsky N, Konety BR, et al. Cancer of the prostate strategic urological research endeavor (CaPSURE). Treatment failure after primary and salvage therapy for prostate cancer: likelihood, patterns of care, and outcomes. Cancer. 2008;112:307–14.

16. Chaussy CG, Thueroff S. Transrectal high-intensity focused ultrasound for local treatment of Prostate Cancer. Urologe A. 2009;48(7):710–8. Review. German.

17. Klotz L. Active surveillance for prostate cancer: patient selection and management. Curr Oncol. 2010;17 Suppl 2:11–7.

18. Soloway MS, Soloway CT, Eldefrawy A, et al. Careful selection and close monitoring of low-risk prostate cancer patients on active surveillance minimizes the need for treatment. Europ Urol. 2010;58(6):831–35.

19. Klotz L. Active surveillance for Prostate Cancer: For whom ? J Clin Oncol. 2005;23(32):8165–9.

20. Roemling MJ, Roobol MW, Kattan TH, et al. Nomogram use for the prediction of indolent prostate cancer: impact on screen detected populations. Cancer. 2007;110:2218–21.

21. • Onik G, Narayan P, Vaughan D, et al. Focal nerve sparing cryoablation for the treatment of primary prostate cancer: a new approach to preserving potency. Urology. 2002;60:109–14. The primary idea of carrying out a focal treatment goes back to Onik et al. They used Cryoablation to offer patients a "prostate lumpectomy".

22. Bahn DK, Silverman P, Lee Sr F, et al. Focal prostate cryoablation: initial results show cancer control and potency preservation. J Endourol. 2006;20(9):688–92.

23. Onik G, Vaughan D, Lotenfoe R, et al. Male lumpectomy: focal therapy for prostate cancer using cryoablation. Urology. 2007;70:18–21.

24. Ellis D, Manny TB, Rewcastle JC. ocal cryosurgery followed by penile rehabilitation as primary treatment for localized prostate cancer: initial results. Urology. 2007;70:9–15.

25. Muto S, Takashi Y, Saito K, et al. Focal therapy with Highintensity—focused-ultrasound in the treatment of localised prostate cancer. Jpn J Clin Oncol. 2008;38:192–99.

26. Vallancien G, Prapotnich D, Cathelineau X, et al. Transrectal focused ultrasound combined with transurethral resection of the prostate for the treatment of localized prostate cancer: feasibility study. J Urol. 2004;171(Pt 1):2265–7.

27. • Chaussy C, Thüroff S. The status of high-intensity focused ultrasound in the treatment of localized prostate cancer and the impact of a combined resection. Curr Urol Rep. 2003;4:248–52. Provides outcome data for HIFU with pre-transurethral resection of the prostate compared with HIFU alone and provides the basis for common combination therapeutic options.

28. Lee HM, Hong JH, Choi HY. High-intensity focused ultrasound therapy for clinically localized prostate cancer. Prostate Cancer Prostatic Dis. 2006; 9:439–43.

29. Chaussy CG, Thueroff S. High-intensive focused ultrasound in localized prostate cancer. J Endourol. 2000;14:293–9.

30. Thüroff S, Chaussy C. High-intensity focused ultrasound: complicationsand adverse events. Mol Urol. 2000;4:183–7.

31. Chaussy C, Thüroff S. High-intensity focused ultrasound in the management of prostate cancer. Expert Rev Med Devices. 2010;7:209–17.

32. Thüroff S, Chaussy C. High-Intensity focused ultrasound for prostate cancer. In: Li-Ming Su, Young Stephen C, editors. Early Dignosis and Treatment of Cancer: Prostate Cancer, Chapter 9. Philadelphia: Saunders Elsevier; 2008. p. 177–92.

33. Shoji S, Nakano M, Nagata Y, Usui Y, Terachi T, Uchida T. Quality of life following high-intensity focused ultrasound for the treatment of localized prostate cancer: a prospective study. Int J Urol. 2010;17:715–19.

34. Murat FJ, Poissonnier L, Rabilloud M, et al. Mid-term results demonstrate salvage high-intensity focused ultrasound (HIFU) as an effective and acceptably morbid salvage

treatment option for locally radiorecurrent prostate cancer. Eur Uro. 2009;55:640–7.

35. Berge V, Baco E, Karlsen SJ. A prospective study of salvage highintensity focused ultrasound for locally radiorecurrent prostate cancer: early results. Scand J Urol Nephrol. 2010;44:223–7.

36. Chaussy CG, Thueroff SF. HIFU treatment of locally advanced prostate cancer. J Endourol. 2010;24 Suppl 1:PS12–2.

37. Chaussy C, Thuroff S, Nanieva R. Hormone resistant prostate cancer treated by robotic high intensive ultrasound. J Urol. 2010;183(Suppl):e262.

38. • Wu F, Wang ZB, Lu P, et al. Activated anti-tumor immunity in cancer patients after high intensity focused ultrasound ablation. Ultrasound Med Biol. 2004;30(9):1217–22. Research looking at the potential of HIFU to have an immunogenic role in prostate cancer.

39. Wu F, Wang ZB, Cao YD, et al. Expression of tumor antigens and heat-shock protein 70 in breast cancer cells after highintensity focused ultrasound ablation. Ann Surg Oncol. 2007;14 (3):1237–42.

40. Hu Z, Yang XY, Liu Y, et al. Investigation of HIFU-induced antitumor immunity in a murine tumor model. J Transl Med. 2007;5:34.

41. Lu P, Zhu XQ, Xu ZI, et al. Increased infiltration of activated tumorinfiltrating lymphocytes after high intensity focused ultrasound ablation of human breast cancer. Surgery. 2009;145(3):286–93.

42. Donnelly BJ, Saliken JC, Brasher PM, et al. A randomized trial of external beam radiotherapy versus cryoablation in patients with localized prostate cancer. Cancer. 2010;116:323–30.

43. Bill-Axelson A, Holmberg L, Filén F, et al. Radical prostatectomy versus watchful waiting in localized prostate cancer: the

Scandinavian prostate cancer group-4 randomized trial. J Natl Cancer Inst. 2008;100:1144–5.

44. Young HH. The early diagnosis and radical cure of carcinoma of the prostate: Being a study of 40 cases and presentation of a Radical operation which was carried out in four cases. Bull Johns Hopkins Hosp. 1905;16:315–21.

APPENDIX—12

A Brief Description of the Ultimate Prostate Scan (UPS)—Targeting Disease . . . 'One Patient at a Time'

3.0 TESLA MAGNETIC Resonance Imaging with Diffusion **(MRI-D) and DCE (Perfusion)** featured by the Diagnostic Center for Disease™ represents a **"state of the art"** comprehensive scan of the prostate. The diagnostic features seen with this scan are not seen with any other diagnostic modality including Color 'Power Doppler' Ultrasound, PET scan, Prostascint scan or CAT scan. The MRI scan powered by a 3.0 Tesla magnet, provides a spectacularly detailed image of the prostate that has never been seen in a clinical setting. As some have said, this scan allows us to establish a **"road map" to disease detection**, thereby, allowing us to do for the patient and the disease what is required and nothing more. Furthermore, this scan enables our Physician staff to evaluate the extent of disease including whether the disease, when present, has escaped the capsule of the prostate or whether the disease has invaded the Seminal Vesicles. **For men who have been diagnosed previously with prostate cancer, this scan may change the selected treatment choice as it so commonly does.** There is little point, as example, in having your prostate removed (Robotic Prostatectomy) when it is established that the cancer has escaped the capsule of the prostate. Additionally, the MRI technology allows us to **target a lesion** in question rather than expose a patient to "prostate mapping" or saturation biopsies. The risks are high and varied when the prostate gland is biopsied at half centimeter intervals during a saturation biopsy procedure including 'needle tracking', extensive bleeding, sepsis and even death. **This is not a procedure we endorse!**

At the **Diagnostic Center for Disease™**, we understand that when biopsies are performed . . . the process can spread cancer cells so we encourage a **pre-biopsy protocol** that disables and weakens cells that "needle track" through the prostate capsule making it virtually impossible for the locally escaping cells to become a focal site of metastatic cancer. Clearly, **we see value in a patient avoiding needless biopsies** or limited targeted biopsies (if we must) guided by the MRI images to enhance our decision making process relevant to treatment (if required). In effect, based on how we see the prostate, we are able to avoid the **"shot in the dark" approach, commonly seen in conveyor belt medicine**, thereby, taking the guess work out of the biopsy procedure. In cases where no cancer is found on MRI, despite an elevated PSA level, a needless biopsy can certainly be avoided while the inflammatory disease encountered can be treated. **We think you will appreciate the way we think and embrace the way we care for you.**

Spectroscopy, when utilized, represents a unique investigative sequence that allows us to look into the prostate cell at the by-products or metabolites of cell function. Based on the make-up of these metabolites, we are able to assess the health of the cells. Cancer cells, as example, are represented by a high level of Choline while normal cells are represented by high levels of Citrate. MRI and Spectroscopy as an additional sequence are complementary to each other enhancing our diagnostic capabilities albeit not embraced worldwide.

While many sequences of image acquisition are performed routinely during the course of your MRI scan, we are looking for a concordance of factors that enable an improved diagnostic commentary. To this end, we have recently added an additional scan sequence called **Dynamic Contrast Enhancement (DCE or Perfusion)**. This exciting scan sequence allows us to capture and subsequently validate how cells process a safe and well studied injectable called Gadolinium. **When regions of interest are identified on MRI, the application of DCE with Diffusion may be the difference maker between calling a region of interest cancer or non-cancerous.** We charge a global fee for this service representing all sequences pertinent to your comprehensive exam priced competitively. At the Diagnostic Center for Disease™, we value the health of every person we meet and treat all patients with the utmost dignity and respect. **In the event of questions or comments, please feel free to visit our center or have a 'conference call' with Dr. Ronald Wheeler, our Medical Director. We believe that knowledge is power; enabling you, the patient, to have the decision making tools you need to define a healthier future.**

APPENDIX—13

Chronic Disease Management may be the best "first choice" when prostate cancer is diagnosed and if quality of life is important to you!

Facts to live by:

1) Chronic Disease Management (CDM) always works, with virtually 100 percent success, versus a 40-60 percent failure rate when utilizing traditional therapy.

2) Chronic Disease Management is a "patient friendly" approach that controls the disease expectantly and supports quality of life issues. In other words, men do not need to give up their sexual abilities or invest in Pampers with conservative management.

3) The Chronic Disease Management treatment approach does not preclude the use of traditional "definitive" therapy at some later point in time.

4) Patients do no need to experience treatments that predictably fail and unpredictably succeed. In other words, why guess about the possibility of success with radical prostatectomy or radiation therapy, while risking impotency and incontinence, when you

can live with the disease, much like patients live with diabetes or rheumatoid arthritis?

5) As healthcare practitioners, **we should never want to do more for a patient's disease than is necessary or required.**

6) As healthcare practitioners, **we should never want the treatment to be worse than the disease itself.**

7) Chronic Disease Management avoids a rush to judgment, while allowing the educational process to take place. The longer a patient succeeds with CDM therapy, the more confident he will become. Remember, at any point when a patient feels 'it is my lucky day', he can "switch gears" and go for a cure. A calm, informed patient will always make better treatment decisions.

8) If a patient is unsure about what to do, a final decision can wait. Patients with a Gleason Score of 7 or higher should consider anti-androgen therapy during the educational interval, to ensure stability of the disease, especially if the PSA value is approaching 10.0 ng/ml. Too many patients are not advised by their physician of the need to suppress the disease during the educational process. While I am certain there are no studies to guide this process, medical intellect and common sense suggests there may be an opportunity to control cancer over a period of several months to a year or more; conservatively. During this time, patients are encouraged to have a monthly PSA blood test, to monitor disease activity and keep learning. Metaphorically speaking, how many people advocate walking away from a smoking campfire?

9) Chronic Disease Management should be considered if a patient's PSA is higher than 10 ng/ml at the time of diagnosis. Individuals with this level of PSA have a high risk for extracapsular disease (disease outside of the prostate) associated with concern for treatment failure. Based upon statistical data for organ confinement or extracapsular disease, it is my opinion that these patients are better candidates for Chronic Disease Management.

APPENDIX—14

Why HIFU Fails

PROSTATE CANCER REMAINS "public enemy number one" as men age. It is commonly stated that if men live long enough, we will all get prostate cancer. Put another way, if we live to be 100 years old, 100% of men will have contracted prostate cancer. Epidemiologically, it is estimated in excess of 230,000 men will get prostate cancer in 2011. This amounts to a new case of prostate cancer diagnosed every 3 minutes. According to the Surveillance, Epidemiology, and End Results (SEER) Data from the National Cancer Institute (NCI), more than 500,000 men will contract prostate cancer yearly by the year 2020. **Clearly prostate cancer is epidemic, if not pandemic while representing one of the most unpredictable, yet potentially deadly, diseases men face.**

"3.0 Tesla MRI Scan Predicts and Confirms the Presence of Prostate Cancer"

Once the diagnosis of prostate cancer has been made by a concordance of diagnostic techniques including: Prostate Specific Antigen (PSA), digital rectal examination (DRE) and a 3.0 Tesla Magnetic Resonance Imaging scan (with or without spectroscopy), the decision making process for treatment is expedited without undue risk to the patient for 'needle tracking'.

In centers of excellence like the Diagnostic Center for Disease™ in Sarasota, Florida, biopsies are discouraged based on the aforementioned 'needle tracking' tied to an unacceptable cancer recurrence rate by 7-10 years post treatment. Based upon the ability of MRI (at the 3.0 Tesla strength) to localize a cancer, no more than 6 targeted biopsies are ever necessary (assuming the patient accepts the risks germane to biopsy) to find the most aggressive prostate cancers that pose the greatest risk to men. It is now common knowledge that 50-60% of prostate cancers diagnosed can be treated conservatively as they are associated with a Gleason 6 pathologic grade. **What this means for the future is that the Urologist or Radiation Oncologist will be inclined to treat fewer cancers more aggressively with something other than Active Surveillance or Chronic Disease Management (CDM), once the facts are universally understood.**

Assuming organ confinement of a cancer (validated by an MRI scan), a PSA value of less than 10.0 ng/ml and an absence of digital rectal findings in association with a Gleason Score of 6 (3+3), an individual currently qualifies as a surgical candidate to the Urologist or Radiation Oncologist, who tries to make the case for cancer cure. While many of these patients would be excellent candidates for a CDM protocol, the majority of men with this clinical presentation of cancer (at the urging of their doctor) will often times choose a definitive form of cancer treatment, like a radical prostatectomy or radiation, rather than treat the disease conservatively. Lost in all of this is the fact that 30-56% of all prostate cancers diagnosed are over-treated. In 2011, the primary list of "definitive treatments" include: Robotic Prostatectomy, Prostatectomy without the robot, Radiation Seed therapy (Brachytherapy), Intensity Modulated Radiation Therapy (IMRT), Cryosurgery and Proton Beam therapy. While there are variations in the application of the techniques mentioned, there is one glaring omission! High Intensity Focused Ultrasound (HIFU), while available outside of the USA for more than 15 years is not yet FDA approved and, therefore, not on the list of reimbursable treatments available in the USA! The prolonged delay in approval of this therapy is an unconscionable mystery when it is realized that HIFU is approved for uterine fibroids, (a benign disease) in women. Complicating the controversy further, HIFU is the most patient friendly treatment for organ confined prostate cancer in the world.

"HIFU is an Effective Therapy but as with any Cancer Treatment, Patient Selection is Critical to the Outcome"

Specifically, a study evaluating High Intensity Focused Ultrasound in Radiation failure patients is currently in a Phase III Trial format under the auspices of the FDA. Therefore, approval of HIFU (Ablatherm or Sonablate 500 technologies) in the USA is not anticipated until at least 2012 or 2013. Presently, men who choose HIFU are able to make a judgment as to the relevance of this form of therapy based upon European and Japanese data which boasts cure rates upwards of 80-87% at more than 5 years. The most significant obstacle is that men must agree to leave the country to receive this novel, if not quintessential prostate cancer treatment. The majority of men with the diagnosis of prostate cancer will make their treatment decision based on multiple reasons including their personal extensive research, excellence in side effect profile, cost, entitlement, family pressure, gut opinion, fear, venue of operation, insurance reimbursement, ease of application, time necessary to rehabilitate, speaking with friends and various other educational tools. **Without question and assuming that money is not a determining**

factor in making a decision, the best first choice in any disease treatment will always be the form of therapy that expeditiously allows a man to get back to living life to its fullest within the shortest amount of time while minimizing morbidity like incontinence, rectal wall injury and sexual dysfunction.

The procedure that ranks number one in virtually every definable category for men, who don't have to depend on their insurance coverage to pay for their healthcare, is High Intensity Focused Ultrasound (HIFU). The most compelling reason for men to choose this therapy is quality of life interests; thereby, ensuring the best percentage chance of remaining sexually potent and continent of urine and bowel function. HIFU is a procedure that uses acoustic energy (sound waves) to generate a thermal energy that is delivered with unparalleled precision to the prostate. Assuming there was no risk for extracapsular extension of disease or definitive invasion of the Seminal Vesicles as determined by the 3.0 T MRI scan, the focused energy emanating from the treating transducer will treat the prostate tissue methodically with pinpoint accuracy allowing a block of cells of varying size to melt under intense heat measured at 70-90 degrees Centigrade. While no procedure is perfect, HIFU predictably ensures that if appropriate energy is delivered to the tissue, prostate cancer cells and benign cells that encounter the thermal energy will die. Equally appealing beyond a scalpel-less outpatient procedure is that the operation typically takes approximately 2 to 4 hours to complete (dependent on the technology chosen with Ablatherm typically taking 2 hours), as well as the ability to walk away with urinary continence and sexual capability. This is the reality for the majority of carefully selected patients.

"Sexual Potency is maintained by Design as the Neurovascular Bundles are identified prior to initiating the Treatment Plan"

The ability to visualize in real time the location of the sphincter mechanism that allows a man to remain dry and free from urine leakage and understand the location of the neurovascular bundles that enable the process of erectile function assures the vast majority of men with organ confined disease that functional social skills have been additionally protected from the acoustically generated thermal energy. The ability to treat the prostate with virtually no disruption of the prostate capsule avoids unnecessary spillage of cancer cells that is common to radical prostatectomy and Brachytherapy. Equally important is the ability to avoid rectal injury common to radiation delivered by IMRT, Brachytherapy (with or without External Beam) or Proton Beam therapy. Unlike cryosurgery, an equally destructive ablative therapy, the nerves, arteries and veins associated with the neurovascular bundle are proactively spared with HIFU from trauma allowing erectile ability to remain intact. Despite all of the fanfare associated with HIFU, there are a significant number of failures nonetheless. To date, there is not a HIFU treating physician who has not experienced failure. As I previously stated, no therapy is perfect. So when and why does HIFU fail? **As a practicing HIFU Physician of many years, it is my experienced opinion that HIFU fails when we try to apply the technology to all patients rather than patients who qualify. In other words, to achieve the level of success with HIFU (or any procedure for that matter); patient selection is critical to the outcome.** This is consistent with the application of any technical skill intended to cure prostate cancer. Therefore, we must not use the 'one size fits all' mentality with HIFU that commonly occurs with radical prostatectomy and radiation therapy. As skilled surgeons, we must be able to accept that not all men with prostate cancer will be viable candidates for HIFU for a variety of reasons and therefore, must be encouraged to treat their disease in some alternative manner.

"Why HIFU Fails to Cure Prostate Cancer"

So what clinical prostate characteristics preclude the success of the HIFU procedure? **In a few words, prostate size, stones, and density of tissue ; as these three anatomic observations represent the three most critical issues to be considered to assure the HIFU procedure to be performed effectively, assuming organ confinement of the cancer and an absence of obvious cancer into the Seminal Vesicles as noted preferentially by a preoperative 3.0 T MRI scan.** Relevant to prostate size, there is an expectation for the gland intended for treatment, to be no larger than 30-40 grams or cubic centimeters. Ablatherm, a truly robotic procedure favors smaller prostate size while the Sonablate 500 technology can accommodate larger prostates. Prostate stones on the other hand, are equally problematic to both technologies. Calcification or stones are believed to be formed in the prostate tissue in association with prostate inflammation, a phenomenon common to all prostates that note a PSA value of greater than 1.0 ng/ml. There is a concern that stones or calcification may prevent the focused energy emitted from the transducer from getting beyond a calcified acoustic barrier to the tissue on the other side; thereby, absorbed by the stones, or worse; reflected back toward the rectal wall. While rectal wall injury is not common with HIFU, we always anticipate what may occur and prepare a strategy to prevent it. It has been my experience that calcification (prostate stones) that fail to generate a significant acoustical shadow are not likely to alter the delivery of energy in any meaningful way. This statement has been validated as correct in hundreds if not thousands of cases! The most common location for prostate calcification is along the tract of the urethra (urine tube) as it passes through the prostate from the bladder as well as at the junction of the Peripheral zone and the Transition zone. Regarding the prostate size, the anterior to posterior diameter (A-P diameter) should not be greater than 4.0 centimeters (40 millimeters) ideally, consistent with the maximum distance the focused ultrasound beam must travel from the treating transducer to the prostate limit, anteriorly. The A-P diameter must be less when the Ablatherm technology is utilized.

Tissue density would also be a factor that jeopardizes the success of the procedure if the thermal energy cannot penetrate effectively in all regions. It is my belief that higher grade prostate cancer cells are more dense than lower grade lesions. Additionally, if cystic structures are encountered there is a possibility of a 'heat sink' effect. Heat sink in this instance is the dissipation of thermal energy by a cluster of blood vessels (vascularity) or cystic structures that prevent a killing temperature from being delivered to the targeted tissue. A determination of vascularity, calcification, cysts and prostate dimensions can be routinely evaluated by the implementation of the Gray scale ultrasound and Color Flow Doppler Ultrasound during the pre-treatment assessment. The success with HIFU relies on the fact that effective energy can be delivered to the Peripheral zone where 70% of cancers live. Unfortunately, 30% of prostate cancers are located in the Transition or Central zones, making this area a tougher target to hit when this area is compromised by calcified tissue. This becomes more significant as the sophisticated consumer understands that upwards of 65% of prostate cancer is multifocal and multi-zonal, establishing the possibility that treatment failure may become a reality. It is the under-educated patient who becomes enamored and swept away by a cancer treatment process that allows him to hit a golf ball within 24 hours of a major technical procedure who may overlook the critical clinical points of due diligence that may compromise the intent of the prostate ablative procedure.

"Spectroscopy can validate whether Prostate Cells are Alive or Dead"

Beyond an expectation for success with every procedure performed, HIFU failure is objectively validated by a PSA value of greater than 0.2 ng/ml and identification of live tissue on a 3.0 Tesla MRI scan. Alternatively, a random needle biopsy, replete with the threat of spreading residual cancer cells beyond the prostate capsule, remains an option but unacceptable in my opinion. When spectroscopy is utilized, an absence of metabolites at the cellular level is tantamount with an absence of live cells and consistent with an EKG that is flat lined or in this case; no evidence of disease or living prostate tissue.

While prostate disease in general and prostate cancer specifically continues to enjoy expanded press coverage, men will improve their chances of being diagnosed with less disease earlier by having PSA testing beginning at age 30 as I routinely suggest. This generation of men will have the opportunity to consider focal therapy that will be performed in concert with Magnetic Resonance Imaging technology to isolate the lesion in question as well as guide the delivery of thermal energy to a fraction of the prostate, while retaining healthy functional tissue. To be able to deliver thermal energy to a patient's prostate in an outpatient setting over a lunch hour will become a very appealing concept to an upwardly mobile and educated society.

Men interested in learning more about the excitement of HIFU and why it will alter the treatment landscape once approved, are invited to visit our website at www.PanAmHIFU.com or contact the Diagnostic Center for Disease™ in Sarasota, Florida at 1-877-766-8400 to visit with me personally on a conference call whereby we can discuss the particulars of your clinical history.

References:

1. Yoon S, Wang W, Osunkoya A, Lane Z, Partin A, and Epstein J: Residual tumor potentially left behind after local ablation therapy in prostate adenocarcinoma. Journal of Urology 2008; **179:** 2203-2206.

2. Villars A, McNeal JE, Freiha FS, and Stamey TA: Multiple cancers in the prostate. Morphological features of clinically recognized versus incidental tumors. Cancer 1992; **70:** 2313

3. Truskinovsky AM, Sanderson H, and Epstein JI: Characterization of minute adenocarcinomas of prostate at radical prostatectomy. Urology 2004; **64:** 733.

4. Epstein JI, Walsh PC, Carmichael M and Brendler CB: Pathologic and clinical findings to predict tumor extent of non-palpable (stage T1c) prostate cancer. JAMA 1994; **721:** 368. Edited: 12/07/11

APPENDIX—15

Heidelberg Working Group for biopsy-free diagnosis established: Decreasing the risks of prostate cancer diagnosis

~Punch biopsies associated with a high risk/New task force established as an interdisciplinary podium I Network of German specialists in Heidelberg~

HEIDELBERG (6 MAY 2009)—Last week saw the foundation of a working group in Heidelberg by renowned experts from the field of urology and diagnostics, whose aim is to network various medical specialties in promoting the development of new methods and the exchange of experiences in the biopsy-free diagnosis of prostate disorders. Prostate carcinoma (PCa) is a malignant form of cancer occurring in the glandular tissue of the prostate. In Germany, nearly three of every one hundred men die of prostate cancer. The early diagnosis of the disease reduces the risk of dying of such a tumor. As a measure to gain conclusive proof as to whether the prostate has been afflicted by a carcinoma, as a rule blood investigations are performed and the area is screened ultrasonically, after which a biopsy specimen is taken. This concept involves an invasive removal of tissue; albeit a standard procedure, it is nevertheless subject to controversial medical debate. In many cases three or even more punch biopsy specimens, selected from as many as 30 specimens punched from the prostate, are necessary to securely diagnose prostate carcinoma. "This may lead to the influx of bacteria into the bloodstream, which in worst-case circumstances can result in life-endangering septicemia", Dr. Joachim-Ernst Deuster, the Heidelberg-based urologist, warns. **"And if the biopsy needle hits a prostate carcinoma, this bears the risk of spreading tumor cells in the body. What's more, so-called cytokines may be released that are capable of enhancing the growth and metastasis of the prostate carcinoma."** The urologist is director of the private Clinic for Prostate Therapy and has specialized in the gentle treatment of prostate disorders. "Gentle treatment of the prostate should also be accompanied by just-as-gentle diagnostic procedures", says Deuster. He sees an enormous deficit of information related to the topic. For this reason, in Heidelberg last week he established the "Arbeitskreis biopsiefreie Diagnostik" **(Biopsy-free Diagnosis Working Group)**, that was attended by renowned experts from the areas of cytodiagnosis, molecular pathology, and magnetic resonance spectroscopy from throughout Germany. Together with experts from the area of laboratory medicine, they discussed the options available to reduce the risks associated with biopsy-taking procedures—for example by using entirely new and promising methods. These include so-called real-time choline PET/CT (choline positron-emission tomography / computer tomography) of the prostate—a novel, combined imaging method made possible by nuclear medicine—and MR spectroscopy. "Our wish is to offer experienced practicing specialists an informational podium", is how Dr. Joachim-Ernst Deuster explains one of his major aims. "By creating a closely meshed network, urologists and specialists from the cytoanalysis field and in the proven imaging techniques, such as computer tomography, want to join forces to identify ways to improve the accuracy in diagnosing prostate carcinomas or, as the case may be, of being able to exclude a carcinoma with a high degree of probability", adds Dr. Thomas Dill, a urologist from Heidelberg. **The principal aim is centered on the ability to avoid having to take biopsy specimens wherever possible as a measure to minimize the risk for the patient.**

The Working Group will be meeting regularly in the future, and warmly invites specialists from other areas to take part. **(Dr. Wheeler's Commentary: It is heartening to see the academic enthusiasm for biopsy avoidance whenever possible! Dr. Deuster clearly understands our ability to cure patients with prostate cancer is dependent on improved technology while pushing aside, the need for an antiquated obsolete diagnostic exercise like biopsy!)**

APPENDIX—16

Long-Term PCa Control with RP is 'Excellent'

~Radical prostatectomy (RP) for clinically localized prostate cancer achieves "excellent" long-term patient survival, according to researchers~

HENDRIK ISBARN, MD, and collaborators at University Hospital Hamburg Eppendorf, Hamburg, Germany, examined long-term rates of biochemical recurrence (BCR), cancer-specific mortality, and overall survival (OS) in 436 patients who underwent RP between 1992 and 1997 at their institution. None of the men received adjuvant or salvage treatment in the absence of BCR.

At 10 years, 60% of patients were free from biochemical recurrence, the overall survival rate was 86%, and only 6% died from prostate cancer, the researchers noted in *BJU International* (2009; published online ahead of print). Preoperative PSA level, RP Gleason sum, lymph node status, surgical margin status, and pT stage independently predicted BCR, according to investigators.

Dr. Wheeler's Commentary: While I appreciate the honesty and integrity of Dr. Isbarn's research team, **a 40% recurrence of PSA (the world's marker for biochemical failure) following Radical Prostatectomy is an abysmal outcome!** Only 6 out of 10 men achieved biochemical success at 10 years.

While I do not know the specifics of this particular study, most reviewers of this body of work would give it nothing more than a 'D' on the 'A through F' grading system. The most likely scenario in a National Health Care system (NHS) model is that very little attention was given to discrimination of disease. In other words, non-specific imaging tools were utilized (CT scan as example) that failed to accurately stage the patient. This **lack of discrimination for extent of disease commonly leads to a high failure rate**. In my mind, it is sad that men had to go through such a radical procedure that predicted an extremely high failure rate! Hopefully, our German colleagues have learned from their failures and have made adjustments!

NOTES:

APPENDIX—17

Chronic Disease Management (CDM) is a unique treatment concept that integrates traditional medicine and complementary medicine

(Dr. Wheeler goes on the record)

CDM THERAPY IS associated specifically with the least invasive, least traumatic, yet equally effective form of prostate cancer stabilization and/or suppression. Peer Reviewed Literature supports this concept in men with Gleason scores of 5 or 6 (50-60% of all prostate cancers). The key points to CDM therapy include proper diet, appropriate nutrition, adequate exercise, stress reduction, and continued education. CDM Therapy is also associated with a multi-modality, multi-mechanistic approach that utilizes today's scientific breakthroughs to tackle the most dominant type of cancer that men face.

While diet and nutrition alone have been shown to be beneficial for patients with Gleason 6 cancers primarily as a stand-alone protocol, the use of an anti-androgen (Flutamide or Bicalutamide), as a monotherapy, is also offered intermittently, in the event the PSA begins to progressively rise. Notwithstanding the success of this protocol, all men continue to be candidates for a chance at cure through the more well—known concepts of radical prostatectomy, brachytherapy, with or without external beam therapy, cryosurgery or high intensity focused ultrasound (HIFU). **While I favor HIFU, I realize patient selection will best define success or failure regardless of the procedure performed.** Anti-androgens are generally reserved for a patient with a progressively rising PSA that reaches 10 ng/ml or above while being discontinued when the PSA reaches 1.0 ng/ml or lower.

Metaphorically speaking, if cancer of the prostate is compared to a family dog that cannot be trusted with strangers or neighbors, the dog that roams the yard is attached to a leash or chain, allowing him to run only so far before he is restrained. By the same token, prostate cancer activity is not allowed to proliferate beyond what occurs with a PSA number of 10.0 ng/ml. In this clinical scenario and by design, the PSA will decrease sharply over the initial 30-60 days of anti-androgen monotherapy, allowing the cancer process to be suppressed. Based on Quality of Life issues as well as an issue of refractivity (resistance to the therapy), this treatment is commonly discontinued when the PSA reaches 1 ng/ml or lower.

During this time, multiple mechanisms of action are encouraged, including, but not limited to: Anti-angiogenesis associated with drugs such as Lipitor, Zocor, Pravachol or Noscapine, 5-Alpha Reductase Inhibition (Avodart or Proscar [Finasteride]), high dose Vitamin D-3, in an effort to decrease cellular proliferation, COX II Inhibitors, including Celebrex (associated with cyclo-oxygenase inhibition), Omega 3 fatty acids (an anti-proliferative nutrient) as well as the patented prostate nutritional formula, Peenuts®, utilized versus cellular oxidative stress, as defined by a reduction in white blood cells associated with the Expressed Prostatic Secretion (EPS).

Beyond this list of medications, the "Wheeler/Prostate Diet", associated with a modified Mediterranean approach, specifically discourages dairy and animal fats. Integral to the success of this program is the use of red wine, as a powerful anti-oxidant associated with resveratrol. Beyond the anti-oxidant benefit, red wine also serves as a source of phyto-estrogens, a natural antibiotic, and is a potent inhibitor of Endothelin-1. Interestingly, red wine has also shown to be of benefit to heart health, consistent with a daily intake of 1-2 (6 ounce) glasses per day.

Independent of our prostate health program, there is a need to address heart health as well. For this reason, Omega-3 Fatty Acids decrease plaque formation as well as modify the EPA (Eicosapentaenoic acid)/Arachidonic Acid/Ratio, HDL/Total Cholesterol Ratio, and LDL/HDL Ratio. Through the use of this proactive approach, expectation is noted to show a decrease in LDL, an increase in HDL, and a decrease in total cholesterol and triglycerides. Ultimately, through this approach, the heart risk assessment associated with lipids (fats) improves markedly. Lipids should be monitored with the Vertical Auto Profile blood test available through this office and Atherotech.

The American Association of Cancer Research (AACR), an organization that is comprised of some of this country's most brilliant micro-biologists and geneticists, presented research in December 2001 that has revolutionized the treatment of nonbacterial prostatitis. Specifically, the inflammatory process of prostatitis was shown to be associated with cellular oxidative stress, in conjunction with cellular dysplasia and subsequent free-radical formation. A loss of the enzyme Glutathione-S Transferase may play a pivotal role in diminishing an important cellular defense mechanism, allowing for proliferative inflammatory atrophy with cellular mutation to take place. Prostatic Intra-epithelial Neoplasia (High Grade PIN) is commonly associated with prostate cancer and may lead to its evolution.

Utilizing the number of white cells in the Expressed Prostatic Secretion (EPS) as the most accessible and well-understood marker, consistent with the disease process of non-bacterial prostatitis, the Peenuts® prostate nutritional formula has been shown to effectively decrease the degree of prostate inflammation over time. EPS, in effect, becomes a validated clinical test that can be performed at all urology clinics. The inability to utilize the EPS as a valid biologic marker, in concert with the use of the Peenuts® formula as the only patented prostatitis product, potentiates a level of academic ignorance that is unacceptable. Data consistently notes that a reduction in the white blood cell count in the prostate secretion is associated with a reduction in PSA. Maybe a reduction in PSA using the chronic disease management protocol highlighted by the Peenuts® formula (3 capsules daily) should be the primary goal to avoiding a more extensive evaluation for prostate cancer. Clearly, a point to ponder with an elevated PSA!

Dr. Ronald Wheeler Goes on the Record

Case History:

Jim Little, was 50 years old when first seen by me in Sarasota, Florida in June, 2005. By history, Jim had a PSA value of 5.1 ng/ml with digital rectal findings present consistent with cancer on both sides of this prostate. Jim's clinical cancer stage was T2c. Prior to seeing me, Jim had a biopsy in February 18,1999 at age 44, confirming the presence of prostate cancer, while noting a Gleason Score of 6 (3+3). Two of six cores were positive noting one core with 82% cancer involvement (Left Apex) while a second core from the Right Apex noted 27% involvement. According to the Partin Prediction tables (referencing Dr. Alan Partin's Prostate Cancer Prediction Tables), Jim had a 55% chance his cancer was organ confined. Better stated, Jim had a 45% chance his cancer was beyond the capsule of the prostate (extracapsular). Wanting to avoid surgery for multiple reasons, Jim embarked on a 6 year journey that included various alternative modalities including the use of PC-SPES (an Estrogenic Compound), Progesterone, Co-enzymeQ10, Barlean's brand Greens, Modified Citrus Pectin, Alpha Lipoic Acid, Flax (ground seeds and oil with cottage cheese) and Neo-Prostate (a Betasitosterol product for prostate health). **Nothing seemed to be working against Prostatitis which continued to provide a resource to the evolution of Prostate Cancer as noted by a white blood cell count in excess of 100 cells per high powered microscopic field (range: 100-180 white blood cells/400X); notwithstanding the use of Neo-Prostate continuously for 6 years.** Neo-Prostate has been touted incorrectly as a product that decreases inflammation in prostate. **Patients should not use Neo-Prostate as a supplement when prostatitis is suspected.**

Despite Jim's best efforts, bolstered by Physician guidance; as well as his support group consensus opinion and a normal AMAS (Anti-malign in the Antibody Sera) test result his **PSA was 8.2** when he arrived at my door step. Concerned for a rising PSA, that suggests enhanced cancer aggressiveness, if not a possible mutation, consistent with his previous strategy, I recommended we re-tool his treatment regimen to reflect my Chronic Disease Management strategy. The first part of his experience with me included a trial of Casodex (an anti-androgen) as a Monotherapy at 150 mg daily. Minimally, I want to suppress his disease while utilizing various disease altering modalities and mechanisms of action that had been proven to have an impact on prostate cancer. Relevant to Casodex, I recognize the high dose had not been approved by the FDA, but I knew the prescription drug was commonly used in Europe without incident when applied intermittently. Additionally, I had a long track record of success with the formula. With this background information, the following commentary that Jim provides to the support group is enclosed below. **Jim's comprehensive case presentation and report may be reviewed elsewhere in the Appendix.**

—Original Message—

From: James Little
To: pralt-discuss@prostate90.com
Sent: Monday, December 26, 2005 4:27 PM
Subject: [pralt-discuss] PEENUTS

Jim's Commentary: For those of you interested. My PSA continues to drop 4 months after discontinuing Casodex. The latest number is 1.6. I am taking 4 Peenuts capsules a day and have been for the last 6 months. I eat a low fat Mediterranean diet and take Avodart, fish oil, and vitamin D. I take no other supplements and I engage in regular exercise. It will be interesting to see on my follow up visit to Dr. Wheeler this spring if the use of Peenuts has affected the EPS white cell count and prostatitis. All indications at this point suggest a positive response! Jim Little

In a message dated 12/26/2005 7:13:09 A.M. Eastern Standard Time, jnl72254@yahoo.com writes to Dr. Wheeler for his input:

Jim's Commentary: While I am thrilled that my PSA continues to drop while off of Casodex, I have no clue as to why. My expectations were for the PSA to drop while on the Casodex and then start to rise again when the drug was stopped. The continued decline over the last 4 months has been a pleasant surprise and makes me wonder what is actually happening with the cancer. I do not think for a minute that the cancer is in remission or shrinking. Am I wrong about that? What I think more likely is that the production of PSA has been affected by the drugs and that the cancerous condition still exists, despite the drop in PSA. Please clear this up for me.

Dr. Wheeler's response: Casodex (Bicalutamide), an anti-androgen is a very good first line drug for prostate cancer when the PSA has risen to 8.0 ng/ml or higher as it is desirable to reduce the number while suppressing the disease. The lowering of your PSA number beyond a nadired value has not been commonly described and is not the same as 'androgen withdrawal syndrome'. PSA is a well known dependable marker of Prostate Cancer disease activity in a patient such as yourself who is hormone sensitive; validated by your response to the high dose Casodex. When we get the MRI Scanner in Sarasota, Florida; we will be able to objectively show the activity from the cancer and then do a comparative a year later. Until such time, you will always be suspicious that what you see is not true. A part of your opinion is jaded by the previous opinions that you have learned (incorrectly in many instances, I might add) in the trial and error program associated with your chat group. Any drop in PSA is a good thing when you know you have a hormone sensitive cancer process. As you will recall, I have a group of Gleason 6 prostate cancer patients who are in a study to show the benefit of diet and nutrition on the cancer process. I am confident you have this data. In this study, none of these patients have ever been exposed to an Antiandrogen, an LHRH Analogue or antagonist. Nonetheless, a review of 23 patients shows that 87% of these men have shown a decrease in cancer activity in association with a mean surveillance period of 38.5 months. To restate, this group of known cancer patients has never been exposed to any hormonal manipulation. The most sentinel event with all of these patients (as with you) is that Prostatitis is being

or has been resolved as a key initiator to prostate cancer evolution. As I have stated often, Prostatitis is the main highway to prostate cancer evolution and possibly growth. This is supported by the American Association of Prostate Cancer (AACR), David Bostwick, M.D., me and others. The objective response to the Peenuts® formula is a fact that has been validated in 4 separate clinical studies. If I wasn't somewhat concerned for your rise in PSA to the 8.2 ng/ml mark and your previous unknown disease contamination from the estrogenic effect of PC SPES, I may have avoided the initial trial of Casodex. I wasn't willing to subject you to possible failure, so I went with a program that I knew had the best chance to put your cancer process into remission. Please remember that you are a Gleason 6 and in my opinion took PC SPES prematurely and inappropriately. This is the message that you need to share with your chat room friends and why they need to be on Peenuts for the proven benefit versus prostatitis, the number one reason PSA rises. As you may know, you have not come to grips yet with the validation and meaning of prostatitis relevant to your clinical disease presentation based on your initial belief Neo-Prostate was working.

Jim's commentary: I had a brief period a while back when my libido increased and I became more sexually active. During this time I had fewer problems with erections (although still not much stamina). Now I seem to have gone back the other way and have lost interest in sex and have more problems with erections. At this point I cannot have one without the use of Cialis. Before treatment started I could always achieve an erection sufficient for penetration. So I have to ask you if this is a normal occurrence after 6 months of treatment or not. I also have to ask you for a prescription for Cialis as mine has expired. I would rather not see another doctor about this.

Dr. Wheeler's response: I would be happy to send you a prescription for Cialis. The process of erectile ability is dependent on so many factors that make it difficult to state with certainty why you now have a dependency on this class of drug (5-PDE Inhibitors). At this point, even your concern for the PSA drop (a good thing) may have caused you to have increased anxiety which will affect your sexual ability. For the record, anti-androgens, are not associated with predictable erectile dysfunction. As you know, Estrogens and chemical castration with the use of an LHRH Analogue like Lupron or Trelstar will have a predictable negative impact on your abilities to perform sexually. I have had many patients on anti-androgens with no significant sexual dysfunction in the past, while the same would go for Avodart (a 5-Alpha Reductase Inhibitor).

Jim's commentary: I re-read your report the other day and was reminded of your recommendation to get an MRI to establish a baseline image of the cancer. This is something that I never had done and would like to have. I had considered going to see Duke Bahn as his ultrasound scans are favored by the Pralt group, but I have not had the time and you prefer MRI over power Doppler ultrasound. Where would I have this procedure done? I am sure I would need a prescription for that as well.

Dr. Wheeler's response: An MRI (Magnetic Resonance Imaging) study is what I want you to have! The best study in my opinion uses a 3.0 Tesla magnet as well spectroscopy. Unfortunately spectroscopy for the prostate has not caught on in the world's market place and is currently available

in selected cities across the USA. Peter Scardino, M.D. (Chairman of Urology at Sloan-Kettering), stated that "MRI-S is the next greatest diagnostic tool for prostate cancer". We expect to get the 3.0 Tesla magnet (MRI-S unit) by mid-year in 2006, while we expect to be affiliated with University Centers in the evaluation of patients such as yourself. This is an academically exciting diagnostic test that evaluates the levels of cellular metabolites including: Creatine, Choline, Polyamines, and Citrate. In effect, a fingerprint of disease is created through the various multi-parametric sequences that are unique to you and your disease process. While I have an interest relevant to cancer, I also have a keen interest from a prostatitis standpoint relevant to the early signs of cancer detection. To state the obvious, the 3.0 T MRI technology (with or without spectroscopy) is much better than a 1.5 T MRI while also excluding the need for future ultrasounds under any technique including Color Flow "power Doppler" with or without contrast agents, AMAS tests and the like. The goal in all that we do is to avoid the need for future prostate biopsies, which as you know, may be associated with spreading prostate cancer when present.

Jim's commentary: I just received a letter from your office about a follow up visit. I did not plan on doing that until 1 year but would not be opposed to going to Florida in the winter! Do you want me at 6 month intervals or yearly? What is done at your follow up visits and how much are they? I am assuming you do the same tests.

Dr. Wheeler's response: Your time frame for seeing me is 6-12 months. I only want to see you if there is something meaningful that we need to address. I will let you decide

exactly when, based on how you are currently doing. The follow up visit will undoubtedly include a digital rectal exam, a repeat Uroflow test, a Post void residual (a test that measures the amount of urine in your bladder following the act of urination) and a repeat comparative EPS. We will spend more than 1 hour in this review. I would suggest that you get with our Clinic Coordinator after the first of the year to discuss the fees. None of this is terribly expensive but required to ensure that you are performing clinically as expected (assuring your quality of life).

Per usual, I am here to assist you with your questions. At some point in time when your questions require extensive explanations, we may want to resort to a conference call.

As you know, your health is just as important to me as it is to you!
Warm regards,

Ronald E. Wheeler, M.D.
941-957-0007
"Zero Tolerance for Prostate Disease"

Subj:
Re: Bob Bond's PSA Jumped from 5.1 to 6.4 in Last 90 Days
Date:
12/23/2005 4:30:44 P.M. Eastern Standard Time
From:
PROSTADOC
To:
bobbond@houston.rr.com
BCC:
johnkane1@verizon.net, jarensmith@sbcglobal.net

In a message dated **12/23/2005** 3:55:34 A.M. Eastern Standard Time, bobbond@houston.rr.com writes:

Hello Dr. Wheeler and Staff, Can you give me an overview of how I should manage my disease?
Dr. Wheeler's response to the questions is noted below:

Bob, Given your Gleason 7 (4+3) cancer status, you must not be surprised about movement in the PSA. On the other hand, there is clear data to suggest that a great diet is neutral to prostate cancer growth while a poor diet will assist the exacerbation of the disease process. For this reason, I urge you to do the best you can from a dietary and exercise standpoint. The reason you are on the CDM Protocol is based on the fact that any "definitive treatment program" is subject to failure. As you know, you will not add an antiandrogen such as Casodex until your PSA typically reaches 10.0 ng/ml or higher. If I were you, my next PSA would be in 60 days. Additional testing that would be recommended for you would be a 3.0 Tesla Magnetic Resonance Imaging Scan (with or without spectroscopy). This is brand new technological advancement to a concept that has been around since the early 1980s. We expect to have this technology in Sarasota in Mid July, 2006. As you know from a personal perspective, it is absolutely imperative to know the status of your disease at any given time through PSA and imaging. In many patients, the MRI scan is expected to negate the need for additional biopsies while in others it will assist a decision making process as related to an attempt at a cure or a continuance of the surveillance process. Beyond this, I will try to address the questions below.

Bob Bond's commentary: You should have received a fax report yesterday from Lakewood Family Physicians, showing that my PSA has jumped 25.5% in the last 90 days from 5.1 to 6.4. Needless to say, that came as a jolt to me!

Dr. Wheeler's response: I am not surprised by the change in PSA, notwithstanding the previous drop. Remember that a Gleason 7 is characterized as a volatile cancer; therefore, unpredictable and commonly aggressive.

Bob Bond's commentary: With it having gone down from 5.5 in early July to 5.1 in mid-September, I was expecting at least a slight drop from 5.1 even though I have not been as strict on my diet or done as much exercise per week in the last 90 days as I had in the prior 60 days. However, I do not believe that it would have kept going down below 5.1 even if I had replicated the first 60-day period.

Dr. Wheeler's response: Please realize that your commitment to Prostate cancer stabilization or suppression is a full time job and must be taken very seriously. The bonus will be a better quality of life while predictably controlling the cancer.

Bob Bond's commentary: I will outline below what I am taking in medication and food supplements, what I am eating, and my exercise program. Please let me know if there are any more tests that should be run at this time or any changes or additions to the medications that I am taking, or any changes in other areas.

I noticed, upon re-reading your excellent and very extensive report of July 11, 2005 that you mentioned a couple of things that relate to an elevated PSA reading: "in the event there is an elevation in the PSA Result, the necessity for heightened surveillance will dictate a repeat PSA on monthly intervals."

Question #1: Would you like me to begin having PSA tests run monthly?

Dr. Wheeler's response: While you could always go to monthly PSAs, I think it may be premature to do this at this very moment. I would recommend another PSA in 2 months and then we will reassess. If the PSA jumps significantly again, we will move to a monthly schedule.

"While the patient appears to be best suited for CDM protocol, additional viable consideration include: Radiation Therapy, with or without Seed Implantation, or Cryosurgery." **Question #2:** Am I correct in assuming that it is still too early to go to one of these Radiation Therapy options? **Dr. Wheeler's response: As you consider treatment choices is always best to be cautious! What you must realize is the distinct possibility that the radiation may not assist a curative process. As you visit with Radiation Centers, they will put the best "spin" on this form of therapy in an effort to attract you. Be aware that radiation imparts a risk of bladder cancer and colon cancer that is twice that of the normal population. At this point, I am a bit more cautious. If you choose to make a run at success with any form of therapy, a 3 Tesla MRI scan must be done first; but then you must realize the possibility that any procedure may fail. Once you are comfortable with this**

thought, you will be best prepared to make the
next move.

Bob Bond's commentary: In the event the conservative
approach outlined by you fails to suppress and/or stabilize the
PSA, is the patient instructed to add an anti-androgen (Casodex
or Flutamide) as a monotherapy; specifically, if the PSA reaches
10 ng/ml or above? In other words, will the patient begin the
anti-androgen, at the appropriate dosage, and continue that
therapy until the PSA reaches 1 ng/ml or below. **Dr. Wheeler's
response:** I like your thought process! You are correct that we
do not want your PSA to rise to a level higher than 10.0 ng/
ml as we try to maximize disease stabilization while avoiding
risk of metastasis. **Bob Bond's Question #3:** Am I correct
in assuming that it is still too early to go to one of these two
anti-androgens? **Dr. Wheeler's response: Anti-androgens
given as a monotherapy has been proven very successful in
my practice model. We have had success with every stage
and grade of cancer. While an LHRH Analogue such as
Lupron, Trelstar or Zoladex could also be an option, it may
be more than what you need to control the cancer process.
Surveillance and a trial of an anti-androgen when your PSA
reaches 10.0 ng/ml or above will assist our understanding of
your specific case requirements. In your case, (if and when
your PSA reaches 10.0 ng/ml or above), I would recommend
high dose Casodex (150 mg per day) as the anti-androgen
of choice. The avoidance of the LHRH Analogue predictably
avoids: bone loss, hot flashes, muscle wasting, lethargy,
mood swings, depression, weight gain, and etcetera. As you
can see, if you don't need this testosterone suppressing
agent in your Chronic Disease Management Protocol, there
is a tremendous benefit to you as a patient. To restate, we do
not want an intended treatment to be worse than the disease**

itself and/or to create a host of side effects that could have been avoided if we had only considered a more conservative approach in the first place. It is my expressed opinion, that far too many Gleason 6 prostate cancer patients are exposed needlessly to an LHRH-Analogue as an anti-androgen alone may have addressed the disease appropriately as validated by our success in this group of patients. In an effort to enhance the patient's comfort level that the disease process of Prostate Cancer is not becoming more aggressive, recommendation is made for the patient to have an Alkaline Phosphatase and Prostatic Acid Phosphatase (PAP) at 6-12 month intervals.

Bob Bond's Question #4: Since we can clearly see that the Prostate Cancer is becoming more aggressive, is there a reason for having this test run now? **Dr. Wheeler's response: The above mentioned laboratory tests can be performed at any point in time. While neither test is sensitive or specific enough to make unequivocal statements relevant to your disease process, they may provide another dimension to our understanding. If for example, the Alkaline Phosphatase is elevated, it may be prudent to evaluate the bone skeleton for signs of bone disease. A total body Scan associated with the 3.0 Tesla MRI scan would likely be my best first test in this scenario while avoiding unnecessary radiation associated with the typical bone scan.**

Bob Bond's Question #5: After reviewing the data shown below as to the medications and supplements that I am taking, do you have any recommended changes in the amount, frequency or combination in which I am taking any of these drugs or supplements? If so, please elaborate. **Dr. Wheeler's response: No changes Bob! Stick to the script!**

Question #6: After reviewing the data shown below as to foods I am eating, are there any foods that should be added to my diet, and are there others that should be reduced or eliminated? If so, please specify. **Dr. Wheeler's response: As you become more familiar with the extensive report from this clinic, you will realize that all of the dietary comments relate to a modified Mediterranean Diet, reviewed extensively in the book. This diet is not difficult to understand. Specifically, you need to avoid saturated fats associated with red meat and dairy products (milk, cheese, ice cream and eggs). Acceptable sources of protein are multiple including egg whites, breast meat of chicken, breast meat of turkey, fish (example: tuna, halibut, salmon, mackerel, and sardines), beans, and peanut butter. Beyond these sources of protein, you are encouraged to eat fresh fruits and vegetables including but not limited to the Brassica group highlighted by: Brussels sprouts, cabbage, kale, kohlrabi, broccoli, collard greens, mustard greens, and cauliflower. The oil of choice is olive while a glass of red wine or two daily is very beneficial for multiple reasons, not the least of which is to relax you. Simple carbohydrates such as sugar, white pasta, and white bread should be minimized, if not avoided. Snacks may include nuts realizing that nut meats contain healthy vitamins and minerals. Nuts that I specifically endorse are peanuts (dry roasted), almonds, walnuts, hazel nuts, pistachios, and Brazil nuts. Water is a key component to any dietary program as 85% of our body is composed of water. Any selection of water must meet certain standards of preparation including filtration. I recommend highly a product associated with reverse osmosis filtration. You would be surprised at the amount of contaminants contained in a typical glass of water from the tap. While they may meet the very basic standards set forth by Federal, State, and local guidelines for water quality earning it a** label of potable, it doesn't mean it meets the standards set forth by our program or that it is not too contaminated for your personal consumption. Beyond what I have presented, you should avoid processed foods including canned goods whenever possible based on a notable absence of flavor and nutrients while avoiding preservatives including sodium. Other foods to avoid are hot dogs, chili, canned meats, kielbasa, bratwurst, barbeque, meat balls, bologna, sausage, bacon and ham. As you will recall, pork (touted as a white meat) is a red meat like beef, lamb, and wild game. Until someone compares the level of saturated fats in red meat, showing an absence of saturated fat, these types of meats are to be avoided. As I always point out, the "South Beach Diet" is not prostate friendly or prostate healthy. Pickles, popcorn (popped in an air popper), pretzels (non-fat), mustard, and non-fat cheese are OK. Trans fat, commonly found in baked goods to extend the shelf life, is to be avoided. Brown rice is great while white rice is out. Honey is a simple sugar and should be avoided. Soft drinks and soda pop should be avoided whenever possible. Fruit juice is a carbohydrate and should be consumed in moderation while juicing of carrots is discouraged based on the high sugar content and concern for the possibility of osteoporosis. While I don't disagree that confirmatory studies are needed relevant to osteoporosis, I am concerned about vitamin A (beta-carotene becomes vitamin A) toxicity as well. Sandwich spreads are to be avoided as well as mayonnaise and cream sauces. Half and half is out but skim milk is OK. Tomato and tomato-related products are OK but one must remember that there is a significant amount of sugar and corn syrup in catsup and barbecue sauce and adjust accordingly. Spices including pepper are generally just fine. Egg beaters make great omelets when sources of quercetin such as onions, peppers and spinach are added. As a snack on a "once in a while schedule" is dark chocolate which contains stearic acid, favorable to assisting the battle versus prostate cancer. Relative to liquor, there is not a lot of merit in recommending any of this but the sedative effect may assist; especially for a fellow with all of these questions. Just kidding! Caution is placed relevant to Cirrhosis of the liver when moderation of alcoholic beverages is not observed.

Question #7: Any other thoughts or suggestions? All comments are encouraged and much welcomed.

Medications and Supplements:
My medications and Supplements are all taken together, washed down with a glass of 75% "light" grape juice and 25% red wine, followed by another glass of 20% lemon juice and 80% "light" grape juice, followed by a cup of green tea. These are usually taken within 15 minutes after eating breakfast or late dinner.

Taken each morning around 11AM: 2—Healthy Heart Omega 3's, 2—UroStar, 1—Peenuts, 1—315 mg Green Tea capsule, 1—0.5mg Avodart, 1—80mg Diovan, and 1—500 mg Vitamin C tablet. **Dr. Wheeler's response: So far so good!**

Taken each evening around midnight: 3—Healthy Heart Omega 3's, 2—UroStar, 1—315 mg Green Tea capsule, 2—0.5 mcg Hectorol, 1—5mg Terazosin, 1—1,250 mg Garlic supplement, and 1—500 mg Vitamin C tablet. **Dr. Wheeler's response: You are still doing well!**

Question #8: Do you see any problem with taking all the capsules at one time? If so, which one(s) should be taken separately and how long before/after taking the others in the morning or evening group? **Dr. Wheeler's response: While I don't see any specific problem relative to the absorption, I would probably set the Avodart apart and take it with lunch or an empty stomach. I am merely trying to ensure that you get the maximum response desired from the medications and nutritionals ingested although without further study, this is merely a hypothesis.**

Question #9: Knowing that I am taking this medication within 15 minutes of completing a meal, is this the best time to be taking the medicines and supplements, when their contents are not only being mixed with each other but also mixed with all that I have just finished eating? If I should wait longer after eating to take the pills, then how long should I wait? **Dr. Wheeler's response: There is no specific reason to vary your technique here as I prefer you to take nutrients with a meal whenever possible. While there may be an exception, I would keep doing what you are doing thus far.**

Foods Eaten:
Note: It might be helpful to know that I usually go to bed around 2:30-to-3:30AM, and get up around 10-to-11AM. (Cathie goes to sleep around 9PM and gets up around 5AM.) **Dr. Wheeler's response: Suit yourself with your sleep pattern. I merely encourage adequate rest to allow you to perform the daily activities without taking a nap. As you might suspect, if you take a nap, you may not sleep well the following night!**

Breakfast around 11AM: ½ Breakfast bowl of half Crunchy Nuggets (like Grapenuts cereal) plus half Maple Pecan Crunchy whole grain cereal with Soy milk. I then usually eat around 7-10 raw almonds and 7-10 roasted almonds, usually one of each together, for better taste. I then eat around 10-12 non-salted peanuts that were in their shells. Occasionally I substitute for the cereals, eggbeaters with either veggie sausage or turkey sausage. Around once every 10 days, I get up early for some reason and we go out to eat breakfast, wherein I usually eat 2 scrambled eggs, 2 sausage patties and a strip of bacon, plus some grits and 3 pancakes with syrup, all of which are on your "don't eat" list. **Dr. Wheeler's response: Now we have identified a culprit in the diet. You must be strong, steadfast and unwavering in your ability to say no when the waitress asks you if you will have your usual. If the waitress doesn't get the message either leave no tip or change restaurants. She will miss you but your health will improve!**

Lunch (for me), dinner for Cathie around 4:30-to-6PM: This one varies. If we go out to eat, I usually try to get either chicken or fish as the meat, and frequently eat Salmon or Tuna steak if available. If a salad is served, I will usually get a small one. I sometimes get Chick-Fil-A chicken strips and cole slaw. **Dr. Wheeler's response: No Chick-fil-A based on the lack of quality of the oil it is fried in. Also the breading on the chicken strips should be avoided. I am not picking on this restaurant chain but fast food chains should be avoided whenever possible. When this can't be done, get a salad and/or a grilled chicken breast. Avoid French Fries, bread and soda!** When eating at home, we frequently eat grilled chicken and some frozen vegetables that can be warmed up quickly. **Dr. Wheeler's response: You are now back on track! Congratulations!** If eating at home and I already have a large salad made (designed to last about 3 days), I will usually eat a medium-large bowl of salad with either chicken strips, grilled chicken or a small can of tuna mixed in with the salad. **Dr. Wheeler's response: What is it about the chicken strips that you don't understand? Obviously, I am**

consistent with my thought and the chicken strips are not good for you!!

The salads that I make usually consist of romaine lettuce, mixed lettuce, tomatoes, cucumber, cauliflower, broccoli, red or yellow bell pepper (usually red), red onion, finely chopped kale, celery, olive oil, raspberry vinaigrette, and low-fat ranch dressing. **Dr. Wheeler's response: Avoid the low-fat ranch dressing and continue to use the raspberry vinaigrette. Until you got to the dressing part, I thought we were back on the same page. I am looking for dedication from you as you move forward. Remember, I also want to prevent heart disease whenever possible as related to any dietary decision process.**

In between meals, I will usually eat a few peanuts and a few almonds. Sometimes I will eat a part of an apple, or some grapes, or strawberries or blueberries, or an orange or nectarine, usually depending upon what is in season and what is on sale at the time. **Dr. Wheeler's response: You are back in the favorable column again. I can see that you do know how to eat a healthy snack.**

Dinner (for me), usually around 11:30PM to 1:00AM: Usually some of the salad I have previously made, along with some turkey or a small can of tuna, though, since Thanksgiving, it frequently involves less healthy left-overs from various eating events. **Dr. Wheeler's response: Here we go again . . . Don't take home the leftovers; this is a sign of weakness. Leave them to someone much younger to eat; with no known disease!** Also, I will sometimes eat a half 14 oz. can of warmed up diced tomatoes that include garlic and onions. I was eating a half can every night, but have been neglectful in recent weeks. **Dr. Wheeler's response: To summarize, you have some** good habits and some bad habits. At your age, I would have expected you to have known better but you will learn, I am confident. Remember, the prostate healthy diet is also heart healthy!

Question #10: What are your recommended changes, if any, in what I eat or when I eat? **Dr. Wheeler's response: I have already commented on what you eat at great length. The time you eat is up to you but a healthier approach is to avoid a big meal that includes leftovers prior to going to sleep. The best time to eat the biggest meal of the day is lunch time. Beyond this comment, you can make adjustments as you feel are within your capacity to change.**

My son and I have joined Life-Time Fitness, a very elaborate fitness facility near our home, and plan to get back with the program several times a week after having slacked off the last couple of months. During that period, I also gained an extra 10 pounds, now up to an unhealthy weight of 222 lbs. **Dr. Wheeler's response: Bob, if you would have started this email with this statement, I would have been a little easier on you. The scale does not lie and reflects the sins that you have committed. I expect the requisite number of Hail Mary's and a more generous offering next time you are at church (just kidding of course; well, maybe not). Make the necessary changes and take everything I have said in this email to heart. I thank you for allowing me permission to include this email in my book as it memorializes that I have spent 3 hours on an email with a dear patient. This experience tells me that I shall never do it again and speaks volumes on why the book must come out. For you my friend, I did it this time but a conference call will always be the best way to handle the topics covered. I am making this point, just in case you have** any close friends who may have the same idea as you. As a closing remark to a prostate cancer survivor . . . you must get your son on Peenuts® and get his PSA checked prior as a baseline. Please compare his number to mine. My PSA is 0.3 ng/ml and it has been for the past 7 years.

Blessings to you, my brother, as you continue to travel down life's highway.

I posed questions, Dr. Wheeler, so that you could just list the Question Number, and state your answer, rather than having to repeat everything I asked. **Dr. Wheeler's response: Now you tell me!** Also, do you feel a need to recommend some medical procedure or change in medication just to "calm me down". It was indeed a psychological blow to see that my PSA had not only not gone down from the previous 5.1 but had actually quit going down and had gone up by more than 25% to 6.4 in the last 90 days. However, I am over the shock now, and eagerly await your reply. **Dr. Wheeler's response: As for the future, please list the rules of the email at the start of the email, not at the end. Per usual, I thank you for the opportunity to make a point to others who will read this in my book. At this point, it is my best advice to continue to monitor your PSA at monthly intervals. We will reconsider a treatment option at some later time but there is no hurry here!**

Best regards to a loyal patient!

Ronald E. Wheeler, M.D.

APPENDIX—18

Is VB3 an Acceptable Diagnostic Alternative to EPS?

Direct Comparison of EPS to VB3 (Post Massage Urine Analysis)
EPS is Diagnostic for Prostatitis when ≥ 10 WBCs/HPF (400X)

Patient	EPS	UNITS	DX	VB3	UNITS	DX
FG	30-50	WBCs	Yes	2-4	WBCs	No
JH	10-30	WBCs	Yes	6-8	WBCs	No
WJ	30-200	WBCs	Yes	1-4	WBCs	No
DJ	100-TNTC	WBCs	Yes	10-30	WBCs	Yes
JK	200-400	WBCs	Yes	2-8	WBCs	No
DK	20-100	WBCs	Yes	3-6	WBCs	No
JN	250-350	WBCs	Yes	60-70	WBCs	Yes
RW	100-500	WBCs	Yes	7-20	WBCs	Yes
TS	20-TNTC	WBCs	Yes	3-8	WBCs	No
KC	80-TNTC	WBCs	Yes	6-8	WBCs	No
DM	60-250	WBCs	Yes	6-12	WBCs	Yes
TD	5-25	WBCs	Yes	0-1	WBCs	No
NC	4-80	WBCs	Yes	6-14	WBCs	Yes
GW	5-30	WBCs	Yes	1-4	WBCs	No
DC	20-80	WBCs	Yes	4-8	WBCs	No
DV	20-60	WBCs	Yes	0-4	WBCs	No
PL	20-60	WBCs	Yes	1-3	WBCs	No
JK	200-400	WBCs	Yes	2-8	WBCs	No
GH	30-120	WBCs	Yes	20-80	WBCs	Yes
WM	20-400	WBCs	Yes	3-8	WBCs	No
DN	40-250	WBCs	Yes	1-4	WBCs	No
MM	5-20	WBCs	Yes	2-6	WBCs	No
MH	100-TNTC	WBCs	Yes	8-12	WBCs	Yes
DW	10-100	WBCs	Yes	1-3	WBCs	No
JN	80-TNTC	WBCs	Yes	1-5	WBCs	No

Patient	EPS	UNITS	DX	VB3	UNITS	DX
RC	100-400	WBCs	Yes	2-80	WBCs	Yes
PG	20-80	WBCs	Yes	2-7	WBCs	No
TH	60-120	WBCs	Yes	60-500	WBCs	Yes
BG	40-60	WBCs	Yes	2-3	WBCs	No
SH	20-80	WBCs	Yes	0-2	WBCs	No
JL	10-350	WBCs	Yes	0-3	WBCs	No
RC	100-200	WBCs	Yes	6-20	WBCs	Yes
DF	100-400	WBCs	Yes	3-7	WBCs	No
RP	200-300	WBCs	Yes	10-20	WBCs	Yes
JF	6-40	WBCs	Yes	1-2	WBCs	No
RN	160-300	WBCs	Yes	3-8	WBCs	No
RB	120-TNTC	WBCs	Yes	5-8	WBCs	No
WD	40-140	WBCs	Yes	3-6	WBCs	No
RN	100-250	WBCs	Yes	20-160	WBCs	Yes
RO	10-100	WBCs	Yes	1-3	WBCs	No
GG	10-300	WBCs	Yes	2-8	WBCs	No
DM	20-250	WBCs	Yes	3-15	WBCs	Yes
WS	15-40	WBCs	Yes	15-20	WBCs	Yes
AW	60-250	WBCs	Yes	4-12	WBCs	Yes
FW	30-TNTC	WBCs	Yes	6-10	WBCs	Yes
TM	175	WBCs	Yes	10-15	WBCs	Yes
JK	35-TNTC	WBCs	Yes	5-8	WBCs	No
DH	25-250	WBCs	Yes	10-12	WBCs	Yes
DM	3-50	WBCs	Yes	7-18	WBCs	Yes
N=49	Mean: 151		100%	Mean: 16.7		39%
	Median: 145			Median: 5.5		
	Mode: 300			Mode: 5		

Legend:

EPS & VB3 Represented as Range of White Blood Cells per Microscopic Evaluation (400X)

VB3 was evaluated immediately following EPS per Standard Urologic Protocol; TNTC=500 WBCs

EPS=Expressed Prostatic Secretion, the Diagnostic test for Prostatitis (Stamey & Meares)

30 Microscopic fields (minimally) were evaluated at (400x) to determine the WBC range

NOTES:

IPSS—INDEX
AUA (BPH) SYMPTOM SCORE

Patient: _____ Date:	Not At all	Less than 1 time in 5	Less than half the time	About half the time	More than half the time	Almost always
INCOMPLETE EMPTYING 1. Over the past month, how often have you had a sensation of not emptying your bladder completely after you finished urinating?	0	1	2	3	4	5
FREQUENCY 2. Over the past month, how often have you had to urinate again less than 2 hours after you finished urinating?	0	1	2	3	4	5
INTERMITTENCY 3. Over the past month, how often have you found you stopped and started again several times when you urinated?	0	1	2	3	4	5
URGE TO URINATE 4. Over the past month, how often have you found it difficult to postpone the urination?	0	1	2	3	4	5
WEAK STREAM 5. Over the past month, how often have you had a weak urinary stream?	0	1	2	3	4	5
STRAINING 6. Over the past month, how often have you had to push or strain to begin urination?	0	1	2	3	4	5

URINATING AT NIGHT

7. Over the past month, how many times did you most typically get up to urinate from the time you went to bed at night until the time you got up in the morning?

0	1	2	3	4	5

SYMPTOM SCORE: 1-7 Mild Symptoms, 8-19 Moderate Symptoms, 20-35 Severe Symptoms

Total Symptom score: _____

BOTHER SCORE DUE TO URINARY SYMPTOMS

	Delighted	Pleased	Mostly satisfied	Mixed	Mostly dissatisfied	Unhappy	Terrible
QUALITY OF LIFE DUE TO URINARY SYMPTOMS How would you feel if you had to live with your urinary condition, the way it is now, for the rest of your life?	0	1	2	3	4	5	6

NOTES:

APPENDIX—20

CIGNA HEALTHCARE COVERAGE POSITION

Subject Prostate Saturation Biopsy

Revised Date..**5/15/2007**
Original Effective Date...................................**5/15/2006**
Coverage Position Number **0450**

Table of Contents

Hyperlink to Related Coverage Positions
Gene-Based Testing for Prostate Cancer
Screening, Detection and Disease
Monitoring
Prostate-Specific Antigen (PSA) Screening for Prostate Cancer
Transrectal Ultrasound (TRUS)

INSTRUCTIONS FOR USE

*Coverage Positions are intended to supplement certain **standard** CIGNA HealthCare benefit plans. Please note, the terms of a participant's particular benefit plan document [Group Service Agreement (GSA), Evidence of Coverage, Certificate of Coverage,*

*Summary Plan Description (SPD) or similar plan document]
may differ significantly from the standard benefit plans upon
which these Coverage Positions are based. For example, a
participant's benefit plan document may contain a specific
exclusion related to a topic addressed in a Coverage Position.
In the event of a conflict, a participant's benefit plan document
always supersedes the information in the Coverage Positions.
In the absence of a controlling federal or state coverage
mandate, benefits are ultimately determined by the terms of the
applicable benefit plan document. Coverage determinations in
each specific instance require consideration of 1) the terms of
the applicable group benefit plan document in effect on the date
of service; 2) any applicable laws/regulations; 3) any relevant
collateral source materials including Coverage Positions and;
4) the specific facts of the particular situation. Coverage
Positions relate exclusively to the administration of health
benefit plans. Coverage Positions are not recommendations for
treatment and should never be used as treatment guidelines.
©2007 CIGNA Health Corporation*

Coverage Position:
**CIGNA HealthCare does not cover prostate saturation biopsy
because it is considered experimental, investigational or
unproven.**

General Background

Prostate cancer is the most common cancer diagnosed in
North American men, excluding skin cancers. It is estimated that
in 2007, approximately 218,890 new cases and 27,050 prostate
cancer-related deaths will occur in the United States (National
Cancer Institute [NCI], 2007a). Prostate cancer is the second
leading cause of cancer death in men, exceeded only by lung
cancer. It accounts for 29% of all male cancers and 9% of male

cancer-related deaths. Prostate cancer is rare in men younger than age 50, and incidence rises rapidly with each subsequent decade. The age-adjusted incidence rate is higher in

African-American men compared to white males. Mortality from the disease is higher in African-American males, even after adjusting for access-to-care factors. Risk factors for prostate cancer include family history, as well as age and race. Other possible risk factors include alcohol consumption, vitamin or mineral interactions, and other dietary habits (NCI, 2007a).

Screening of asymptomatic men for prostate cancer has become a widespread practice in the United States.

Screening procedures used for prostate cancer screening include digital rectal examination (DRE) and prostate-specific antigen (PSA). In situations of an abnormal DRE and/or elevated PSA, a transrectal ultrasound (TRUS)-guided prostate biopsy is usually performed. Prostate biopsy is used to diagnose prostate cancer, as well as in staging of the condition. In general, prostate biopsies are considered safe and are usually performed in an outpatient setting. The more common complications from prostate biopsies include: hematuria, hematospermia, and hematochezia. Other complications are rare and are more severe, including: severe bleeding, prostatitis, sepsis, urinary retention, and vasovagal reactions.

The prostate biopsy samples the areas of the prostate gland where tumors are most frequent, in a systematic manner. The biopsy is not lesion directed. The ultrasound is used to guide the biopsy needle into different areas of the gland rather than identifying lesions. The traditional prostate biopsy was the sextant biopsy, which involves taking six biopsies in a parasagittal line drawn halfway between the lateral border and midline bilaterally, from the base, mid-gland, and apex, with a

20–25% positive biopsy rate (Raja, et al., 2005). It was thought that the sextant technique was inaccurate mainly because it undersampled the peripheral zone of the prostate. Modifications of the sextant biopsy have been developed and reported on in the literature. The modified sextant biopsy protocol involves moving the middle biopsies of the standard sextant laterally and the biopsy trajectories angled anterolaterally so that mainly the peripheral zone is sampled. This method appeared to improve the cancer detection rate (Raja, et al.,2005). Extended biopsy techniques that utilized additional cores directed to the peripheral zone have been developed. It has been noted that the sensitivity of prostate cancer screening may be improved by taking 10–12 cores rather than six cores. Taking 10 to 12 tissue cores has become the standard of care (Wilson and Crawford, 2004). Sextant and extended biopsy with 10–12 cores is generally performed with local anesthesia. It has been estimated that up to 31% of all non-palpable prostate cancers diagnosed with needle biopsy and treated with radical prostatectomy are potentially insignificant tumors, with volumes less than 0.5 cm3 (Djavan et al., 2003). In some situations, there may be a continuing suspicion of prostate cancer even with repeated negative prostate biopsies. The prostate saturation biopsy has been proposed for circumstances where the patient is considered high-risk for prostate cancer, but biopsies have been negative. The saturation biopsy involves taking between 20 to 40 core biopsies. Additional cores may be taken for larger prostates. It is theorized that the saturation biopsy may detect cancer that was not detected with a prior biopsy. The technique is similar to the sextant or the extended biopsy in that it is performed during a TRUS, utilizing the core needle biopsy device. Some type of regional or general anesthesia or intravenous sedation is typically used. Another method of performing saturation biopsy involves utilizing a transperineal, grid-based method using a brachytherapy template. This method is theorized to be more systematic and allows for improved sampling of the area immediately anterior to the urethra (Raja, et al., 2006). The saturation biopsy is based on the assumption that the cancer is small and/or located in one of the deeper reaches of the gland (Raja, et al., 2006). The whole gland is sampled without following any particular zonal pattern. It is thought that the larger number of evenly distributed samples increases the probability of detecting an underlying cancer, regardless of the tumor size or location. Increased bleeding is generally noted with an increased amount of core biopsies (Routh and Leibovich, 2005). A concern with this type of biopsy approach is the possibility of an increased risk of detecting clinically insignificant cancers which may lead to unnecessary treatment.

It has been noted in the literature that controversy exists regarding which zones of the prostate to sample during a biopsy and how many cores to obtain that will minimize the diagnosis of clinically insignificant cancers. Various interrelated factors are involved in the decisions of when to biopsy and when to perform a repeat biopsy. These factors include: the PSA level, age of patient, family history, size of prostate, and the location and type of prior biopsies. It has been noted in the literature that, although prostate needle biopsy is considered the gold standard for cancer diagnosis, it is impossible to verify the absence of cancer in the prostate in vivo; as a result, the true false-negative rate remains unknown (Chrouser and

Lieber, 2004). It appears that increasing the number of biopsies may be associated with increased risk due to an increase in complications (Raja, et al., 2005). Review of the literature does not indicate that the prostate saturation biopsy is more effective than an extended prostate biopsy for the detection of clinically significant prostate cancer or that use of this test will lead to an increase in survival or prognostic yield.

Literature Review

Stewart et al. (2001) conducted a study based on the hypothesis that markedly increasing the number of cores obtained during prostate needle biopsy may improve the cancer detection rate in men with persistent indications for repeat biopsy. Saturation TRUS-guided biopsy was performed in 224 men. The mean number of previous sextant biopsy sessions was 1.8 (range one to seven). The median years from the first biopsy until the saturation biopsy was performed were 2.4 years. A mean of 23 saturation biopsy cores (range 14–45) were distributed throughout the whole prostate including the peripheral, medial and anterior regions. Indications for repeat biopsy included persistently elevated PSA levels in 108 cases and persistently elevated PSA and abnormal rectal exam in 27 patients, and persistently abnormal rectal examination in four patients, high grade prostatic intraepithelial neoplasia (PIN) in the previous biopsy in 64 patients, and atypia in the previous biopsy in 21 patients. In 112 of the 224 men (50%), it was noted that they had only a single set of negative biopsies before undergoing the saturation biopsy. It was noted that cancer was detected in 77 of the 224 patients (34%). Of the 77 patients in whom cancer was detected, 52 underwent radical prostatectomy. The location where the cancer was detected with the saturation biopsy was not reported. The complication rate for saturation biopsy was 12% and hematuria requiring hospital admission was the most common event. The authors concluded that saturation needle biopsy of the prostate is a useful diagnostic technique in men at risk for prostate cancer with previous negative office biopsies. Grossklaus et al. (2001) conducted a retrospective case review of the results from 135 consecutive patients who underwent radical retropubic prostatectomy (RRP). Needle biopsy data, including the number of cores, percentage of positive cores, laterality of the positive cores and Gleason sum were compared with the pathological data of the RRP specimen. The data was further separated into those with six or fewer cores (96 men) from those with more than six cores (39 men). It was noted that there was no significant relationship between the number of cores obtained and the predicted pathology of the RRP specimen. There did not appear to be a difference in the number of positive cores, bilateral positive cores or percentage tumor in the cores between men with more or less than six biopsies. It was noted that the percentage of positive cores may be the best predictor of pathological stage and tumor volume.

The authors concluded that taking more prostate needle biopsy cores seems to improve the detection of prostate cancer, but there appears to be no major improvement in prognostic information over that gained with traditional sextant biopsies. Fleshner and Klotz (2002) conducted a study to determine the role of saturation prostate biopsy among selected men with unexplained worrisome PSA parameters. The study involved 37 men who underwent saturation biopsy. This involved obtaining 24 peripheral zone cores, six to 12 transition zone cores and two lateral lobe transurethral samples. All of the men had previously undergone at least three prior sets of TRUS prostate biopsies. The median PSA level and the percent-free PSA level was 22.4 ng/ml (range 7.8–73.8) and 0.11 (range 0.04–0.17), respectively. The specimens were sent for pathologic examination in sets of six in order to determine the marginal benefit of additional sampling. After pathologic examination, it was noted that five patients (13.5%) had detectable carcinoma. In all cases, the carcinoma was detected in the 18 peripheral zone cores. Acute prostatitis was noted in 19% of the specimens. The study concluded that most men with multiple previous biopsies and increasingly worrisome PSA parameters do not have cancer and that the marginal utility of the saturation biopsy is low. It was noted that although rare additional cases may be detected using this technique, 18-core peripheral sampling is recommended for those difficult diagnostic cases. Sur et al. (2004) conducted a prospective randomized study to compare standard prostate biopsy to extensive biopsy utilizing intravenous conscious sedation (IVCS). Initial biopsy patients (n=197) were randomized to either standard biopsy (i.e., 6–12 biopsies, mean 10.1) using intrarectal lidocaine gel, or extensive biopsy (i.e., 20 biopsies) using IVCS. The objective was to determine if the extensive biopsy technique resulted in a higher rate of cancer detection and/or improved patient tolerance of the biopsy procedure compared to a more standard biopsy technique. Eighty-eight patients (48%), underwent the standard biopsy, and 94 (52%) underwent the 24-core extensive biopsy, with 15 patients withdrawing from the study. The authors note that while the sextant biopsy with six core samples may not be sufficient, the optimal number of biopsies required to maximize cancer detection without over-detection of clinically insignificant cancers is still uncertain. It was noted that the extensive prostate biopsy with 24 cores did not improve cancer detection rates compared to a standard biopsy technique in which an average of 10 cores was obtained. The IVCS technique was well tolerated and associated with significantly less pain and greater patient satisfaction than the rectal lidocaine gel alone. The authors note that the results imply that saturation biopsy is not necessary in patients undergoing initial prostate biopsy so long as extended biopsy that includes 8–12 cores is utilized.

Rabbets et al. (2004) reported on the diagnostic yield of office saturation biopsy in patients at increased risk for prostate cancer and at least one negative prior biopsy. Saturation prostate biopsy was performed on 116 patients with at least one prior negative biopsy and with certain risk factors, including persistently elevated prostate specific antigen, abnormal DRE, or prior atypia or PIN on a prior biopsy. A total of 34 cancers were detected for an overall diagnostic yield of 29%. In this series, only 22% of the patients had undergone prior sextant biopsies. In a small cohort, it was noted that there was a 64% cancer detection rate (seven of 11) in patients who had undergone a previous sextant biopsy. The authors concluded that saturation biopsy has a significant cancer detection rate even in patients who have undergone prior biopsies with more extensive lateral sampling.

Epstein et al. (2005) conducted a review of 103 men who had been predicted to have insignificant cancer in their radical prostatectomy (RP) specimen. The aim of the study was to determine whether saturation biopsy of the prostate could reliably predict insignificant and significant cancer in men who were candidates for watchful waiting. Candidates were identified based on the preoperative needle biopsy pathologic findings and serum PSA levels. The patients had limited cancer on the routine needle biopsy: no core with more than 50% involvement; Gleason score less than seven; and fewer than three cores involved. Saturation biopsy with an average of 44 cores and an alternate biopsy saturation scheme with one half of the number of cores were performed in the pathology laboratory on the RP sections. Of the tumors, 97% were organ-confined. The RP Gleason score was less than seven in 84% of the cases. Of the cancer specimens, it was noted that 71% were insignificant, and 29% had been incorrectly classified before surgery using standard biopsy schemes. Using the full saturation biopsy scheme, and where significant cancer was predicted, the probability of having insignificant cancer appeared to be 11.5% (i.e., false-positive rate). If the algorithm model predicted insignificant cancer, the significant cancer was also only 11.5% (i.e., using the alternate biopsy sampling scheme, the false-positive rate was 8%, and the false-negative rate was 11.4%).

The authors note that the results of the current study need to be prospectively evaluated to determine their validity. In addition, further testing would be required of the algorithm with saturation biopsy of patients in vivo. It was also noted that the classification of insignificant and significant cancer did not necessarily predict the biologic behavior of cancer long-term.

Jones et al. (2006) reported on results of a sequential cohort study that compared office-based saturation prostate biopsy to traditional 10-core sampling as an initial biopsy. A 24-core biopsy was performed on 139 patients undergoing initial prostate biopsy. Indication for the biopsy was an increased PSA of 2.5 ng/dl or greater in all patients. The results were compared to 87 patients who had undergone 10-core initial biopsies. Cancer was detected in 62 of the 139 patients (44.6%) who underwent the saturation biopsy and 45 of the 87 patients (51.7%) who underwent 10-core biopsy. The study notes that breakdown by PSA level failed to show benefit to the saturation technique for any degree of PSA increase. The authors concluded that the saturation technique did not appear to offer benefit as an initial biopsy technique and that further efforts at extended biopsy strategies beyond 10–12 cores are not appropriate as an initial biopsy strategy. Meng et al. (2006) investigated the impact of the greater number of prostate biopsies on the nature of cancer identified. **The authors noted that increasing the number of cores obtained at the time of TRUS-guided biopsy has increased the number of cancers identified; however, there is also increasing recognition that many men with prostate cancer may not benefit from early aggressive intervention**

and that over-detection of prostate cancer has resulted in over-treatment.

The Cancer of the Prostate Strategic Urologic Research Endeavor database, a longitudinal disease registry of men with prostate cancer, was utilized to identify 4072 men with six or more prostate biopsies obtained at initial diagnosis. Of these patients, 30%, 47% and 24% underwent 6, 7 to 11, and more than 12 biopsies, respectively.

There was a significant correlation noted between the biopsies and numerous sociodemographic and clinical variables, including PSA, comorbidities and income. It did not appear that there was a difference in disease characteristics as assessed by Kattan and Caner of the Prostate Risk Assessment scores among men with a biopsy number between six and 17. In a subset of 1548 men who underwent radical prostatectomy, no differences were observed regarding biochemical-free survival at a follow-up of 2.2 years.

The authors concluded that, "The increasing number of prostate biopsies obtained at diagnosis increases cancer detection but the impact on disease characteristics remains unclear. Our data suggest that the risk stratification of prostate cancers is independent of biopsy number (6 or greater) in a contemporary cohort of men." Bott et al. (2006) reported on a case series to describe a modified saturation biopsy technique and results of extensive transperineal template prostate biopsies in men with a high risk of prostate cancer for whom repeated transrectal biopsies were not diagnostic. The study included 60 men who had a rising PSA level and had at least two sets of benign octant biopsies or two or more prior biopsies containing high-grade prostatic intraepithelial neoplasia or atypical small acinar proliferation. In a transverse image, the prostate was divided into six regions. Three to five transperineal biopsy cores were taken in each of the six regions with the use of a brachytherapy template. Cancer was detected in 23 (38%) men. Of this group, cancer was detected in the anterior region of the prostate alone in 12 men (60%). One patient required overnight admission for hematuria, and two developed urinary retention. There were no reported cases of sepsis. The authors concluded that, "In men with a clinical suspicion of prostate cancer, but benign or equivocal prostate biopsies, extensive transperineal template biopsy of the prostate is a useful diagnostic tool. It allows sampling of the whole prostate in a systematic and safe fashion." Walz et al. (2006) conducted a study of 161 men who underwent saturation biopsies to explore the yield of saturation biopsy and developed a nomogram to predict the probability of prostate cancer on the basis of saturation biopsy. The biopsy involved obtaining an average of 24 cores and was performed in men with persistently elevated PSA levels. All had at least two previously negative, eight-core biopsies.

Prostate cancer was detected in 41% (n=66). Positive cores were found mainly in the far lateral zone (79%), the medio-lateral zone (36%) and the transition zone (18%). It was reported that the rate of insignificant cancers was 15.6%, or five of the 32 men treated with radical prostatectomy; however, the assessment of clinical significance could only be assessed for those who underwent prostatectomy and could not be assessed for the remaining 34 patients. The complication rate was noted to be 2.5% and included two acute urinary retentions, one acute prostatitis and one reactive syncopal episode. Two hospitalizations for intravenous antibiotics were required. The results indicated that PSA density and transition zone volume were the most significant predictors of prostate cancer. The authors concluded that saturation biopsy may be indicated in men with a persistent suspicion of prostate cancer. Merrick et al. (20006) reported on a study of 102 patients to determine the prostate cancer incidence, anatomic distribution, Gleason score profile, and tumor burden in patients diagnosed by transperineal template-guided saturation biopsy. All but one of the patients had undergone at least one prior negative TRUS biopsy. On average, patients had undergone 2.1 prior negative TRUS biopsies with a mean of 22.4 core biopsies. The prostate gland was divided into 24 regions for the biopsy, and the median number of cores taken was 50. Prostate cancer was diagnosed in 43 patients (42.2%). It appeared that there was considerable anatomic variability in prostate cancer distribution, with no anatomic region of the prostate without cancer. Complications included urinary retention in 38% of the patients who required a urinary catheter overnight, six for two days, and three for six days. Hematuria was noted in one patient who required overnight hospitalization. In their analysis, the authors noted that transperineal template-guided saturation biopsy "results in promising diagnostic yields for patients with prior negative TRUS biopsies. However, ideal patient selection, optimal transperineal saturation biopsy technique, number of biopsy cores, and regions to be sampled remains to be clarified."

Eichler et al. (2006) conducted a systematic review to compare the cancer detection rates and complications of different extended prostate biopsy schemes. Eighty-seven studies were analyzed with a total of 20,698 patients. Data was pooled from 68 studies that compared a total of 94 extended schemes with the standard sextant scheme. It was noted that increasing the number of cores was significantly associated with the cancer yield. Laterally directed cores appeared to increase the yield significantly, whereas centrally directed cores did not appear to. Biopsy schemes with 12 cores that took additional laterally directed cores detected 31% more cancers than the sextant scheme. Biopsy schemes with 18 to 24 cores did not detect significantly more cancers. Adverse events for schemes up to 12 cores were similar to those for the sextant pattern. Adverse event reporting was poor for schemes with 18 to 24 cores. The authors concluded that prostate biopsy schemes consisting of 12 cores that add laterally directed cores to the standard sextant scheme strike the balance between the cancer detection rate and adverse events and that taking more than 12 cores does not add significant benefit.

Professional Societies/Organizations

National Comprehensive Cancer Network (NCCN): The NCCN published clinical practice guidelines for early detection of prostate cancer. The guidelines include an algorithm for follow-up of TRUS-guided biopsies. This algorithm includes recommendations for when extended-pattern biopsy, defined as 12 cores, is to be performed for initial and repeat biopsies. The recommendations include the following (NCCN, 2006):

- The number of cores in extended pattern biopsy includes:
  ❑ Sextant (6 cores)
  ❑ Lateral peripheral zone (6 cores)
  ❑ Lesion-directed at palpable nodule or suspicious image
- Transition zone biopsy is not supported in routine biopsy. However, the addition of a transition zone biopsy to an extended biopsy protocol may be considered in a repeat biopsy if PSA is persistently elevated.
- After two negative extended TRUS biopsies, prostate cancer is not commonly found at repeat biopsy.
- For high-risk men with multiple negative biopsies, consideration can be given to a saturation biopsy strategy.

U.S. Preventive Services Task Force (USPSTF): The USPSTF published clinical guidelines: Screening for prostate cancer: Recommendations and rationale. The guidelines do not discuss prostate biopsies, but includes the following statements regarding biopsies: "DRE and PSA are the two principal tests currently used in the United States to screen for prostate cancer. Determining test characteristics of any screening test for prostate cancer is difficult because clinicians disagree on which cancers are "clinically important," and thus disagree on an appropriate target for early detection. The gold standard often used in screening studies—needle biopsy—may miss cancers that are present. Conversely, needle biopsy may serendipitously detect cancers unrelated to abnormal screening results. Especially in asymptomatic older men, screening with DRE and PSA may detect cancers that appear clinically significant based on size and tumor grade, but which would not have progressed to clinical symptoms during the patient's lifetime."

Summary

The prostate saturation biopsy has been proposed as a diagnostic tool for a subgroup of high-risk patients in whom prior conventional prostate biopsies have been negative. The aim of this technique is to improve cancer detection rates in these individuals. It has been proposed that the larger number of evenly distributed samples may increase the probability of detecting an underlying cancer, regardless of the tumor size or location. The role of prostate saturation biopsy in the detection of prostate cancer has not yet been established. It is not known whether this method improves the health outcomes of individuals.

There is a concern with this type of biopsy that there is an increased risk of detecting clinically insignificant cancers which may lead to unnecessary treatment. It appears that there may be an increased risk associated with an increase in the number of cores obtained. There is no consensus regarding which zones of the prostate to sample during a biopsy and how many cores to obtain that will minimize the diagnosis of clinically insignificant cancers. It has not been demonstrated in the published peer-reviewed literature that the prostate saturation biopsy is more effective than an extended prostate biopsy for the detection of clinically significant prostate cancer, or that use of this test will lead to an increase in survival or prognostic yield.

References:

1. Taneja SS. Prostate biopsy: targeting cancer for detection and therapy. Rev Urol. 2006 Fall;8(4):173-82.

2. American Cancer Society Guidelines for the Early Detection of Cancer. Revised: 02/28/2006. Accessed March 29, 2007. Available at URL address: http://www.cancer.org/docroot/ped/content/ped_2_3x_acs_cancer_detection_guidelines_36.asp? sitearea=ped

3. American Cancer Society. Detailed Guide: Prostate Cancer—Can Prostate Cancer Be Found Early? Revised: 03/10/2006. Accessed March 29, 2007. Available at URL address: http://www.cancer.org/docroot/CRI/content/CRI_2_4_3X_Can_prostate_cancer_be_found_early_36.asp

4. Boccon-Gibod LM, de Longchamps NB, Toublanc M, Boccon-Gibod LA, Ravery V. et al. Prostate saturation biopsy in the reevaluation of microfocal prostate cancer. J Urol. 2006 Sep;176(3):961-3; discussion 963-4.

5. Boczko J, Messing E, Dogra V. Transrectal sonography in prostate evaluation. Radiol Clin North Am. 2006 Sep;44(5):679-87, viii.

6. Bott SR, Henderson A, Halls JE, Montgomery BS, Laing R, Langley SE. Extensive transperineal template biopsies of prostate: modified technique and results. Urology. 2006 Nov;68(5):1037-41. Epub 2006 Nov 7.

7. Chrouser KL, Lieber MM. Extended and saturation needle biopsy for the diagnosis of prostate cancer. Curr Urol Rep. 2004 Jun;5(3):226-30.

8. Cookson MM. Prostate cancer: screening and early detection. Cancer Control. 2001 Mar-Apr;8(2):133-40.

9. Djavan B, Remzi M, Marberger M. When to biopsy and when to stop biopsying. Urol Clin North Am. 2003 May;30(2):253-62, viii.

10. Descazeaud A, Rubin M, Chemama S, Larre S, Salomon L, Allory Y, et al. Saturation biopsy protocol enhances prediction of pT3 and surgical margin status on prostatectomy specimen. World J Urol. 2006 Dec;24(6):676-80. Epub 2006 Nov 7.

11. Eichler K, Wilby J, Hempel S, Myers L, Kleijnen, J. Diagnostic value of systematic prostate biopsy methods in the investigation for prostate cancer: A systematic review. York, UK: Centre for Reviews and Dissemination (CRD): 2005.

12. Eichler K, Hempel S, Wilby J, Myers L, Bachmann LM, Kleijnen J. Diagnostic value of systematic biopsy methods in the investigation of prostate cancer: a systematic review. J Urol. 2006 May;175(5):1605-12.

13. Epstein JI, Sanderson H, Carter HB, Scharfstein DO. Utility of saturation biopsy to predict insignificant cancer at radical prostatectomy. Urology. 2005 Aug;66(2):356-60.

14. Fleshner N, Klotz L. Role of "saturation biopsy" in the detection of prostate cancer among difficult diagnostic cases. Urology. 2002 Jul;60(1):93-7.

15. Grossklaus DJ, Coffey CS, Shappell SB, Jack GS, Cookson MS. Prediction of tumour volume and pathological stage in radical prostatectomy specimens is not improved by taking more prostate needle-biopsy cores. BJU Int. 2001 Nov;88(7):722-6.

16. Harris R, Lohr KN. Screening for prostate cancer: an update of the evidence for the U.S. Preventive Services Task Force. Ann Intern Med. 2002 Dec 3;137(11):917-29.

17. Igel TC, Knight MK, Young PR, Wehle MJ, Petrou SP, Broderick GA, et al. Systematic transperineal ultrasound guided template biopsy of the prostate in patients at high risk. J Urol. 2001 May;165(5):1575-9.

18. Jemal A, Siegel R, Ward E, Murray T, Xu J, Smigal C, Thun MJ. Cancer statistics, 2006. CA Cancer J Clin. 2006 Mar-Apr;56(2):106-30.

19. Jones JS, Patel A, Schoenfield L, Rabets JC, Zippe CD, Magi-Galluzzi C. Saturation technique does not improve cancer detection as an initial prostate biopsy strategy. J Urol. 2006 Feb;175(2):485-8.

20. Jones JS, Oder M, Zippe CD. Saturation prostate biopsy with periprostatic block can be performed in office. J Urol. 2002 Nov;168(5):2108-10.

21. Klotz LH. International regional working groups on prostate cancer: results of consensus development. Can J Urol. 2005 Feb;12 Suppl 1:86-91.

22. Matlaga BR, Eskew LA, McCullough DL. Prostate biopsy: indications and technique. J Urol. 2003 Jan;169(1):12-9. Review.

23. Meng MV, Elkin EP, DuChane J, Carroll PR. Impact of increased number of biopsies on the nature of prostate cancer identified. J Urol. 2006 Jul;176(1):63-8.

24. Merrick GS, Gutman S, Andreini H, Taubenslag W, Lindert DL, Curtis R, et al. Prostate Cancer Distribution in Patients Diagnosed by Transperineal Template-Guided Saturation Biopsy. Eur Urol. 2007 Feb 23.

25. National Cancer Institute (NCI) a. Prostate Cancer (PDQ®): Screening. Last Modified: 3/13/2007. Accessed March 29, 2007. Available at URL: http://www.cancer.gov/templates/doc.aspx?viewid=3bd07dce-4376-4dcb-b993-03c3dbe23e6e&version=1

26. National Cancer Institute (NCI) b. Prostate Cancer (PDQ®): Treatment. Last Modified: 3/15/2007.

Accessed March 29, 2007. Available at URL: address:http://
www.cancer.gov/cancertopics/pdq/treatment/prostate/
healthprofessional

27. National Comprehensive Cancer Network (NCCN). Prostate cancer early detection. Clinical Practice Guidelines in Oncology—v.1.2006. Accessed March 29, 2007. Available at URL address: http://www.nccn.org/professionals/physician_gls/PDF/prostate_detection. df

28. National Comprehensive Cancer Network (NCCN). Prostate Cancer. Clinical Practice Guidelines in Oncology—v.1.2007. Accessed March 29, 2007. Available at URL address: http://www.nccn.org/professionals/physician_gls/PDF/prostate.pdf

29. [No authors listed] Prostate-specific antigen (PSA) best practice policy. American Urological Association (AUA). Oncology (Williston Park). 2000 Feb;14(2):267-72, 277-8, 280 passim.

30. Patel AR, Jones JS, Rabets J, DeOreo G, Zippe CD. Parasagittal biopsies add minimal information in repeat saturation prostate biopsy. Urology. 2004 Jan;63(1):87-9.

31. Philip J, Ragavan N, Desouza J, Foster CS, Javle P. Effect of peripheral biopsies in maximizing early prostate cancer detection in 8-,10—or 12-core biopsy regimens. BJU Int. 2004 Jun;93(9):1218-20.

32. Philip J, Hanchanale V, Foster CS, Javle P. Importance of peripheral biopsies in maximising the detection of early prostate cancer in repeat 12-core biopsy protocols. BJU Int. 2006 Sep;98(3):559-62.

33. Pinkstaff DM, Igel TC, Petrou SP, Broderick GA, Wehle MJ, Young PR. Systematic transperineal ultrasound-guided template biopsy of the prostate: three-year experience. Urology. 2005 Apr;65(4):735-9.

34. Rabets JC, Jones JS, Patel A, Zippe CD. Prostate cancer detection with office based saturation biopsy in a repeat biopsy population. J Urol. 2004 Jul;172(1):94-7.

35. Raja J, Ramachandran N, Munneke G, Patel U. Current status of transrectal ultrasound-guided prostate biopsy in the diagnosis of prostate cancer. Clin Radiol. 2006 Feb;61(2):142-53.

36. Routh JC, Leibovich BC. Adenocarcinoma of the prostate: epidemiological trends, screening, diagnosis, and surgical management of localized disease. Mayo Clin Proc. 2005 Jul;80(7):899-907.

37. Schoenfield L, Jones JS, Zippe CD, Reuther AM, Klein E, Zhou M, Magi-Galluzzi C. The incidence of high-grade prostatic intraepithelial neoplasia and atypical glands suspicious for carcinoma on first-time saturation needle biopsy, and the subsequent risk of cancer. BJU Int. 2007 Apr;99(4):770-4. Epub 2007 Jan 16.

38. Silletti JP, Gordon GJ, Bueno R, Jaklitsch M, Loughlin KR. Prostate biopsy: past, present, and future. Urology. 2007 Mar;69(3):413-6.

39. Sur RL, Borboroglu PG, Roberts JL, Amling CL. A prospective randomized comparison of extensive prostate biopsy to standard biopsy with assessment of diagnostic yield, biopsy pain and morbidity. Prostate Cancer Prostatic Dis. 2004;7(2):126-31.

40. Siu W, Dunn RL, Shah RB, Wei JT. Use of extended pattern technique for initial prostate biopsy. J Urol. 2005 Aug;174(2):505-9.

41. Stewart CS, Leibovich BC, Weaver AL, Lieber MM. Prostate cancer diagnosis using a saturation needle biopsy technique after previous negative sextant biopsies. J Urol. 2001 Jul;166(1):86-91.

42. Taneja SS. Optimizing prostate biopsy strategies for the diagnosis of prostate cancer. Rev Urol. 2003 Summer;5(3):149-55.

43. Taneja SS. Prostate biopsy: targeting cancer for detection and therapy. Rev Urol. 2006 Fall;8(4):173-82.

44. U.S. Preventive Services Task Force. Screening for prostate cancer: recommendations and rationale. Am Fam Physician. 2003Feb15;67(4):787-92.

45. Walsh PC, Retik AB, Vaughan ED, Wein AD, editors. Campbell's Urology 8th ed. Philadelphia: Saunders; 2002.

46. Walz J, Graefen M, Chun FK, Erbersdobler A, Haese A, Steuber T, et al. High incidence of prostate cancer detected by saturation

biopsy after previous negative biopsy series. Eur Urol. 2006 Sep;50(3):498-505.

47. Wilson SS, Crawford ED. Screening for prostate cancer: current recommendations. Urol Clin North Am. 2004 May;31(2):219-26.

48. Wilson, S, Glode, ML, Crawford, DE. Prostatic Carcinoma. In: Schrier RW, editor. Diseases of the Kidney & Urinary Tract. Philadelphia: Lippincott Williams & Wilkins; 2007. ch 30.

APPENDIX—21

May 28, 2009
My story in brief:
The Clinical events in the life of Greg O'Haver

I AM AN active healthy athletic white male who turned 49 this past October. In September my family physician, whom I have been seeing for years conducted a PSA blood test on me. He said that he recommends to all of his patients to have a PSA test performed around the age of 50. His information is based on the best recommendation of the American Cancer Society. The test results came back as a 34 with the normal being less than 4.0. Nonetheless, the test result number did not mean anything to me at the time as I felt great. I was however, concerned with the message from the doctor's office which alarmed me, so I decided to have the test performed again. The test came back with similar results. I was referred to a local Urologist and told to schedule an appointment as soon as possible.

I was able to get in to see the Urologist within a week or so. The Urologist explained the serious nature of the high PSA number and informed me that he needed to do a biopsy right away to determine if cancer was present. I was told it was the only way to determine exactly what was going on within my prostate and the procedure was routine and would be performed in his office. I agreed to have it done and had it scheduled within a couple of days. I now know, I should have asked more questions because the biopsy was not what I expected. The procedure involved having 10 needles shot into my prostate through my rectal wall with only a local anesthetic gel applied to the prostate area. The pain was far greater than I had imagined and so were the long lasting effects. I had blood and brown goo in my urine, semen and seepage from my rectum for nearly 6 weeks.

The results from the biopsy came back as cancer noting a Gleason score of 7 (4+3); not favorable to me. Subsequently, a consult with the Urologist and my closest family members was scheduled. During the consult my Urologist informed me that he strongly recommended a radical prostatectomy to be performed in the very near future. Other options were available including radiation, radiation seeds, and cryotherapy however, he explained that the radical prostatectomy was "the gold standard" and it offered me the best chance of cure and for extending my normal way of life. He made a strong case for scheduling the procedure promptly as my disease would most assuredly kill me if I didn't act immediately.

My family and I left the office stunned and in total shock. They urged me to have the procedure performed immediately. Something told me however, that I was not getting the whole story and I should continue searching for more answers. I did not like the statistics that I was given without any meaningful discussion given to the cause of this cancer and real chance for cure. He made me feel like a radical prostatectomy was truly my only option. I felt that there should be something outside the traditional impersonal big money institutional thought process that only looks at you as a statistic. In my search for more information, I finally came across a name from a person I knew at a local health food store . . . his name, Dr. Ronald Wheeler, a Urologist from Florida.

My research and telephone conversions with Dr. Wheeler made me confident it was worth the trip to Sarasota, Florida to let him take a look at me in a second opinion. Once there I quickly saw the Diagnostic Center for Disease as a first class operation with a first class staff. I was treated as a person from the first time I walked in the door. I knew quickly that Dr. Wheeler was committed to giving me the best care and insuring I was well informed. He began with his MRI-Spectroscopy procedure which I learned could have saved me the pain and problems related to the biopsy, not to mention preventing the possibility of needle tracking which can spread the cancer cells during the barbaric biopsy procedure. Dr. Wheeler also started me on a regimen of natural supplements to assistant my body in strengthening itself as well as a protocol to clean up the spill of cells from the needle biopsy procedure. After the MRI-S scan had identified the cancer as confined to my prostate, my wife and I decided to have a new procedure called High Intensity Focused Ultrasound (HIFU) performed. This procedure has not yet been FDA approved and is only in clinical trials here in the United States. I was surprised to hear how long Dr. Wheeler had been successfully performing HIFU, a procedure commonly available around the world.

Dr. Wheeler performed the procedure on me in concert with the International HIFU team in Cancun, Mexico in February. The procedure was well orchestrated and was handled exactly like it was explained to me. I only had mild discomfort from the procedure and was walking around sightseeing the next day with my wife. The only issue whatsoever was a small catheter inserted just above my pubic bone during the procedure that I had to remain in for three weeks until I was urinating normally through the normal channel. There was no removal of body parts or major cutting and/or surgical complications or extended hospital stays that are commonly related to the other options listed for me early on.

Now to the great news! I have just received my PSA results three months after the HIFU procedure was performed. The results showed a PSA value of 0.1 ng/ml, consistent with an absence of disease. I am unbelievably relieved! Clearly, I am on the road to overcoming this devastating disease and hopeful the disease is gone forever. Physically and mentally I feel stronger than ever; thanks to Dr. Wheeler's skill and management decisions. I am so thankful and blessed that I was able to find the best treatment option out there for me and my family. I encourage anyone with questions or concerns related to prostate health to contact Dr. Wheeler and his staff at the Diagnostic Center for Disease in Sarasota, Florida. Their commitment to providing personalized state of the art patient care is a cut above the traditional methods that we have become accustomed to.

Sincerely,

Greg L. O'Haver

Greg L. O'Haver
12824 Old Dayton Pike
Soddy Daisy, TN 37379

Dr. Wheeler's response: I am very pleased with Greg's PSA result after one year using the HIFU technology. As with all patients, we will continue to monitor his progress. Minimally, we have impacted the cancer and improved Greg's chances of living a normal healthy life! In the event the PSA rises, over the next months or years, a repeat MRI scan will be performed to determine the next best step in his care. **Concern is noted for his high initial PSA associated with a subsequent biopsy without controlling for needle tracking prior to the biopsy.** Additionally, I have concern for the natural history of his disease! Without question, this case represents a scenario too often seen! Without symptoms, Greg had no idea the severity of his disease until the PSA was drawn. If the US Preventative Task force was in charge of Greg's care, he would not have had a PSA. Hopefully, Greg will continue to do well post operatively. We assume nothing and will continue to inspect the disease at 3 month intervals using the PSA, the venerable marker of disease activity!

APPENDIX—22

MY BATTLE TO SURVIVE PROSTATE CANCER

My name is Donald T. Huang, a retired engineer from Boeing Company in Seattle, WA. On September 7th, 1995, I was diagnosed with prostate cancer with a Gleason score of 10 and PSA of 17.5 at the University of Washington Medical Center. A UW Urologist wanted to treat me with radical prostatectomy (RP). He told me to have an RP for cure because hormonal therapy is not a cure. I almost believed him. Additionally, he added, "I know what is best for you. If you go for surgery, I will give you twenty years to live. If you take hormone therapy, I will give you two years to live. If I were you, go for broke..." I almost went for surgery until he wanted to remove my bladder too. TWO YEARS TO LIVE??? I was only 63 years old. My golden years had just begun. I was so shocked, numb and scared, as I had no sign or symptom other than a rising PSA. The urologist also pressured me to make a decision in a month because my cancer cells were a fast growing type. I called my two brothers-in-law for advice. One is Dr. Shun Hung Ling (Obstetrician-Gynecologist). He favored surgery from surgeon's viewpoint but no bladder removal. That is too radical for me. The other one, Dr. Shun Mei Ling (Endocrinologist in Los Angeles) researched extensively for three weeks. He phoned and said, "Don, I have found the right treatment for you. It is called Total Androgen Blockade. It provides you a good quality of life. The surgery is way too aggressive. If I had the disease, I would want to be treated this way." I was so relieved to hear those wonderful words. Both sent me stacks of prostate cancer papers for surgical and non-surgical procedures. Despite the fact that I am an educated man, I felt helpless for the first time in my life as I had no medical knowledge. With their help, I managed to take a crash course in short time to learn the medical terminologies.

After I studied all the research materials, I contacted Dr. John Thompson (Oncologist at University of Washington) and requested Total Androgen Blockade for treatment. However the UW Cancer Review Board recommended radical prostatectomy or radiation therapy as standard treatment from a medical establishment point of view. I rejected both and felt confident that TAB would be my best choice. They were skeptical and cautious in the beginning, but finally they honored my request.

Dr. Bob Leibowitz (Oncologist in L.A.) had popularized Total Androgen Blockade (now called Triple Blockade) in the early 1990s. The treatment consists of Lupron, Flutamide, & Proscar, a combination Dr. Leibowitz thought could cure prostate cancer. Feeling comfortable, I began an extended treatment that would last 14 months. At 3 months into the treatment, my PSA dropped from 17.5 to 0.1. During the course of treatment, both Dr. Leibowitz and Dr. Edwin Jacobs (Oncologist of Sherman Oaks, CA) had given me invaluable advice and encouragement. The first cycle of therapy enabled me to avoid any additional treatment for almost 7 years (from 10/5/1995 to 9/11/2002).

During that time, I attended many prostate cancer conferences and learned as much as I could about different treatments regarding this dreadful disease. In 1996, I went to a PAACT (Patient Advocates for Advanced Cancer Therapy) sponsored Prostate Cancer conference in Grand Rapids, Michigan. I met Drs. Fernand Labrie, Bob Leibowitz, Charles Meyers, Stephen Strum, Ronald Wheeler and several others. It was an eye opener for me. Hormone therapy alone has so many variations for use according to this group of experts. Some doctors use one drug, some use 2 or 3 drugs. The length of treatments were also different, some use 6 to 9 month, some use 12, 14, or 24 month and up to 6 years. It was so confusing! It was a very difficult task to figure out the right treatment for me? One can ask 5 doctors the same question and you will get 5 different opinions. One will wonder which one is the right one.

In 1999, I read an article about prostatitis in the PAACT newsletter written by Dr. Wheeler, a member of their medical advisory committee. I subsequently contacted Dr. Wheeler and through him I learned about the PEENUTS® treatment for prostatitis. As I learned, as men age, virtually all men will get prostatitis. Also prostatitis has been shown to evolve into prostate cancer. Since I have both diseases, there was no way to know which one contributed what percentage to the PSA rise. Now I am taking PEENUTS® with confidence as I know through experience it will keep prostatitis at bay. The PEENUTS® formula has made a very impressive impact on how I empty my bladder as well as contributing to the resolution of prostatitis. Because it has been so helpful to me, I recommend it to all my friends in the U.S. & Taiwan.

During the time that followed the 14 month TAB therapy (12/5/96 to 9/11/02), my PSA kept rising; PSA was 0.5 in 1997, 4.7 in 1998, 11.2 in 1999, 13.4 in 2000, 19.1 in 2001, & 32 in 9/4/02. My original plan was to begin taking the PC-SPES treatment when my PSA reached 20. Unfortunately, the California Health Board and FDA forced PC-SPES off the market in June 2002. I was now in limbo and wondering what I would do next. Meanwhile my PSA rose to 32. My Oncologist suggested me to go on chemotherapy with Taxatere or Mitoxantrone as the only option left because he feared that Triple Blockade would not work again for me because of my aggressive Gleason 10 cancer. Dr. Lings (my two brothers-in-law) did not approve of the chemotherapy because they didn't have a lot of confidence in Taxatere or Mitoxantrone with an aggressive cancer. Even with chemotherapy, there is confusion and disagreement among doctors. Some doctors use 1 or 2 drugs, some use a cocktail of 4 or more drugs. How do I know which one is right one for me?

After a long discussion with my two brothers-in-law, I decided to take TAB treatment for second time. Since I am an engineer and a fighter, not freedom fighter but jungle fighter, I don't give up easily. My logic is now very simple; the TAB worked for me the first time, so maybe it will work for me the second time. After all, I have been off TAB for almost 6 years. As I remember the treatment's title is "Intermittent Triple Androgen Blockade" as published in New England Medical Journal a few years ago. It means you can go back on TAB multiple times until you become hormone resistant or refractory. In my case, if and when it fails, I will then seek other options like chemo. I restarted treatment on 9/11/2002 and completed in 1/2/2004 with Lupron + Casodex (50mg) + Proscar + Celebrex + PEENUTS®. The PSA results were just like 7 years ago. Everyone was surprised and pleased with the results. Who said that Triple Blockade couldn't work second time?

Through my stressful journey over the past nine and half years, I learned that many patients are not well informed about treatments other than radical prostatectomy. Many of them who had surgery became incontinent or impotent. All expressed that if they had only known there were other options; they may not have undergone surgery in the first place. Because of those comments, I realized that I am very fortunate to have two knowledgeable brothers-in-law, Dr. Wheeler, Dr. Leibowitz, and Dr. Thompson to advise me throughout this ordeal. Also, I know that a patient must take the time to become well informed and be comfortable as well as confident with such a critical decision. There is no cure for prostate cancer because I believe it is a systemic disease; but it can be controlled and lead to a good quality of life. Survival in my case required the support of my family and friends for which I am grateful.

Dr. Wheeler's Commentary:

Donald was lucky to have a support team to allow him to step back from the heat of the moment when the diagnosis was revealed, to shun an expert's opinion to remove his bladder and prostate while learning an unknown language (medicine) at a rapid pace in order to assess his best option. The opinion offered to him by the surgeon was one that would be supported by most Urologists; however, it would have been the wrong choice. Most patients with this grade of cancer would wilt under the anxiety and pressure that the diagnosis creates and do most anything the doctor said for any chance of success. **In this particular case, surgery had little to no role as the literature shows that 85% of all cancers return within 5 years regardless of the therapy offered and performed.** Donald did not want to become a statistic! This case represents the best use for triple blockade in my opinion. Donald made himself available to some of the world's experts, making his case a sentinel case where everyone wanted to provide their expertise to allow him success as measured by continued quality of life as well as an extension of life. His success with a Gleason 10 cancer is truly remarkable. Donald did for this disease what was required and nothing more. Despite all the good that we had done, Donald's disease reared its ugly head with a progressively rising PSA. In effect, Donald (like virtually every patient with prostate cancer) became resistant to all that was offered him and was sent to hospice for pain management and inevitable death. Then along came Zytiga™ (Abiraterone Acetate) taken at 1000 mg per day in the absence of hepatic insufficiency. **Donald's progressively rising PSA which had reached 1600 ng/ml decreased with**

a one month supply of Zytiga™ to less than 10.0 ng/ml and less than 5.0 ng/ml following two months. This was indeed, pretty remarkable! Needless to say, Donald's pain has abated and he graduated from hospice to the real world of the alive and kicking! **To graduate from Hospice is indeed a rare event and noteworthy!** Donald is happy to be back to his loving family and will be monitored closely for additional signs of metastasis or disease progression!

APPENDIX—23

Bryce Zender's Story

INSTEAD OF WRITING the usual cancer memoir where a person's life is defined narrowly in terms of the disease and efforts to combat it, let me offer a broader perspective. My life did not just begin with the diagnosis of prostate cancer and will not end with it. Perhaps by initially sharing a few of the many defining moments in my life, I can put my struggle with cancer in the larger context of my life. In turn this view may help the reader understand who I am and why I chose certain courses of action in my bout with prostate cancer.

Like most young people, I felt almost invincible early in my life until I was confronted with the possibility of death for the first time. It happened while crawling through an infiltration course at Fort Polk in Louisiana. As part of basic training, young recruits like myself, were required to crawl on their stomachs under barbed wire while machine guns were rattling live bullets a foot or so above our bodies. Some men froze with fright while others conquered their fears and completed the course. Then this realization occurred to me; letting fears dominate is common place and expected while overcoming them is hard, requiring discipline and faith.

A few years later, I had an epiphany while making a career choice. My decision was to enroll in graduate school and pursue an advanced degree. These studies led to a Fulbright scholarship and a brief academic career. More importantly, my education set me on a path of lifetime learning marked by respect for scientific knowledge and disciplined thinking.

Perhaps the most defining moment in my life happened when my wife Mary Ann agreed to marry me. After marrying in San Francisco, we were blessed some years later with a daughter, Kira. From my life with these two women, I have gained the gifts of unconditional love and a wonderful family. Obviously, there were other decisive moments where my choices determined the path of my life, but these events were most critical. Also these experiences influenced greatly my choices in my ensueing struggle with prostate cancer.

In December of 1999, at age 64, I became aware of the importance of prostate cancer when my primary care physician, Dr. Samoy, noted a high PSA number among the results from my annual physical examination. She explained to me briefly that a number of 5.0 ng/ml indicated a possible problem ranging from an enlarged prostate to a cancerous one. Furthermore, she recommended I see a Urologist. 3 short months later, in March of 2000, I had an appointment with a Urologist in Lakeland, Florida where I now make my home. He recommended and performed an ultrasound and a biopsy. Fortunately for me the biopsy was negative but the experience won't soon be forgotten. Clearly, this was a wakeup call for me.

In December of 2001, my routine physical with Dr. Samoy again noted an elevated PSA blood test result of 6.0 ng/ml and again suggested I follow up with the Urologist. Rather than return to my former Urologist who wanted to perform another biopsy, I decided I needed a second opinion. Through my extensive research on the internet, reading medical journal articles and books, my choice was Dr. Ronald Wheeler at the Diagnostic Center for Disease in Sarasota, Florida. In August of 2001, Dr. Wheeler and his assistant spent more than 2 hours conducting tests on me that I had never experienced anywhere else. In addition, his comprehensive visit included another hour or so with my wife and I discussing the entirety of my case while answering all of our questions. Collectively we decided to treat the inflammation in my prostate in a conservative attempt to avoid another biopsy. This included Dr. Wheeler's patented formula called Peenuts; an all natural formula intended to lower the PSA if no cancer was present. While I believed this should have been the initial course before the previous biopsy, I was surprised my previous Urologist did not know what Dr. Wheeler knew about inflammation in the prostate. Heartened by what we heard from Dr. Wheeler, we set out on a journey where Dr. Wheeler would be the Coach and we would be loyal players on the team. Winning for us would be me improving my overall health and achieving a healthy prostate.

Despite our best efforts, including improvement in my urinary symptoms and decreasing the prostate inflammation, my PSA continued to climb to 10.8 ng/ml by January of 2002. Given my rapport with Dr. Wheeler and my confidence in him, I returned to his clinic where an ultrasound and biopsy was scheduled using a relatively new technology at the time called Color Flow Doppler to guide the needle placement aimed at suspicious blood vessels. A short time later, Dr. Wheeler contacted me with news that the biopsies indicated that I had a Gleason score 6 prostate cancer. In concert with Dr. Wheeler's strategy, we would control the disease predictably with an anti-androgen medication called Flutamide. Fortunately, this medication would not diminish my Testosterone or my abilities sexually as a male but rather would temporarily disable, weaken and suppress the cancer disease process resulting in a lower PSA. I had taken the Flutamide for only 3 short months, with minimal side effects, until May 23, 2002 when it was stopped based upon a PSA blood test result of 0.5 ng/ml. Over the next several months, I read everything I could get my hands on regarding prostate cancer and it various treatments. Based on the fact there is high variability in the success of cancer treatments based on a multitude of factors, I was content to continue the course outlined by Dr. Wheeler. In the back of my mind, I remained concerned about the potential aggressiveness of cancer while concerned that it could escape to other parts of my body. Here again, I experienced yet another epiphany relevant to my cancerous condition. Like most individuals who are faced with their own mortality, I was fearful yet hopeful. The fact that the anti-androgen Flutamide had reduced my PSA to 0.5 indicated a glimmer of hope. Through my readings, I realized my approach was one of many to stop the progression of cancer. With this knowledge in hand and the confidence that Dr. Wheeler provided, my fears were eased as I now had hope in combating my cancer.

In late spring of 2002, I decided to get yet another opinion on what I should do. I returned to the Urologist who performed my first biopsy. After a review of what Dr. Wheeler had recommended, his thought was that I should have a radical prostatectomy. Concerned that I may be missing an opportunity to cure my cancer if I did not heed the advice of this doctor, I began to seek the opinions of men who had the procedure. I personally knew some men from Civic organizations who had the surgery who were less than pleased with their results. Some mentioned incontinence while others mentioned impotency while still others mentioned both. While I realized these complications were not intended with the procedure, I nonetheless, realized they represented a condition I must be prepared to live with. Through my readings, I also learned that the radical procedure was extremely complex and depended highly on the skill of the surgeon as well as the biology of the disease. I learned of Pat Walsh from Johns Hopkins who carefully screened his patients, treating only the best candidates for the surgical procedure. Based on my understanding of my problem, I opted to defer surgery or other definitive treatments for the immediate future.

In the summer of 2002, I again visited with Dr. Wheeler to discuss his best plan. Based on everything he knew, the most conservative yet predictable way to control prostate cancer was through a protocol he developed, called Chronic Disease Management. This would allow me to resume my life without issues of incontinence or impotency. In effect, his strategy would allow me to live with the cancer much like men and women live with diabetes or arthritis. His plan called for a modified Mediterranean diet, nutrition versus prostate inflammation, exercise, stress reduction and continue to be proactive educationally. He also prescribed Finasteride, a medication that blocks the conversion of Testosterone to Dihydrotestosterone, Zocor, a medication to lower my cholesterol and Vitamin D3 to slow down prostate cancer cell growth. I was also instructed to continue my meditation schedule and take my multiple vitamins every other day. As my wife and I are essentially vegetarian, the program did not appear to be a challenge. My exercise routine would be running a couple of miles every other day and a weekly tennis outing. Dr. Wheeler also cautioned me that while he was confident my disease would remain quiescent, he would be prepared to use an anti-androgen intermittently if the PSA approached 10.0 or higher. Dr. Wheeler assured me that this protocol would not preclude the use of another type of treatment at a later time. PSA testing would be monthly until we achieved a better understanding of the disease activity. Once this was established, I would perform PSA testing at two month intervals while every 3 months would be implemented as the best timetable for my active surveillance program, assuming stability of the number. It was still my responsibility to schedule my PSA testing with my local doctor while he received all results including an Alkaline Phosphatase and Prostatic Acid

Phosphatase at 6 month intervals. Now for more than 4 years, my PSA has remained remarkably stable with my most recent PSA being 4.1 ng/ml. **It is amazing how stable my cancer has been over the past 4 years under Dr. Wheeler's guidance.** I often think about how my life would have been altered if I had agreed to a radical prostatectomy. The stability of my disease has since been confirmed by his 3.0 T MRI-Spectroscopy scanner to be organ confined allowing me the confidence that what I have been doing for all these years—made sense. Additionally all of this great information has allowed me the chance that I needed; to treat this disease as a chronic disease while maintaining my active lifestyle without interruption. I should add that Dr. Wheeler's involvement of my wife proactively in all that has been done has assisted her anxiety level, while very much appreciated by her.

I hope that the preceding account of my struggles with prostate cancer will help others and their loved ones who are faced with similar issues. In this brief history, there are, in my opinion, a few important insights that emerge from my personal experience and perhaps noteworthy to others. **First**, all of us have sentinel moments in our lives that determine the path our lives will take. We have control of these processes if we will only take the initiative. We can't leave these important decisions to anyone, even our doctor. **Second**, prostate cancer, though a life altering disease and potentially life threatening is just another sentinel or critical moment in our lives about which we must make careful decisions so that we do not become fatalistic victims of disease. Dr. Wheeler's protocol was the right approach for me as it conservatively managed my disease while allowing me the opportunity to better educate myself for the road ahead. **Third**, although fear is a normal reaction or response when faced with prostate cancer, knowledge instead of fear must prevail to empower your decision process enabling you to what is right first. This process includes your choice of physicians and treatment. **Fourth**, sharing knowledge and insights with immediate family and loved ones in the decision process will tend to reduce their fears and resulting anxieties. **Fifth**, sometimes prostate cancer patients are defined narrowly only in terms of disease and thus marginalized by others, bluntly put, who hold ignorant views about cancer. Thus, prior to this commentary, I chose not to reveal my struggle with prostate cancer beyond my immediate family. Dr. Wheeler has allowed me and my family to see this disease as it really is as opposed to joining the 'urge to treat with surgery' rhetoric. **Sixth**, facing the prospects of death is something everyone must consider sooner or later in life but prostate cancer forces us to consider our mortality at the moment the diagnosis is made. With Dr. Wheeler involved as my Coach, I never felt that I was alone with any decision I had to make. To be sure, looking at death frankly and honestly is not a negative process but a positive one that can aid us to free ourselves from the trivial and focus us on the more important aspects of life.

Finally, every reader of my account, who is faced with the diagnosis of prostate cancer, needs to decide what is best for their specific situation, but not until they have had adequate time to become sufficiently educated. **In my case, Dr. Wheeler was there for me and continues to be there for me!** How he finds time to micro-manage a case like mine with a myriad of responsibilities is beyond my comprehension. I can only say, I can't thank him enough for what he stands for, his success and his dedication to me and the fortunate ones who know him.

Dr. Wheeler's Commentary:

Everyone with the diagnosis of prostate cancer deserves to be treated with respect, dignity and a resolve to do for the disease what is required and nothing more. Treating an elevated PSA, as example, with our patented Peenuts formula as the best first response, allows us to delay or possibly eliminate an unnecessary biopsy if the PSA blood test result decreases. Doctors who fail to understand this simple concept will soon see a shortage of patients to treat as patients will not tolerate the prostate biopsy rhetoric. I believe patients will intuitively understand the advantage of a nutritional formula over an invasive biopsy. In Bryce's case, his cancer responded nicely to conservative measures establishing one more time that treatment should be individualized and conservative when possible. Clearly Bryce's disease qualifies as a disease that would have been over-treated with surgery or radiation. In his case, I was prepared to do more but didn't have to. To treat prostate cancer with 3 months of an anti-androgen and then discover a hiatus from disease for more than 4 years is academically stimulating and excites me to continue to study the biology of this unpredictable disease. Excepting the short course of the anti-androgen, Bryce's clinical course matches nicely to patients who are achieving success in our prospective prostate cancer study group using primarily diet and nutrition to contain their disease. While our clinical experience is quite dramatic with Bryce; the discovery that his disease is organ confined using the 3.0 T MRI-Spectroscopy scan is even more gratifying. Because Bryce chose quality of life over quantity of life, he has received both. While our research continues, I encourage all men with a Gleason 6 cancer to consider treating prostate cancer as a chronic disease. Bryce and others are living proof that it works.

APPENDIX—24

Ray Cunningham's Story

My story began with acute Prostatitis and a fever of 105 degrees. A Urologist treated me with an antibiotic enabling my fever and chills subside. Later, I received a digital examination, a PSA blood test and a urinalysis but according to the doctor, all were normal. Over the next 5 years of checkups (every 6-12 months), my PSA ranged from 2.5 to 6.1 ng/ml. Once the PSA reached 6.1 ng/ml a biopsy was ordered and performed in June 2004. The biopsy revealed an infiltrating adenocarcinoma with a Gleason score of 5(3+2)/6(3+3) involving both sides of my prostate. My clinical stage was noted to be a T1c, meaning the cancer was not detected on the digital exam.

Once the cancer was diagnosed, I was moved along as if I was on "a conveyor belt to the operating room." At age 72, the only option given to me was the knife, no alternatives. Even doctors at Vanderbilt recommended the radical prostatectomy. The doctor stated, "Let's cut it out and get rid of it so you can get on with your life." No discussion was given to what I am going to do about impotency or incontinence, if this occurs. Am I going to be doomed to wearing diapers the rest of my life? I was fearful about a radical prostatectomy as the urologist was sharpening his knife. I had nowhere to turn; I just wanted to run but I did not know where to run. I had requested and received a second opinion which was the same as the first opinion. I had talked to men who had the operation with bad outcomes. I had never met anyone who was totally satisfied with a radical prostatectomy. Faced with gloom and doom, I did not know what to do until in casual conversation, an unexpected bit of advice was given to me. I was asked to speak with a man named John Frye from Colorado. At this point in time, with no place to turn and no alternatives, I was only a week away from a scheduled radical prostatectomy.

When I spoke with Mr. Frye by phone, I explained what was going on; he suggested that I speak with Dr. Ronald Wheeler about my case. John said, he thought Dr. Wheeler would advise me not to have surgery and that there would be a good chance he could treat me for this condition in a non-surgical manner called Chronic Disease Management. I was thrilled with what I had heard and contacted Dr. Wheeler immediately. I would later learn that Dr. Wheeler was one of a few specialized, leading edge, clinical and research urologists in the country. **In a 30 minute conversation with Dr. Wheeler, I had learned more about my condition than I had learned from all of my doctors in more than 5 years.** Based on this conversation, I knew I had to go to Sarasota, Florida and meet with Dr. Wheeler and learn more about his exciting research that would include me.

Man, was this exciting! In the space of a 30 minute conference call, my life had changed. The concern, the anxiety and my desperation had turned to hope, confidence in a solution and jubilation that my life would not change radically. While I was hopeful from the moment I entered Dr. Wheeler's clinic, I was confident in his strategy after 15 short months when my PSA had dropped from 6.1 to 0.9 ng/ml. My success was based primarily on the Wheeler Diet and nutrition. My voiding symptom score had improved by 56% and my EPS (white blood cell count associated with the expressed prostatic secretion) had improved by 84%. I have seen definite improvement and feel strong, healthy and very thankful.

I believe Chronic Disease Management has been shown to be a viable treatment option, allowing men to have an alternative to radical prostatectomy when prostate cancer is detected. This program encouraged me to change my diet, introduced me to the patented Peenuts® formula for prostatitis resolution and provided a prescription medication. It was that simple.

With all my heart, I want to say that I believe my Heavenly Father intervened when he put me in touch with Dr. Ronald Wheeler. I do not believe it was merely accidental. The direction I received came in a totally unexpected way for which I am most grateful.

Ray Cunningham 02/16/06

Dr. Wheeler's Commentary:
It was a pleasure and privilege to assist the health of Ray Cunningham. Ray is prototypical of men who are shocked, disturbed and confused by the diagnosis of prostate cancer. Based upon my research which is discussed throughout this book, I have demonstrated that prostate cancer can be treated conservatively. To be sure, I want to do for the disease what is required and nothing more. Men who employ the Chronic Disease Management approach can expect success though a program of diet and nutrition primarily while preserving sexual, bowel and bladder function. Rather than monitor the disease activity with a repeat biopsy as many Urologists suggest, our center features a very sophisticated 3.0 Tesla MRI scan that can compare a

baseline image sequence to a follow up scan sequence with high confidence. **Based on the fact that traumatic biopsies spread prostate cancer cells (if encountered), the preference is to compare disease states with imaging rather than a biopsy procedure that suffers from sampling bias.** Based on exciting new research, **there is data to suggest that biopsies actually cause cells to mutate based on inflammation from the needle stick with the possibility of creating a cancer that may not have been present initially.**

After 4 years on this program, Ray's PSA is now 2.2 consistent with stability of disease. While we continue to monitor this number at 3 month intervals, Ray's success is primarily based on the reduction in prostatitis as an inflammatory disease. Based on the 3.0 T MRI scan, Ray has no evidence of disease beyond his prostate capsule or into the Seminal Vesicles. What this really means to Ray is that he remains a candidate for a definitive treatment such as high intensity focused ultrasound or some other potentially exciting new therapy that preserves quality of life while ablating the cancer. **In my Urology practice, success is measured one patient at a time.**

APPENDIX—25

Chronic Disease Management—A Worldwide Prostate Cancer Strategy

~Ross McVeigh's story as told by his wife Carol~

HI, MY NAME is Carol McVeigh and my husband Ross has prostate cancer. I would like to tell you what it was like being told Ross had prostate cancer and how we found the information we needed to make a decision that ultimately led us half way around the world to Dr. Ronald Wheeler at the Prostate Center (now the Diagnostic Center for Disease™), in Sarasota Florida. I hope that in telling our story, others will realize that it's alright to think **'outside the box'** and challenge established medical beliefs. I believe that ultimately the outcome for Ross has been more positive because of our joint efforts.

Dr. Wheeler had asked me to tell Ross' story from my perspective as a wife and a nurse. I am a registered nurse with over 35 years experience in nursing as a midwife and have a PhD in Nursing. Ross is an aircraft Engineer, an independent contractor and for many years he has been involved in Defense Department activities. We have been married for 37 years; live a comfortable lifestyle on the Gold Coast in Queensland, Australia while our two adult children work overseas. Despite our background and education nothing prepared us for Ross being diagnosed with prostate cancer. Our life changed forever on February 20th 2003 . . .

I remember sitting in the specialist's office with Ross, watching the doctor review his results, and being informed that five of the eight biopsies were positive for cancer. Aged just 60, his PSA was 19.6, Gleason score 6 and he had **no symptoms; none at all**. The specialist carefully outlined the possible treatment options, which in Ross' case were radical prostatectomy, external beam radiation, and watchful waiting. I also remember being told that there was perhaps a 50% chance of 'getting it all' and that damage from the surgery could be extensive (i.e. impotence, urinary incontinence, bowel damage). Additionally, we needed to wait two weeks before an MRI and bone scan could be done in an effort to define the extent of disease. This waiting period, as the specialist explained, was needed to allow the prostate to heal following the biopsies. I felt like I had been hit with a baseball bat as I walked out of the Doctor's surgery in shock, fighting back the tears and thinking 'this can't be happening to us' and 'I have to be strong for Ross'.

We drove home in silence and had two long weeks ahead of us to do nothing but think; why us, why Ross and what could we do? While we assumed from what the specialist had said the cancer was outside the prostate. What we didn't know was if it had spread to other parts of Ross' body and to what extent. I think we had a couple of stiff drinks and met with friends to share our news. Almost immediately Ross started to search the Internet for information about treatment options, outcomes and anything that could help us make an informed decision. In addition to that, I also activated the resources of one of the largest nursing organizations in the world. We needed all the help we could get . . . now!

The next two weeks were a bit of a blur. Although I continued to work outside the home, my waking hours were filled with personal thoughts of what this diagnosis would mean to us as a couple and to Ross in particular. Our time was spent searching for information, telling family, friends and colleagues and being lost in thought about how will this change our lives and also wondering how long Ross would live. I had always expected to spend a few years alone at the end of my life, however, this was the first time I had actually considered that Ross might die and leave me alone for more years than I cared to contemplate. My initial shock was accompanied by an inability to concentrate, a serious problem with insomnia, as it was nothing for me to wake up at 2AM and remain awake for the rest of the night. My GP prescribed sleeping pills but they simply made things worse. I really thought I should have coped better as a nurse; I thought I should have been more resilient as a wife, but with so many things going on in my life I began to question my ability to deal with this crisis!

With all of this going on Ross still managed to review over 2,300 articles and numerous web sites. I read much of what he found of value and everything suggested there was a continuing inability on the part of medical practitioners to cure men of prostate cancer using established radical surgery and external beam radiation. Neither of these traumatic therapies had demonstrated significant survival benefits compared to more conservative medical approaches. The only procedures to emerge from the literature as potentially curative, given Ross' bleak clinical picture, were cryosurgery and seed implants. Unfortunately in Australia cryosurgery is viewed as experimental, only offered as 'salvage treatment' while the only cryosurgery unit in this country was closed due to equipment failure and lack of funding. Furthermore, he was not a candidate for seed implants because this procedure was not funded in Australia for men with PSA levels higher than 10.0. Armed with this information, Ross had no difficulty coming to the realization that he wanted to aim for quality of life—not longevity. Based on potential side effects, he rejected radical prostatectomy and external beam radiation as viable options. He said he would rather have five good years than ten bad years and I supported his decision.

Two weeks later Ross had his MRI and bone scan. I remember watching Ross walk down the hall with the technician while I was instructed to sit in the waiting room. I wondered why they exclude me, his primary support person; it just seemed so unnecessary and certainly added to my level of frustration and concern. I was tempted to protest but past experience had taught me not to intervene. I wanted to support Ross; however, I decided to remain silent and do as I was told. Once we had all the information we were faced with one sealed envelope after another. I don't know why they insist on sealing the envelopes, they were his results, it was his body, and we already knew he had cancer . . . what could possibly be worse!? Needless to say we opened the reports, reviewed them carefully and made arrangements for a follow-up consultation with the urologist.

During our return visit the urologist revised the possible cure rate downwards to perhaps 25 to 30 percent. Although the bone scan and MRI results failed to show obvious spread of the disease, it was most likely outside the prostate capsule anyway. Once again the specialist reviewed the available treatment options and offered to refer Ross to a radiologist for assessment. Ross declined that offer but asked about seed implants (a form of radiation), cryosurgery and the possibility of medical treatment prior to a treatment choice. As we tried to negotiate alternate treatments to radical prostatectomy the responses we received were less than encouraging. Ross was not a candidate for seeds, cryosurgery was unavailable, and the urologist said medical treatment would make his job harder. When I asked how it could possibly make his job harder if the prostate was smaller in size, his response was "well it's not going to put it back in the capsule"! **The surgeon assured Ross that he would do his best "to get it all" but there would inevitably be some residual damage, including a high probability of being totally impotent and incontinent of urine.** We left the specialist's office feeling dissatisfied, frustrated and depressed, yet even more determined to take our time making a decision. Although we arranged a follow-up visit in approximately two weeks, we didn't return as planned.

Dissatisfaction with the treatment options available to Ross in Australia meant we had to continue our search. Working as a team Ross continued to explore the Internet focusing on cryosurgery while my job was to write e-mails to a number of cryosurgery units in the USA and Canada. Although the replies we received did not always tell us what we wanted to hear, all but one clinic responded to our requests for information. Unfortunately in the short-term Ross was not a candidate for cryosurgery, his prostate was simply too large. It was about this time that Ross discovered a number of articles about medical protocols used in the treatment of prostate cancer. One of those articles was written by Dr. Ronald Wheeler, introducing for the first time the idea that prostate cancer could be treated as a chronic disease. While not a cure, this approach seemed to offer Ross the prospect of quality of life without the damage associated from surgery or radiation. Just three weeks after Ross was diagnosed with prostate cancer, we contacted Dr. Wheeler via e-mail and spent hours looking at information on his web site. I was amazed at how quickly Ronald (as we came to know him) replied to our e-mail requests for information and within two weeks of our first communication we had decided to travel halfway around the world to Sarasota Florida. Just three e-mails and two telephone conversations later we were arranging what would, in retrospect, become one of the best decisions we had ever made.

Upon reflection I am amazed at what we accomplished. During the five weeks since Ross was first diagnosed, we had been forced to put aside our fears and make decisions that would inevitably affect us for many years to come. Our computer skills and use of the Internet had proven as invaluable as the support we received from family and friends. One friend asked permission to include Ross in the prayers at a local prayer group, another did his own search of the web and shared information with Ross, others simply offered words of support and asked if there was anything they could do to help. Invaluable during this time was also the support and information provided by many of my colleagues both within Australia and overseas. Knowing that we had the support of so many people was wonderful. Along the way we also tried to inform our friends and family about the importance of knowing your family history and of PSA testing. Most, including Ross' brothers saw their doctors and had their PSA checked but many failed to obtain the actual results and accepted their doctor's report that 'it was normal'. We would later learn that men must **"know the number!"**

Although it would take another five weeks for us to organize our trip, we had lots to do. We met with Ross' GP to enlist his support. Although he didn't understand why we were going to the United States, and insisted Ross would require surgery anyway, he agreed to support the protocol when we returned. Armed with in-principle medical support, free airline tickets arranged through our mileage plus program, the knowledge that our daughter had arranged accommodations and rental cars, as well as with the assistance of our son who had booked air travel within the USA . . . we were on our way.

Once in Florida we had two days to rest following our long and exhausting flights. Our time with Ronald had finally come. I remember arriving at the clinic, helping Ross fill out the forms, standing up to accompany him into the rooms, but being told to wait in the waiting room. I was really getting tired of waiting rooms and despite Ross asking if I could be present I was told I could join him later. A full battery of tests were completed, some of which had not been carried out in Australia; the examination phase over, I was invited to join Ross in Dr. Wheeler's office. Ronald discussed Ross' clinical picture and outlined the medical protocol he recommended. He was obviously passionate about his work and offered us hope, something that had been missing when considering surgery and/or radiation. The protocol seemed to make perfect sense to us and we wondered why Doctors in Australia were not offering the same treatment. I remember feeling overloaded with the amount of information provided and despite my nursing background, I didn't understand why he was prescribing some of the medications. Despite that, with Ronald as our 'Coach' we believed we could make this work.

When we returned to Australia we fully expected support from Ross' doctor as he had pledged, that monthly PSA blood tests would not pose a problem, and that the prescription medications needed to make this treatment work would be available. **Think again!** Although we provided the GP with a copy of Ronald's extensive report he was less than supportive. When asked to order certain medications he said "what do you need this for?", "never heard of Avodart . . . Proscar would have to do" but the last straw was when Ross was told that three month PSA testing would have to do. The GP saw no reason to do the PSA monthly and refused to provide the necessary requisitions. It think it was following that particular consultation that I came home to find Ross had had a few drinks, not like Ross at all! I think I probably joined him for a few more drinks and we quickly considered our options. For the first time we began to wonder if we could make this work given that the protocol was driven by monthly PSA results.

Faced with this unexpected hurdle my first step was to consult with my personal GP. He was in the same group practice as Ross' doctor and I told him that I was really angry that Ross' doctor was less that cooperative. Despite this unacceptable professional attitude, I provided him with yet another copy of Dr. Wheeler's report. Seems the first one had not made its way into Ross' file. We didn't have to wait long for a reply from my doctor. He phoned us at home and asked to talk with Ross. He wanted permission to send the report to a group of researchers, and although there were some aspects of the treatment he didn't understand, he assured us that he would support the protocol. In addition to gaining his support, I also called the lab to find out how we could arrange regular PSA tests without a requisition. The lab told us what they needed and we quickly obtained a letter from Ronald that would allow Ross to have his PSA done on demand.

I think it was during this period of time that my initial shock, disbelief, and frustration was replaced by anger. I told Ross I wasn't angry with him, I was actually angry that he had prostate cancer; I was angry that PSA testing was not routine in Australia; I was angry that despite my education and experience as a nurse, I remained unable to make the medical system work smoothly for him. I couldn't believe that medical practitioners in Australia were less than proactive in trying to prevent prostate cancer and I was enraged when one of my nursing colleagues said we were lucky "it's only prostate cancer". I certainly didn't feel lucky. Didn't she know that men actually die of prostate cancer!? I can't remember ever being so angry. I felt my life had been turned upside down and unfortunately sometimes Ross was on the receiving end of my rage. I wanted my old life back but I knew that wouldn't happen.

For the next few months my life seemed to revolve around organizing Ross' medication, trips to the lab for blood tests, consultations with the GP, waiting anxiously for results, and sharing our excitement as Ross' PSA number dropped rapidly. It took only three months on Flutamide (an Anti-androgen) for his PSA to drop from 19.6 to the magical number one. Each time we had new results, I would e-mail Ronald and he would reply with words of wisdom and encouragement. I remember when I reported that the PSA had finally reached one and I asked if that was low enough? Ronald's reply was," yes one was low enough, so Ross could come off the Flutamide but should remain on everything else." Although we celebrated this victory, we were still on a steep learning curve and wondered how long it would take for Ross' PSA to climb back up to 10.0 or higher?

And so life continued ... there were monthly PSA tests, regular visits to the GP and an ongoing struggle to obtain Avodart on a regular basis. Although Avodart was licensed for sale, the drug company was not currently marketing it in Australia. Once again, we were faced with an obstacle and had to find an alternate way to obtain a regular supply. On two occasions we had it sent to us but unfortunately the second package was ceased by Customs and only released when we provided detailed documentation about the drug, Ross' condition, and proof of the drug's status in Australia. When the package finally arrived, we found most of the capsules were stuck together; presumably due to exposure to high temperatures or perhaps even x-rays. I was left wondering if the quality of the drug had been affected but there was simply no way of knowing and it was the only supply we had. Following that experience we decided to use a different approach and brought a larger supply back with us following an overseas trip.

Ross has followed Ronald's protocol since May 2003 and in June 2004 we returned to Sarasota for a follow-up visit. At that time Ross' PSA was still only 5; he had completed just one round on Flutamide, and he remained symptom free. We discussed the protocol with Ronald, who discussed future plans, including an adjustment to the upper limit for PSA. Given Ross' clinical picture we joked that he was going for the world record for **'Flutamide Free Days'**! I came away from that consultation believing that with Ronald's continued support and guidance, the involvement of our local GP, and our own determination Ross was going to continue to enjoy good quality of life for many years to come.

As we approach two years since Ross was diagnosed with prostate cancer, Ronald's protocol has at last become part of our daily life. Although we must plan in advance when you are going away on a trip, Ross now organizes his own medications, his PSA remains low at just 7.1 (world record, here we come), and while his prostate remains enlarged, he is symptom free, while his urinary flow and residual urine have returned to normal. Even though we continue to be challenged by a system that controls access to PSA testing, Avodart, and proprietary supplements like Peenuts®; experience has taught us that even those obstacles can be overcome. As our journey continues I am pleased to say that the feelings of frustration, depression, and anger that once filled my days have been replaced with a sense of hope and confidence. Somehow Ross and I have managed to 'normalize' something which was truly abnormal. For that, we now have our life back and we are thankful to Dr. Wheeler as a professional, a friend and most of all his confidence, compassion and expertise.

Dr. Wheeler's Commentary:

Clearly, I am very pleased with the success experienced by Ross. The validation for success with the Chronic Disease Management (CDM) strategy was achieved by an evaluation of Ross' prostate using the 3.0 Tesla Magnetic Resonance Imaging scan. The images obtained during the scan demonstrated unequivocally that the cancer process was organ confined. Not only does this finding validate the decision, to treat Ross' cancer as a chronic disease, it also highlights CDM as a viable treatment alternative for patients with prostate cancer while preserving quality of life. Interestingly, the original commentary by the Australian Physicians suggesting the disease was extracapsular was incorrect; even though statistically, historical data suggests they should have been correct. **This is really the basis for the scan!** The strength of this finding is not to show doctors were incorrect but rather to get it right for the patient with the disease. The point of any diagnostic modality is to improve the confidence of treatment decisions. While we didn't have 3.0 Tesla MRI scanning in 2003, we have it now, enabling difficult cases like Ross' to be evaluated with an improved margin of Predictability that the decisions made are more likely to be correct than incorrect; not left to an educated guess. More importantly, for Ross McVeigh and his family, their decision to make the long trip to the USA appears to have paid them back in spades to this point. Interestingly, the choice to remain conservative with the CDM approach or to try to cure the disease will now become the dominant topic of discussion. **Ross ultimately underwent HIFU under my direction and has reported excellent PSA results consistent with a cure for the disease!**

APPENDIX—26

Benign Prostatic Hyperplasia (BPH)

BPH STANDS FOR benign prostatic hyperplasia. Hyperplasia indicates an increase in number of cells rather than an increase in cell size. Reportedly, benign prostatic hyperplasia affects 30-50% of 50 year old men. Similar to other prostate diseases including prostatitis, urinary symptoms are the most common complaint among men with BPH including the number one reason men seek medical advice through a doctor's appointment. Later in this educational vignette, you will learn that prostatitis is the primary reason that urinary symptoms exist. Interestingly, among the urinary symptoms, Nocturia (the need to empty the bladder during a nighttime sleep cycle) is arguably the most common symptom expressed by patients in association with an enlarging prostate. A far more sinister process associated with BPH, (that commonly goes unnoticed), is urinary retention. In a typical urology practice setting, a significant percentage of men evaluated for urinary symptoms, also have urinary retention. **While it is the symptoms that drive the patient to the doctor, few if any patients can identify urinary retention, when present. This is very troubling and puts the patient at added risk!**

The inability to empty the bladder completely is associated with its own problem set including but not limited to bladder wall weakening, bladder stone formation, infection and Renal (Kidney) Insufficiency or failure. Of these clinical issues, a bladder infection is likely the most significant concern. As stated earlier, urinary retention is uncommonly recognized by most patients; establishing further reason to maintain a healthy prostate as determined by a PSA less than 1.0 ng/ml. As you will see, prostate disease (primarily obstruction of the urethra or bladder tube) is common to this disorder.

Is it necessary to get checked for urinary retention in the absence of symptoms? Probably not, as an isolated event, but on the other hand, any urinary symptoms that prompt a visit to the Urologist is commonly associated with an assessment of how well you empty your bladder. In this scenario, it is not uncommon to experience a *Uroflow test* to measure urine volume voided over time. An expected flow curve in normalcy is bell-shaped while minimally 125 ml of urine is required to validate the test. An accompanying test to the Uroflow test is a *Post-Void Residual* Urine check. Once the bladder emptying phase is complete, a bladder ultrasound is performed to determine if all urine has been emptied. When men have between 50 and 100 ml remaining in the bladder following the *Uroflow test*, this is interpreted as moderate urinary retention. In this setting, it is quite common for physicians to offer this patient an alpha blocker such as Uroxatral, Rapaflo or Flomax. This class of drug is intended to relax the bladder neck enabling the tube from the bladder through the prostate to become less restrictive. While the majority of men with symptoms sufficient to prompt a doctor visit will be offered this class of drug commonly, fewer than 30% of men, in my opinion, actually have significant bladder neck hypertrophy (restriction to urine flow at the bladder neck).

If greater than 100 ml of urine is identified, it is not uncommon for men to undergo an office Cystoscopy (a look into the bladder through the urethra with a flexible lighted tube) to rule out bladder outlet obstruction (BOO). While I think that any test that reveals urinary retention could be repeated before office Cystoscopy is actually performed, the presence of urinary symptoms in the face of significant retention of urine ($\geq$ 100 ml) should prompt the patient to begin the process of educating himself regarding treatment options. The first question that must be addressed is whether the course of action involves the use of medication or the use of surgery. Regardless of how conservative you choose to be, you will want to become familiar with the side effect profile associated with the medications or procedures offered; realizing that any procedure may be associated with scarring (an irregular healing process) and possible failure. Many men who fear the worst, elect to ignore even the best of advice; choose to self medicate. **While it is always preferable to maintain a healthy prostate and avoid all of the preceding discussion, very few men actually take a proactive position but rather choose to take their chances once the disease process has presented itself. All too often, men choose to use herbs associated with sparse to no research in the hopes that the problem that is present . . . just goes away.** Most men cannot differentiate fact from fiction and fall prey to sales gimmicks and promotionals; trying everything from African Star Grass (Hypoxis rooperi) to beta sitosterols to saw palmetto with mixed results.

Once the transition from prostate enlargement to urinary retention has taken place, it is often too late to make an impact with nutrient formulas and/or medications. Mind you, there is nothing wrong with a trial of conservative management, but the percentage chance of success diminishes with advancing disease.

Let's take a look at a classic case that demonstrates unequivocally why the evaluation of urinary symptoms for BPH must include consideration for prostatitis. While this patient was at risk, he was able to avoid the rush to Judgment. Melvin S is a 58 year old Pharmacist who was experiencing intense (severe) urinary symptoms (21/35 on the AUA Symptom Index). He made an appointment with a qualified Urologist in the Tampa/St. Petersburg area who indicated the need to assess the urethra (bladder tube), prostate, and bladder through a Cysto Procedure (Cysto is short for Cystoscopy, whereby the Urologist puts a flexible lighted tube into the urethra to evaluate the lower urinary tract). Following the procedure, the Surgeon stated that the prostate was enlarged—commenting further that the left lobe of the prostate had crossed the midline creating increased resistance to the flow of urine. It was his professional opinion that the symptoms experienced by Mr. S were primarily based on this anatomical abnormality. Based on his findings, he recommended a brief outpatient procedure that would cut away this portion of the prostate allowing for the symptoms to resolve. While surgery had been scheduled, he took the advice of a friend to try our patented product for the prostate, Peenuts®. Within a week the Pharmacist began feeling better. Based on minimal research, he decided to make an appointment at the Diagnostic Center for Disease™ to get a second opinion relative to the need for surgery. His clinical presentation noted a PSA of 14.9 ng/mg; a significant rise from a 3.2 ng/ml reading, a year prior. Prostatitis was noted with an expressed prostatic secretion of 30-150 white blood cells (normal is less than 10 white blood cells). His symptom score had been recorded at 21 while his prostate size was confirmed at 28 grams using ultrasound technology. Within 3 weeks of starting the Peenuts® formula, his urinary symptom score had dropped to 0-1, or a change of 20.5 points. To say the least, the surgery was cancelled. While this reduction in symptom score is extraordinary, it is not unusual as innumerable documented cases are on file that shows improvement. Based on a clinical assessment of all patients who had been initially evaluated and then followed up at some later date, a mean reduction in urinary symptoms was noted to be 70%. While the digital rectal exam noted no evidence of prostate cancer, the patient was advised against a biopsy based on the prostatitis identified and on the fact that if cancer was present, there was high likelihood that the tumor was outside of the prostate and a biopsy would not alter the therapy. Despite the argument to try to avoid the biopsy and deal primarily with the prostatitis, Melvin insisted on a biopsy under color flow Doppler assistance. The result of a 6 core biopsy evaluated by David Bostwick, M.D. noted acute and chronic prostatitis in all cores without evidence of prostate cancer. With continuing treatment of non-bacterial prostatitis with the Peenuts® formula, the PSA was later recorded at 3.4 ng/ml. Melvin S. is now more than 5 years removed from the prostate biopsy and continues to perform well clinically. While this case shows how one patient avoided surgery and improved his urinary health with a patented prostate nutritional formula, it further demonstrates evidence of a viable alternative to surgery when prostatitis is noted to be the most important clinical disease. In a separate study presented at the NIH in 1999, 235 consecutive men with any measure of urinary symptoms were evaluated for prostatitis. 83 men were less than 50 years old while 152 men were 50 years old or older. The EPS was used to validate the presence of white blood cells confirming the presence of non-bacterial prostatitis, noting that 81% of men younger than 50 had prostatitis as the primary cause of urinary symptoms while 88% of men aged 50 and older were noted to have prostatitis (refer to the EPS/AUA charts). To validate the importance of this sentinel study, a review of the literature confirmed that 80% of men with any level of voiding symptoms did indeed have prostatitis based on the EPS analysis. In men 50 years and older, the text books stated that benign prostatic hyperplasia (BPH) was most commonly associated with urinary symptoms. Clearly, this is not the case as the preponderance of data suggests that prostatitis continues to evolve as we age. Minimally, this study points out the need for an effective prostatitis formula such as Peenuts® in the majority of men who present with voiding symptoms. It also points out that men would be wise to try a course of this nutritional formula at the first sign of urinary symptoms in hopes of improving the clinical course. While I realize that prostate cell growth also begins to take place in men in their early to mid forties, the number of men who have pure BPH without evidence of prostatitis is extremely rare. I have challenged my colleagues to repeat my study but to this point 6 years after the NIH presentation, I have no one interested. Until Urologists prove this for themselves, many more men than is necessary will be asked to undergo a potentially needless surgical procedure. If you decide to try a 3-6 months course of Peenuts®, in lieu of a recommended surgical procedure, please allow your Urologist to follow you along. This is the only scenario whereby your surgeon will be able to see for himself the advantage of treating prostatitis with something other than surgery or antibiotics.

When prostate enlargement has been determined to be the most compelling disease based on urinary retention, I would recommend consideration for the following treatments in the order of priority based on ease of application, side effects, out-patient availability, and/or durability of treatment offered (ability to maintain the benefit achieved); laser prostatectomy, transurethral neo-ablation of the prostate (TUNA) and microwave. As you can see, the TURP (transurethral resection of the prostate) is no longer competitive with out-patient procedures. The so-called, "roto-rooter" has been relegated to the do not perform list as it really does not compare favorably with newer and safer technology. While this is my order of preference, I encourage patients to visit with their doctor to learn which procedure is best and why.

In the event that you prefer a medical approach, the next section outlines the various medications and indications for usage.

NOTES:

Nutritional (Peenuts®) Advantages	5-alpha Reductase Inhibitors Advantages	Alpha 1(a) Receptor Blocker Advantages
Reduces inflammation (validated by the reduction in white blood cells in the Expressed Prostatic Secretion (EPS)	Blocks the conversion of Testosterone to Dihydrotestosterone	Relaxes the bladder neck (BN); (seen in 20-30% of population)
Reduces Urinary Symptoms	Contributes to Anti-angiogenesis	Reduces Urinary Symptoms
Reduces PSA Secondary to inflammation resolution	Decreases prostate size by 20-30% in 6-12 months	Contributes to cell apoptosis (Uroxatral only)
Prostate nutritional (all natural)	Reduces Urinary Symptoms	
Works synergistically with 5-ARIs and Alpha 1(a) Blockers	Contributes to cell apoptosis	
Treats signs and symptoms of non-bacterial prostatitis (95% of all cases)	Decreases the incidence of Prostate Cancer by ~25% (PCPT Trial)	
Patented	Patented	Patented
Enhances Sexual Function	Decreases PSA by half in association with Benign Prostatic Hyperplasia	
Disadvantages	Disadvantages	Disadvantages
None Known	Gynecomastia (minimal; 1-2%)	Lethargy
	Sexual Dysfunction (minimal; 1-2%)	Retrograde Ejaculation
	Does not affect EPS	Does not affect EPS
Product Brand Name	Product Brand Name	Product Brand Name
Peenuts®	Avodart®	Uroxatral®

APPENDIX—27

Avoiding Prostate Biopsies is now 'State of the Art'

PROSTATE BIOPSIES HAVE long been sacrosanct when it comes to diagnosing prostate cancer, with little to no open criticism for a procedure that has become obsolete, if not a public health risk. No longer do patients need to depend on a crude application of a traumatic procedure that lacks precision and accuracy to make a diagnosis. Unlike other organ cancers, diagnosed through excellence in imaging utilizing a 3.0 Tesla Magnetic Resonance Imaging scan, the prostate biopsy procedure relies on a less sophisticated system allowing for poorly detailed images generated by acoustic sound waves (ultrasound) to serve as the primary device to locate the organ in question. **Ultrasound is neither sensitive enough nor specific enough to allow clinicians to predictably isolate a region of interest, let alone hit a region of interest with a biopsy needle.** Better stated, ultrasound cannot accurately locate regions of interest independent of far more sophisticated scans like the 3.0 T MRI scan, with or without spectroscopy. While ultrasound diagnostics will continue to play a role in the medical diagnostic arena, a 20-30% yield for prostate cancer suggests there has to be a better system of prostate imaging that allows a more in depth evaluation of an often maligned organ, while tied to a higher yield for cancer. Currently, 10 men with a PSA (prostate specific antigen) value between 4.0 ng/ml and 10 ng/ml are designated to undergo an invasive procedure that yields 2 or 3 cancers. Better stated, 7 or 8 of the men had a procedure they did not need to have. In a time when cost effectiveness and efficacy of technology is critical to disease diagnoses and management, the health system does not have the luxury of spending in excess of two billion dollars a year guessing about a disease status based on a hit or miss proposition.

Performing prostate biopsies is somewhat analogous to throwing darts with a few exceptions. In darts, you can see the bull's eye or target. Interestingly, despite the fact that you see the target clearly, one rarely hits it. In the case of a prostate biopsy, doctors rarely see or have a target; so in effect, we shouldn't be too surprised that they uncommonly hit a target. **Unlike a dart game, where there is no major consequence to missing the target, data out of the University of California at San Diego validates that needles puncturing the prostate promote inflammation that may ironically, 'hasten the progression of metastases' when cancerous or precancerous tissue is hit. 'In effect the proteins produced by inflammatory cells are the 'smoking gun' behind prostate cancer metastases'.** In a review of the literature, additional concerns are revealed that are noteworthy regarding a process called, 'needle tracking'. Simply stated, 'needle tracking' takes place when a biopsy needle punctures the prostate capsule. The process becomes more sinister when thousands of cells exiting the prostate include prostate cancer cells. According to Katsuto Shinohara at the University of California at San Francisco (UCSF), "needle tracking" is rarely seen. **I would agree with Dr. Shinohara in principle, however, the fact remains that "needle tracking" is rarely seen because it is rarely investigated.** The fact that we rarely see this phenomenon does nothing to diminish the frequency of the event which must (minimally) coincide with the frequency of cancer detection. In my opinion, the phenomenon of 'needle tracking' is universally noted and obvious to every patient who is biopsied, while grossly understated by nearly everyone within this 2 billion plus dollar per year industry. Patients will have no difficulty understanding how this happens as it is quite intuitive to even the most untrained among us that a puncture wound allows cells to escape consistent with the organ punctured. A simple prick of the finger gives most of us the necessary visual.

The most graphic representation that validates "needle tracking" is noted in a case study from University of California at San Francisco published in the Journal of Urology in 2002. The case demonstrates a large lesion within the rectal wall, 3.5 years following a previously established biopsy needle tract. When this mass was subsequently biopsied, the findings revealed the cells to be consistent with prostate cancer. For those less familiar with the anatomy or how cells function, prostate cancer cells cannot grow in the rectal wall without being planted there. This graphic image confirms without equivocation, the validation, that the "needle tracking" process, in fact, does exist and that the rectal wall or perineum (the space between the anus and the scrotum) provides a excellent breeding ground that assists the incubation process equally well. This case presents a plausible explanation for how cancer of the prostate can return more than 10 years after surgery when the inked margins of the prostate capsule show no evidence of cancer extension.

While additional research on this topic is suggested, we should never describe a prostate biopsy as a simple, innocuous procedure with minimal side effects. There are consequences which patients must understand and accept including 'needle tracking'; a previously described process that allows cells to drain from mini-tunnels by the hundreds of thousands. **What happens** to these cells is anybody's guess, but to assume that the cells will die and be of no consequence, as some 'experts' suggest, has been proven wrong, is overly simplistic, optimistic and reckless to say the least. As a patient, you must remember that you are the responsible participant who will bear the scars of your indiscretion or lack of forethought; not the doctor.

The 'Traditional' Rationale for a Biopsy

A tissue diagnosis represents the most valued, definitive and venerable piece of scientific evidence that a disease exists. Every other diagnostic test intends to make the point that validates the need for tissue confirmation. Prostate disease is no different in that there are multiple surrogate markers that predict when a biopsy should be considered and/or performed. While imaging dominates the diagnostic milieu throughout the human body, the PSA blood test has proven to be the most reliable and predictable marker of prostate cancer. Unfortunately and ironically, notwithstanding the lack of specificity, physicians, nonetheless continue to encourage a biopsy in virtually every male with an elevated PSA, regardless of the disease present. Success is defined by a cancer diagnosis while a lack of cancer on a biopsy does nothing to deter a subsequent biopsy with more cores. Historically, physicians are reticent to embrace inflammation as the number one cause of PSA elevation and treat proactively the disease process of prostatitis.

Who Qualifies?

According to research from Johns Hopkins, when a PSA blood test result rises above 0.70 ng/ml, the risk of prostate cancer increases by 3-4 times in men aged 40-60 years, when compared to the normal population. When a PSA is noted to be at least 2.5 ng/ml, there are Urologists and Family Practice Physicians who will recommend a biopsy while others will spare you the trauma of a potentially risk laden and often needless procedure until your PSA reaches a number of 4.0 ng/ml or higher. Additionally, men who experience a progressive rise in PSA of 0.75 ng/ml in two consecutive years will be challenged to get a biopsy as the next best step or recommendation based on PSA Velocity change. Only men who maintain a PSA number less than 2.5 ng/ml without evidence of a bump or nodule on digital rectal exam will be allowed to live another day without the threat of a biopsy being discussed or performed.

Traditionally, the identification of cancer requires confirmation with a tissue sample obtained by a Urologist and reviewed by a Pathologist. Unlike most other cancers where imaging of an organ dictates the target from which cells will be obtained, Urologists have taken the liberty and initiative to look for a cancer without a formal "roadmap". Instead, a relatively unsophisticated review of the prostate with ultrasound technology serves to identify this organ's location for random blind biopsies. Unfortunately, despite many years of experience with ultrasound, physicians continue to randomly place biopsy needles into an organ where a visual target is rarely seen. The result is a procedure that lacks the sensitivity and specificity to predictably find a cancer. Efforts to improve the biopsy by using 'microbubbles' and blood flow to create a target or region of interest has not panned out. Early studies from dedicated research centers like Jefferson Medical Center have been disappointing to say the least. Notwithstanding a lack of direction based on current research, most Urologists target the prostate using a traditional sampling pattern or grid. Depending on the Doctor, 6-80 or more biopsies will be performed commonly in one or more biopsy sessions. Until a better marker is established, PSA remains the most important biological marker that dictates who qualifies for a biopsy despite the fact that it also lacks specificity; in other words . . . creating a need to look for something that is not there; therefore, a false positive. Ironically, the number one reason PSA rises is prostatitis, a non-bacterial event in more than 95% of cases; not prostate cancer. This explains in part why only 20-30% of biopsies performed yield a cancer, our current 'gold standard'. To be certain, we are using the wrong marker to identify which men would benefit most from a biopsy. It would be far better to understand that PSA represents a health marker, noting that any PSA number greater than 1.0 ng/ml represents a diseased prostate, minimally associated with prostatitis. **Therefore, using this model, if patients fail to respond to prostatitis treatment with a lowering of PSA common to inflammation resolution, we now have an appropriate group of men who have qualified for a biopsy. Why this concept is not universally accepted, is beyond me.** My early pilot research shows that biopsies performed on men who fail to lower their PSA with our patented prostatitis formula Peenuts®, to less than 4.0 ng/ml, will note a 92% yield for prostate cancer. **While additional studies are encouraged, in the interim, men who see a significant decrease in their PSA, using this diagnostic exercise to reduce inflammation will avoid an unnecessary biopsy.**

What to Expect from the Biopsy

Side effects commonly associated with a biopsy are numerous but include: pain, bleeding from the bladder and bowel, scarring, blood in the ejaculate, bacterial infection, as well as less commonly noted complications of incontinence, impotency and hospitalization secondary to sepsis where an individual experiences high fever, chills and uncontrollable shaking (rigors) including death and 'needle tracking'!

APPENDIX—28

Biopsy Procedures are on the Rise

RECENT DATA FROM Bostwick Laboratories indicates a growing trend in the number of cores taken during a biopsy session has increased from an average of 8 to18 over the past 12-18 months. The most troubling part of a biopsy procedure is that it is a blind procedure, whereby; there are no specific targets to hit. Equally troubling is that biopsies performed in this manner are rife with failure secondary to sampling bias resulting in false negatives. Even more alarming is the fact that saturation biopsies (upwards of 90 biopsies in a single biopsy session) are recommended to determine cancer sites for focal therapy. Saturation biopsy or prostate mapping is a process whereby tissue samples are taken at 0.5 cm intervals throughout the prostate. Given what has been discussed, the rhetorical question needs to be asked, **"Is is possible to cure a patient with focal therapy once saturation biopsies have been performed?"** To Cryosurgeons across the country and around the world, the consensus opinion is astonishingly . . . yes. How can it be that Cryosurgical Physicians around the country preferentially suggest Cryosurgery, a treatment that freezes the prostate with Argon gas, as an acceptable means to ablate prostate cancer cells locally despite the fact that countless cells have escaped the capsule? The unwitting public needs to understand the facts before they will be adequately prepared to accept the consequences inherent in this diagnostic exercise. While only time will tell how well individuals will perform from the implementation of this form of therapy; adding saturation biopsy to the equation adds an additional unacceptable risk of 'needle tracking', likely contradicting the concept for cancer cure.

A far better and therefore more patient friendly approach to the biopsy conundrum would be to allow a 3.0 Tesla MRI scan with its various sequences to evaluate patients preferentially prior to a targeted biopsy. The advantages are many including the ability for up to 70-80% of patients to avoid a biopsy altogether when no suspicion of cancer is identified. These individuals can be treated for prostatitis with the expectation that their PSA levels will remain low and non-progressing. In those individuals where a lesion is found, targeted biopsies can be administered to a specific localized region of interest (ROI) resulting in fewer needle punctures. In my practice, in an effort to decrease, if not eliminate 'needle tracking', I recommend a protocol that utilizes an anti-androgen such as Casodex® (Bicalutamide) at 150 mg per day for a specific time frame. Casodex® blocks a receptor on the nucleus of the prostate cell, preventing Testosterone and Dihydrotestosterone from attaching, thereby, promoting cell death. While further studies are encouraged, this is a good start to an otherwise enigmatic clinical scenario that begins to unravel for the patient biopsied, at the point of needle contact. **Given the fact that High Intensity Focused Ultrasound (HIFU) is approved in the USA for uterine fibroids (a benign condition in women) and ostensibly very safe in the hands of the most skilled, albeit few, Urologists, the HIFU technology should be suitable for biopsy negative patients with a rising PSA (a most common scenario), MRI validated disease (cancer) in patients with a rising PSA or men with intractable prostatitis referencing that Arnon Krongrad is performing**

radical prostatectomy in Miami on men without evidence of cancer but rather longstanding prostatitis only.

Significant Biopsy Related Studies

Given the significant risks of a biopsy procedure to the patient, attention should be placed on doing fewer biopsies while saturation biopsies should rarely if ever be utilized. In a retrospective study, Grosslaus and colleagues evaluated the difference between a sextant biopsy (6 cores) and a greater number of biopsies relevant to the final pathology at surgical intervention. Specifically, 135 consecutive patients who underwent a radical retropubic prostatectomy were studied regarding number of cores, percentage of positive cores, laterality of positive cores and Gleason score. Their findings noted **no significant relationship between the number of cores obtained and the predicted pathology of the radical prostate specimen**. Furthermore, there was no difference in the number of positive cores, bilateral positive cores or the percentage of tumor in the cores when more than 6 cores were taken. While it was noted that the percentage of positive cores may be the best predictor of pathological stage and tumor volume, **there appeared to be no improvement in prognostic information when more than 6 cores were taken.**

Sur and colleagues conducted a prospective study comparing minimal biopsies to a 24 core biopsy. While there was a suggestion that a 6 core biopsy may not be enough in certain cases, **the 24 core biopsy did not improve cancer detection rates**. There conclusion was that saturation biopsies should not be routinely performed preferentially when prostate cancer is suspected and that **24 biopsies did not outperform a 10 biopsy protocol. Fleshner and Klotz echoed the sentiments that saturation biopsy rarely if ever improved the cancer yield**

when they utilized their standard biopsy technique. Using MRI-Spectroscopy to guide where the needles are strategically placed, as few as 1 or 2 biopsies can isolate a cancer, minimizing cost, trauma and risk potential.

Meng and associates have noted that while increasing the number of cores taken at the time of biopsy may increase the number of cancers identified, **there is increasing recognition that many men with prostate cancer may not benefit from early aggressive intervention and that over-detection of prostate cancer has resulted in over-treatment.** Utilizing the Cancer of the Prostate Strategic Urologic Research Endeavor database, 4072 men with 6 or more biopsies were compared. 30% of the men had 6 biopsies, 47% of men had 7-11 biopsies, while 24% of men had more than 12 biopsies. Interestingly, there was a significant correlation noted between the number of biopsies performed and numerous sociodemographic and clinical variables including PSA, comorbidities and income. When this data was assessed by Kattan and Caner for prostate risk assessment scores, **there appeared to be no difference among men with a biopsy number between 6 and 17.** In a subset of men who underwent radical prostatectomy, there was no difference in the biochemical-free survival at greater than 2 years.

An article found on the American Cancer Society's website and published in the Journal of Urology, presents a point-counterpoint debate regarding saturation biopsy. According to Dr. Michael Lieber lead author from the Mayo Clinic study, 224 men who were previously biopsied as negative or with a precursor lesion like high grade prostatic intraepithelial neoplasia (HGPIN) and/or a change in digital findings underwent a saturation biopsy with upwards of 45 needle cores. The results of this biopsy technique resulted in finding 34% patients (N=77) with prostate cancer. Dr. Lieber, speaking for the Mayo Clinic Urologists, states, "our perspective is, if you're going to biopsy them again (referring to the patients in question), why not use a better (more aggressive) technique initially?" Perhaps, neither Dr. Lieber nor his team of physicians recognizes the grave dangers associated with the biopsy technique. Fray Marshall, M.D., Professor and Chairman of the Department of Urology at Emory University School of Medicine had a little different take on the process. **"After a while, it's overkill.** If you have to biopsy every few millimeters of the gland, it seems like **it would be a bit excessive."** Dr. Marshall does not agree with a blanket application of saturation biopsies. Despite the fact that Mayo Clinic's position is that 87% of cancers found were significant, this opens a debate on what constitutes significant? **Certainly, if you can qualify a patient for a radical procedure, it is easier to define the cancer as significant.** Dr. Marshall questions the significance of a cancer that requires 40 plus biopsies to find. **"Because prostate cancer is slow growing, older men with such small cancers could be harmed more than helped by treatment, leading some to choose a "watch and wait" approach."** Similarly, a chronic disease management (**CDM**) approach makes sense as it represents an academic strategy against prostate cancer. Dr. Lieber admits that some small cancers will be found (with saturation biopsies) but believes small cancers may be significant. He admits that saturation biopsies are bound to be more expensive, but he has **"no trouble with insurance (company) reimbursement".** Hmmmm!

The following patient case presentation speaks to the various clinical modalities utilized at our Center relevant to the diagnosis of prostate cancer including how we apply the biopsy procedure. This presentation also introduces 3.0 Tesla

MRI-Spectroscopy as the art form to take the guess work out of the biopsy procedure. In effect, an MRI-Spectroscopy scan will establish an all important roadmap for where disease lies.

Merlyn Freeman is a 51 year male from Canada with a PSA of 2.1 ng/ml. On digital rectal exam (DRE), his physician felt something on his prostate. Concerned, the patient saw his local Urologist who recommended a biopsy. Needing time to research this topic, Merlyn postponed the biopsy procedure, needing verification that a biopsy procedure was absolutely necessary. In need of a second opinion, Merlyn scheduled an appointment at the Scottsdale, Arizona—Mayo Clinic. The Urologist at the Mayo Clinic examined Merlyn's prostate and suggested that there was a 50% chance a biopsy would yield a cancer. As Merlyn's research continued, he utilized the Internet evaluating every aspect of the biopsy procedure. His concern that a biopsy would allow cells to escape the prostate was particularly unsettling to him. **When he spoke with his Physician Consultants, they denied any association of biopsy with the spread of cancer cells, despite a reference to an article in the Urologist's most prestigious journal.** Intuitively, the inability to spread cancer cells (if encountered), made no sense to Merlyn. As his Internet research continued, he ran across an article that identified the Diagnostic Center for Disease™ which believed as he that needle tracking takes place with virtually every biopsy. Following a free 30 minute conference call with the Medical Director, Merlyn scheduled a formal visit to the Center.

Merlyn scheduled a comprehensive visit at the center to review all aspects of his genitourinary system. Due to my keen interest and expertise in prostate disease, I welcomed the opportunity to offer a third opinion. While examples of a comprehensive visit at our Center are available throughout this book, I will elaborate on Merlyn's clinical markers herein. Merlyn's PSA test result was noted at 2.1 ng/ml in March 2007. Historically, his PSA had been recorded at 1.73 ng/ml in June of 2005, followed by a PSA of 1.95 ng/ml in December 2006. A progressive rise in PSA, regardless of how small, is never a good sign and minimally imparts a 20-30% risk for prostate cancer. A family history of prostate cancer in his Father and brother supported a strong genetic link. A Uroflow test noted an adequate, if not normal, voiding trial while emptying 238 milliliters (1cc = 1ml) with a 10 cc per second average flow and a 21 cc per second peak flow rate. The post void residual was 37.4 ccs consistent with normalcy. The prostate exam noted a relatively small prostate with a defined area of interest on the left side. Based on my 20 plus years as a Urologist, it was my expressed opinion the patient had a 95% chance that prostate cancer was present. An expressed prostatic secretion (EPS), produced during the prostate exam, noted white blood cells throughout the specimen ranging from 10 to 160 per high powered field (400X—microscopically), consistent with non-bacterial prostatitis. Fewer than 10 white blood cells per high powered field would be consistent with normalcy. Prostatitis has been demonstrated to lead to the evolution of prostate cancer as noted by the American Association of Cancer Research (AACR), David Bostwick and others.

Next, an ultrasound was performed. Gray scale ultrasound identified a 24 cc prostate with an area of hypoechogenicity laterally in the left hemi-prostate. Areas of hypoechogenicity are areas that are less echogenic or darker. A visual for hypoechogenicity is to shine a flashlight at a tree during the nighttime hours. The beam will transmit well at the tree and on either side of the tree while remaining dark behind the tree. The area of darkness is analogous to a hypoechogenic or hypoechoic area seen in the prostate. In the prostate, areas that are hypoechogenic may be cancerous approximately 20% of the time according to research data from UCSF and others. The remainder of the prostate noted scattered punctate (tiny) calcification throughout as a visual reminder of the inflammation present. Color Flow Power Doppler was then applied to the prostate. Essentially, this application of ultrasound allows us to visualize blood flow patterns. The Power Doppler feature allows us to evaluate a smaller area with greater intensity. In Merlyn's case the prostate exhibited a relative paucity or scarcity of vascularity or hypervascularity consistent with a lack of abnormal blood flow. Nonetheless, a less than dominant blood flow pattern was identified within millimeters of the hypoechoic lesion and remained of some concern. A lack of significant blood flow is suggestive that a cancerous process may be less than aggressive. Subsequently, an MRI scan with Spectroscopy was performed using a 3.0 Tesla magnet, confirming a region of interest in the left peripheral zone of the prostate laterally. The right side of the prostate noted decreased signal intensity as well, consistent with an unhealthy prostate (Prostatitis) but not as significant as the region of interest on the left side. The capsule of the prostate was noted to be intact without evidence of breach while the Seminal Vesicles were free of disease involvement. Spectroscopy, an integral sequence in the MRI scan (according to some experts) allows us the ability to evaluate the spectra of by-products or metabolites of cell function. In Merlyn's case his Choline + Creatine ÷ Citrate ratio was 1.77. Any value greater than 1.0 is suspicious for and therefore consistent with prostate cancer.

Based upon what we know thus far, the risk factors for prostate cancer in this patient include age, family history, PSA total and velocity, digital rectal exam findings, non-bacterial prostatitis, ultrasound imaging and MRI-Spectroscopy findings. In effect, a multi-parametric approach has convinced me that prostate cancer was present. Given the fact that a tissue diagnosis for prostate cancer is the accepted standard of care consideration was given to a targeted biopsy while protecting against needle tracking. To state more clearly, unlike a biopsy performed elsewhere, a biopsy performed at the Diagnostic Center for Disease is one of precision. The MRI scan is expected to provide a road map identifying the target in question. Without a road map, random biopsies provide a hit or miss approach to finding a cancer. Unlike a targeted biopsy that is focused on a particular area in the prostate, a random biopsy procedure must sample all areas of the prostate in quest for the disease. The targeted biopsy is associated with a maximum of 6 defined needle punctures while a random biopsy may include upwards of 20 or more needle punctures routinely. With every needle placed the risk of complication increases. Sepsis, accompanied by fever, chills and rigors requiring hospitalization, bleeding from the Intestinal tract, Urethra and Seminal Vesicles, often times requiring a blood transfusion; pain, impotency and transient incontinence are a few of the side effects that a patient must understand, accept and be willing to endure until the healing process is complete. While the differences between targeted biopsy and random biopsies appear quite clear, there remains the issue of 'needle tracking'. When cancer cells are encountered during a biopsy protocol, cancer cells will also follow the path of the needle. Once cancer cells have escaped the prostate the stage of cancer potentially changes dramatically. To be sure, an organ confined event now becomes a non-organ confined event. **The threat of metastases that may take 10 years or longer to become evident is nonetheless, a very real possibility. Remember, 40-60% of men fail to be cured by 7-10 years (post treatment). The reason could be needle tracking, the dissemination of cancer cells when the prostate is removed or from capsular disruption from**

the placement of Radiation seeds. In an attempt to prevent the cells that escape from proliferating, we incorporate an anti-androgen prior to the biopsy and continue for two weeks post biopsy. The theory is that an all important receptor on the prostate cancer cell nucleus is blocked from accepting the male hormone Testosterone. This process weakens and/or disables the cell hastening apoptosis or cell death. The clinical validation of this event is commonly seen with a drop in PSA; tantamount to a decrease in disease activity.

Merlyn's targeted biopsy revealed the presence of prostate cancer cells associated with a Gleason score of 7 (3+4) located at the left Apico-mid prostate, consistent with the site outlined so vividly by the MRI scan. Using the diagnostic protocol, the disease process (cancer) had been confirmed, while the spread of cancer cells was discouraged, if not eliminated by the Casodex. Based upon the limited disease, this patient has a unique opportunity to treat the lesion in question focally with HIFU, while preserving the remainder of the prostate. The advantage to the patient is that a selective focal treatment modality allows the patient to resume all male related function with limited to no morbidity or collateral consequence. While there is always a risk the disease could develop at a different location, even years later, there is historical data that supports the benefit of various cell specific mechanisms of action associated with the Chronic Disease Management protocol to improve the likelihood this will not take place. As with all individuals with a diagnosis of cancer, routine surveillance testing will continue on a regular basis.

The Battle Lines are Being Drawn

According to the American Cancer Society, a new case of prostate cancer is diagnosed every 3 minutes with a biopsy while men in their 60s, represent the most common decade of presentation and frequency of biopsy. According to the SEER (Surveillance, Epidemiologic, and End-Results) data, as "baby boomers" continue to age, the rate of prostate cancer detection is expected to worsen over the next 20 years increasing the number of men diagnosed to more than 500,000 per year. This fact suggests that we need to get the biopsy conundrum understood and solved sooner than later with a consensus opinion on how best to diagnose the number one health risk that men face.

The argument for performing a biopsy has become contentious. When, how, why and for whom a biopsy should be performed are questions that must always be addressed. **No one wants to miss a cancer anymore than one wants to find a cancer of little consequence. Noting that biopsies suffer from sampling bias, are traumatic and costly, anger cancer cells to become more aggressive and cause needle tracking, should give us reason for concern and reason to pause. Unfortunately, when cancer is found, a cascade of events occurs that may result in doing more for the disease than is required. This suggests that the landscape of prostate biopsy must change, allowing men with minimal risk to avoid the experience while scanning patients preferentially with significant risk factors in preparation for targeted biopsies, while protecting from needle tracking.** No longer are patients going to sit back, keep quiet and consent to whatever a doctor prescribes. Increasingly, patients seem to be getting the message that the person in control is the person who still has a prostate. Once your prostate is gone your options for disease control and management change drastically. Because prostate biopsy has an inherent risk of morbidity and for advancing a stage of cancer from organ-confined to extracapsular (non-organ confined), the best strategy should always be to defer a biopsy in favor of more conservative measures like treating prostatitis, preferentially, whenever possible. This is advice you can live with while allowing you to live a better quality of life with your prostate disease under control and intact. **The decision to treat prostate cancer without a biopsy is not far-fetched when the treatment is HIFU, a treatment for benign uterine fibroids in women. I don't think men will sit back and tolerate a 'double standard' any more than women would.**

What's the future of prostate biopsy?

Hopefully, this discussion will enable more physicians to realize the diagnostic landscape needs to change. The patient can no longer be asked to assume all risks associated with a biopsy procedure where an educated guess prompts an action based on a less than specific PSA result. No longer can Urologists deny that 'needle tracking' takes place or that; biopsy procedures are potentially harmful. It may well be the evidence uncovered thus far, represents the tip of the "iceberg"; giving new meaning to why so many patients fail to be cured, despite our best technical skill. **One thing is for certain, once the biopsy process begins, I generally don't see a lot of good things that follow. Whether it relates to the disease, the biopsy procedure, the PSA that prompted the biopsy or the treatment rendered, there are few patients who are enthusiastic about the process.** If an opportunity to prevent a disease were presented as an alternative to a future biopsy, by a philanthropic group or an invested insurance carrier, I don't think it would be difficult to recruit men to study.

The biopsy associated with a tissue diagnosis will always be the standard by which other diagnostic modalities are judged. Nonetheless, when suspicion for cancer is generated by any biologic or clinical marker, imaging must become the next best test to perform, while reserving biopsy (if ever) for those individuals whose scan is positive. While treatment of prostatitis would be an inexpensive alternative that will spare a significant percentage of men, those that are biopsied should have this procedure performed based on a map created by imaging not a biopsy needle. **Remembering that you can't hit what you can't see, must allow us to transition to a 3.0 T MRI imaging model.** Targeted biopsies can then be carried out in a region of interest to confirm a suspected cancer. While using an imaging scan to create the target that guides the biopsy needle, the number of biopsies performed per patient will decrease. Additionally, the candidates for biopsy will likely increase as the population continues to age. One would hope that Urologists will be encouraged to be more proactive educationally and less aggressive regarding who qualifies for a biopsy and who does not. **Clearly, a less than complete understanding of the facts will no longer be an allowable defense for ignorance.**

APPENDIX—29

Jim Little's Story, a member of the prostate cancer forum, Prostate 90 (email address: Pralt-discuss@Prostate90.com) to its membership—since October 2005

MOST OF YOU probably know that I have been associated with this group for 6+ years. I have been pretty silent lately for several reasons. I have needed time to think as well as a necessity to change my attitude mostly. I have not been inspired to write here much, quite honestly, because the methods I have used, endorsed at this forum, have not worked for me. The purpose of this writing is not to point the finger at anybody or try to persuade anyone to do anything different. While this is a prostate disease forum, it was my belief; the information disseminated was expected to be 100% factual. With that in mind, I thought I would let you know what I have been doing for the last 4 months, as I have had some success with what I will call "The Wheeler Protocol".

First a review: After being diagnosed with prostate cancer (Gleason score of 6 with a Stage T2c) in Jan. 1999, I decided to refuse surgery and started following Larry Clapp's program in April '99. I had performed a fast 2 times per year every year since then. I took PC-SPES (an Estrogen wrapped around Chinese Herbs) for a 4 month period in May thru August 99. I had all my amalgam fillings removed from my teeth and have never had a root canal or implant. I have a dental check up every 6 months without fail and have had panoramic x rays that found no infections. I have followed a very strict Mediterranean diet and eat no junk or white sugar. All meat is organically raised or wild, mostly fish from Alaska, turkey, or chicken. My diet is 75% vegetable and whole grain. I exercise regularly. I don't smoke and I do enjoy a glass of red wine with dinner and an occasional beer. I never supplemented with testosterone because I do not believe that it cures prostate cancer. There just was not enough evidence for me to support this notion that giving testosterone to a man that already has cancer does anything but fuel the cancer.

Supplements: Neo Prostate for 6 years. Folic acid for 6 years; Selenium, mixed tocopherols (Vitamin E), Co-Enzyme Q-10, a multi vitamin, N-A-C, alpha lipoic acid, and Barleans Greens over the majority of those years.

I saw Dr. Robert Bard, a Radiologist in New York, every year for 6 years for multiple scans. Each year, I was given a glowing report and told how well I was doing. He used phrases like "what I am seeing is significant", "congratulations, you are doing very well", "keep doing what you are doing", etc.; until he got his new equipment. Then it was ... "you have a 6mm by 9mm lesion that has probably always been there". "I just couldn't see it with the old equipment". "You need to see a urologist". This statement made so matter of factly by Dr. Bard and delivered without apology both scared and angered me. **Why had I traveled to New York City and spent thousands of dollars to see this guy if his examinations were so unreliable? If he had missed my cancer for 6 years how could I trust what he was telling me now?** So I did see a urologist, and had another biopsy that found 15% of the gland to be cancerous.

After 6 years on the "Clapp" program, the only time my PSA dropped is when I was taking PC-Spes, not unexpected as I was taking an Estrogen. After I stopped taking it, my PSA began a very slow although fairly steady incline. It was 5.7 at the time of my original diagnosis and the PC-Spes took it to .8. From there it rose over a 5 1/2 year period to 8.5. My urine stream also began to slow. I was in denial about this. I did not want to believe I was getting worse. After all, I had Bard's reports and encouragements telling me how well I was doing, or so I thought. The truth was I was not doing well at all. Bard's new equipment, the second biopsy, and my slowing urine stream proved it. My PSA was rising and I couldn't empty my bladder. I scheduled laparoscopic surgery using the da Vinci robotic system at Henry Ford hospital in Detroit. 2 weeks later I had second thoughts; canceled the surgery and saw a Holistic M.D. The first thing he told me was to go and see Dr. Fred Lee. I saw Dr. Lee 6 years ago for a second opinion and he told me I was going to die without definitive treatment. I saw no reason to see him again even though he is one of the best diagnostic ultrasound men in the world for prostate cancer. He won't see you unless you agree to a biopsy and I wasn't having another one. The holistic M.D. started me on an enzyme therapy called **Vitalzyme X**, **progesterone**, and **Flor essence**. I spent close to $1000.00 in his office in 1 afternoon. I gave the treatment 6 weeks to work but my urinary problems continued to worsen.

I had now lost all direction and confidence in everything I had been doing. I had eaten enough flax oil and cottage cheese (the **Budwig Cancer Cure**) to fill a 10 yard dump truck and taken Neo Prostate for 6 years with no appreciable benefit. I had done the fasts, had the dental work, and spent thousands of dollars, while just continuing to get worse. It was at this point, I decided to see Dr. Ronald Wheeler, a Urologist in Sarasota, Florida.

Most of you probably know of Dr. Wheeler because of his herbal supplement Peenuts®. I had never used Peenuts® but I knew of Dr. Wheeler through the articles he had written in the PAACT Newsletter. I went to see him at his office in Sarasota Florida on June 14, 2005. What I got that day was the most complete prostate examination I have ever had. I have seen Fred Lee and Robert Bard. Their exams do not compare. Dr. Wheeler's exam consisted of a prostate massage and a microscopic analysis of expressed prostatic secretion, a urine flow test, power Doppler ultrasound, and a complete explanation of everything along the way. Dr. Wheeler spent over 4 hours with me. I was his only appointment that morning. At the end of my time with him my wife and I were both convinced that this man was truly concerned about my well being and that he was totally committed to making a difference in how prostate cancer is treated. Quality of life is just as important to him as quantity of life. Dr. Wheeler is a urologist and Surgeon but does not believe that surgery or radiation is necessarily the best way to treat prostate cancer. Whenever possible, he treats prostate cancer as a chronic disease and believes it can be controlled without ruining the quality of a man's life.

Dr. Wheeler's diagnosis was locally advanced prostate cancer with hypervascularity at the capsule along with a raging case of prostatitis. It was unclear if the cancer had spread outside the capsule. "Too close to call" were his words deferring an official opinion to his MRI-S technology. Dr. Wheeler believes that prostatitis is a precursor to prostate cancer. The EPS or expressed prostatic secretion shows prostatitis by an elevated white blood cell count. My white blood cell count was 140 with normal being less than 10. **I found it particularly interesting that I had taken Neo Prostate for 6 years and still had a bad case of prostatitis.** I, now question the value of Beta sitosterol for the treatment of prostate inflammation.

The Wheeler protocol consists of hormone manipulation, lifestyle changes, low fat diet (not too different from my own), fish oil, vitamin D, and Peenuts®. How testosterone effects prostate cancer is manipulated with the intermittent use of Casodex. Avodart is used to decrease the size of the prostate by blocking DHT. Since starting his protocol my PSA is now holding at 2.2 to 2.4. I can urinate without problem and my sex drive is better than it has been in a long time. The only side effect I noticed was that the Casodex made me tire easily when I was taking it. I have been off of it for 2 months now and feel fine. This month my PSA continued to decline even though I am not currently taking Casodex. I understand that I am early in this protocol, but when I look back at where I was 4 months ago and where I am now I have to say that this was a good decision and I am happy I made it. Only time will tell if it was the right one.

In closing, I am very happy for . . . the men in this group who have successfully treated their cancer with the methods set forth in Larry's book and supported in this forum. It just wasn't working for me and I had to try something different.

Signed: Jim Little

Dr. Wheeler's Commentary:

While I am pleased that I have been able to assist Jim, it took a man previously committed to another protocol, to realize, he needed to alter his thought process and make a radical change in his personal health management direction, for this to happen. Jim points out from experience that products, programs and professional judgment advertised to benefit are often times associated with more hype than science. Minimally, men need to beware of schemes that capitalize on an individual's fear and uncertainty. While I am not saying my approach is for everybody, it is the rare individual, I cannot help. My protocol is based on sound scientific principles with an expectation to succeed in virtually every case as witnessed by objective outcome data. Jim's MRI-Spectroscopy scan suggests his cancerous process is close to the capsule but has not yet escaped. Fortunately for Jim, he has been given a second chance to control an unpredictable disease. Presently, he has many options for the future including his current conservative approach utilizing Chronic Disease Management or high intensity focused ultrasound (HIFU) under my direction.

APPENDIX—30

Jack Mosier's Story

MY FAMILY DOCTOR became concerned with the condition of my prostate and my PSA level in the early 1990s. In 1993 when my PSA had reached 6.7 ng/ml, I had been referred to a local Urologist. A biopsy was recommended and performed. At that time, no one spoke about any issues with a biopsy except it had to be done. There were no options or so I thought at the time. While I was thankful the results of the biopsy were negative, I became frustrated as I had no idea what I could do to assist my health. I was told to continue to get a PSA blood test and if it was still high, another biopsy would be performed at some later date. In April of 1995, at age 62, I became quite concerned as my PSA had increased to 12.1. A biopsy was again ordered and performed several months later when the PSA had now reached 12.9 ng/ml. This time the biopsy was found to contain cancer with a Gleason score of 6 (3+3)/7 (3+4). With little discussion, my Urologist gave me 3 options: Radical Surgery with a complete removal of the prostate, radiation and watchful waiting. According to the Urologist, the radical prostatectomy procedure gave me my best chance at cure. Radiation therapy, although an option, was not high on his list as it had a low success rate. The third and final choice was a 'watchful waiting' approach. According to my

Urologist, this approach made no sense based on my age, my life expectancy and my otherwise great health.

After much prayer and agonizing thought, I told my Urologist that I was going to try 'watchful waiting'. I had written a song in 1995, based on the Scripture in Job 23: 8-10, and I claimed the promise of verse 10 in this decision. My search for a non-invasive treatment protocol to control my condition would take nearly 10 years. **I would know when I found the right situation but realized I had to be patient and not press the panic button.** In December, 1995, I began a modified Mediterranean diet consisting of 85% raw fruits and vegetables along with 15% cooked food. The diet consisted of no animal products, no dairy products, no white flour, no salt and no sugar. In June, 1996, I had my annual physical with my family doctor. He stated my blood test results and vital signs were the best they had been in years. I had lost 30 pounds and kept the weight off. My PSA at this time had decreased to 11.8 ng/ml.

Despite my best efforts to keep this disease under control, my PSA began to rise by the fall of 1996. Over the next two years I had tried several regimens that had been touted as successful cancer cures including Essiac Tea, Flaxseed oil with cottage cheese as recommended by Joanna Budwig's camp, soy isoflavones and the Gerson diet. Despite my best efforts, I could not get a handle on this disease. By September 19, 1998, my PSA had reached 23.0 ng/ml. At this time I began taking PC-Spes, a formulation of 8 Chinese herbs compounded in California. My PSA after almost 2 months on this formula had dropped to 0.3 ng/ml. My family doctor and I were absolutely amazed. For the next 3 years I had remained on the formula until the California Department of Health pulled the product from the market place as it had been contaminated with controlled substances like Estradiol, a form of Estrogen and Warfarin, a blood thinner. Despite some undesirable side effects from this compound, I believe the benefits outweighed the risks. Once I was forced to stop the PC-Spes, my PSA started to rise again. Frustrated and concerned that I would now have to face radical surgery or radiation, I began to sample whatever was marketed to ward off prostate cancer. I had tried a couple of products that were supposed to be the same or similar to PC-Spes including PC Calm and PC Hope. They did not help. I subsequently tried fermented soy, Graviola, MGN-3 and high dose Beta-sitosterol. None of what I did made any difference in the disease that had me on the run. I continued to pray to God for direction as I had no idea what to do next.

Lost and without direction, my prayers were finally answered. In early 2003 I had heard from my close friend Evangelist, Dr. Hal Webb that I should contact Dr. Ronald Wheeler at his prostate center in Sarasota, Florida. Like me, Dr. Webb had prostate cancer. In his case he had already experienced Dr. Wheeler's successful approach and recommended him highly. In June 2003, I met with Dr. Wheeler and was put through a battery of tests to assess my disease status. Dr. Wheeler's solution to my problems was to implement a Chronic Disease Management approach whereby a variety of strategies or mechanisms would be put in place versus prostate cancer. Included among these concepts was his diet and validated nutritional plan. **He felt that neither radical surgery nor radiation therapy made much sense as the risk of failure was too high.** At this point my PSA had reached 29.07 ng/ml. I had been led to Dr. Wheeler so I felt I needed to give his plan ample opportunity to work. I had been counseled by Dr. Wheeler to make the necessary commitment and maintain that commitment to achieve success. After only 38 short days on Dr. Wheeler's protocol, my PSA had dropped to 0.67 ng/ml. Once again, my family doctor and I were absolutely amazed. Clearly,

I was one of the lucky ones to have found Dr. Wheeler. I believe this only occurred through the 'Grace of God'.

While I was committed to the protocol of chronic disease management, I had learned several valuable lessons from the early 90s to May of 2003. **First, despite claims to the contrary, there is no 'silver bullet' that cures prostate cancer. Men must resist the temptation to do what I did; wasting years and opportunity on pricey products bolstered by sensationalism. Second, I realize that seemingly simple lifestyle change including diet, nutrition and exercise play a significant role in how you feel and how you look. I also realize the body is built to assist the reparative processes of disease with the aid of the immune system. Thirdly, I realize that I could not have done any of this alone. For this reason, regardless of decision choice, we all need a 'coach' to guide us. In my case, I was truly blessed to have found Dr. Wheeler. One can only surmise where I would be today had I not heard of Dr. Wheeler and his clinic. If I couldn't find Dr. Wheeler on my own, how are other men in need going to find this great human being? I am convinced that all things happen under the control and direction of our Creator and Heavenly Father.** We learn so much when we are subjected to trials, tribulations and afflictions. I will always believe that according to Psalms 119:75 that God has been faithful to me in permitting this affliction. I am most grateful to Dr. Wheeler for the confidence he inspired in me to control this condition through his skill, knowledge and experience. I am also most appreciative for the hours Dr. Wheeler spent with my wife and I; explaining, encouraging and exhorting us to take control of this disease and win the battle against this cancer. I am now 75 years old and have no other health problems. I live every day thanking God for my good health and his direction to Dr. Wheeler. Without the contribution made by Dr. Wheeler and his supporting staff at the Diagnostic Center for Disease, I would not be here today. **May God Bless this wonderful man and the incredible work he does.**

Dr. Wheeler's Commentary:

While I am appreciative of the credit bestowed upon me by Jack Mosier, I do not work alone. I am blessed to have a relationship with our Lord almighty while honored to serve in his glory. While getting prostate cancer may be a given, if we live long enough, how we are diagnosed and treated with this disease is incredibly varied and tantamount to opening 'Pandora's box'. The options are seemingly endless on what to do first when the PSA blood test starts to rise. While I always encourage men to treat Prostatitis first and foremost, there are times when a targeted biopsy could be performed so long as the risks are understood and accepted. If we choose a targeted biopsy, I prefer to have the benefit of a 'roadmap' created by a 3.0 T MRI scan to guide me as to where the cancer is located. This minimizes the number of biopsies currently taken in my practice to 6 only. Many men are wiser beyond their years and realize the value of imaging and the need to treat without biopsies. I applaud men who understand the threshold for diagnosing and treating prostate disease least invasively. While I am confident that imaging will minimize the number of biopsies taken by my colleagues on a routine basis, more important is to decrease the number of men who are asked to get in line for a biopsy when the PSA level rises. **In my mind, the best first step is to identify and understand prostate inflammation as the chief cause of PSA elevation. Notwithstanding the fact that Prostatitis leads to prostate cancer, a lowered PSA result will allow thousands of men to delay a procedure (a biopsy) if not avoid one altogether.** The incredible journey that Jack and his family were asked to take is unfortunate. **In time this will change as word will spread to all who choose to listen.** As professionals, we must not forget to apply our incredible educational talent appropriately. This means that we must not treat men who can't be cured with definitive therapy. By doing so, we will be adding to the misery that many of these men will face. These are men who are candidates for a chronic disease management approach, while allowing sexual and bladder function to remain intact. Other men should be guided similarly, recognizing that Gleason 6 cancers respond equally well to conservative therapy like a Chronic Disease Management approach. **The decision to treat this group of men aggressively is fueled by fear and anxiety by the professional community.** With this in mind, the group that needs consideration for definitive treatment is primarily men with a component of Gleason 7 in their biopsy specimen or with evidence of cancer (even a Gleason 6 score) at the capsular margin. Historically, these presentations of cancer are unpredictable at best in their behavior. This group of patients, in my opinion, does not represent ideal candidates to live with their cancer through any conservative protocol. **With approximately 10,000 men turning 60 every day, there will be no shortage of professional assistance that must be rendered. To state further, there is no time to waste as we must arm the unwitting public educationally to the health dangers that lie in front of them. It is with this task in mind, I will ask others to assist me. I thank all men and women who choose to assist this great cause with me!!**

APPENDIX—31

Letter discussing the care of Jerry Deplazes

October 24, 2005
To Whom It May Concern:

Re: Jerry Deplazes—DOB: 07/10/39

I have been directing the care of Jerry Deplazes as related to the diagnosis of prostate cancer since November 2001. Currently Mr. Deplazes is treating his prostate cancer effectively using a Chronic Disease Management (CDM) approach with my guidance. This concept is not indifferent from treating arthritis or diabetes as a chronic disease while understanding how to live with it through proper management.

A Gleason 6—Prostate Cancer was diagnosed February 13, 2001 as the result of 27 biopsies of the prostate based on a PSA (prostate specific antigen) value of 6.0 ng/ml. The severity of the diagnosis, notwithstanding, Mr. Deplazes expressed a preference with treating this disease effectively, yet conservatively. The protocol outlined for Mr. Deplazes involved the use of multiple modalities associated with various mechanisms of action versus prostate cancer at the cellular level. Germane to this program are several FDA supported medications while in other instances the recommendation may be made for products and/or formulas not under the scrutiny of the FDA, like nutritionals. The initial PSA value prompted the use of Flutamide (an anti-androgen) at 500 mg per day in divided dose. **After approximately 4 months of therapy the PSA had nadired at 1.2 ng/ml and the Flutamide was stopped.** For the past 10 years, Mr. Deplazes' cancer has remained stable with the most recent PSA value recorded at 2.9 ng/ml. Tests to validate suppression of the cancer process beyond PSA have included Magnetic Resonance Imagaing (3.0 Tesla MRI), Prostatic Acid Phosphatase (PAP) and Alkaline Phosphatase.

The success of the protocol to control the prostate cancer process has been dependent on the utilization of multiple products and ingredients including: Multi-vitamins, antioxidants, the patented Prostate formula called "Peenuts®", Pharmaceutical grade Omega 3 Fatty Acids, and a diet consisting of organically raised poultry and vegetables where possible. This protocol has been shown to be effective in a Prospective Study intended to show the benefit of diet and nutrition versus Prostate Cancer. The study abstract was recently published in the Journal, Urology (September Supplement, 2005; Vol.66 No.3A). In addition to the above referenced vitamins and supplements, Mr. Deplazes also uses prescription medications Zocor (40 mg daily), Vitamin D3, and a 5-Alpha Reductase Inhibitor, like Avodart.

While the success of this program cannot be questioned, the approach utilized has enabled Mr. Deplazes to enjoy a quality of life not experienced with more commonly recognized treatment modalities such as Radical Prostatectomy, Radiation Therapy, HIFU and Cryosurgery. If there is a need to clarify and/or validate any of the commentary within this document, please feel free to contact me directly. Based on the inherent success that Mr.

Deplazes has shown over the past 10 plus years, the treatment protocol is expected to continue unabated and successfully.

Ronald E. Wheeler, M.D.
Medical Director of the Diagnostic Center for Disease™
www.MrisUSA.com

APPENDIX—32

The 8 Phrases you never want to hear from your Doctor:

1. "A Radical Prostatectomy is the 'Gold Standard' or 'Standard of Care'." I urge you not to fall for this rhetoric!

2. "Radical Prostatectomy is your best chance for cure". Be mindful, your best percentage chance for cure could be very low and not worth the risk!

3. "I'll do everything I can to get the cancer out". This makes no sense at all! If you hear this, run for cover! The enemy could be in front of you!

4. "I will guarantee you that your prostate cancer will not come back". There are no guarantees! The best information to hear is the doctor will guarantee to do the best that he can. That is all he can guarantee!

5. "I will do the best I can or I know what is best for you". Do not fall for this! After reading this book, you will know what is best for you! Knowledge is power!! Don't ever forget that!

6. "Your PSA is normal!" Yes, if it is less than or equal to 0.5 ng/ml. Otherwise, treat the prostatitis which (by the way), is the number one leading cause of PSA elevation. Since when does having a disease called prostatitis represent a normal event? It does not!

7. "Trust me!" I never want to hear that from anyone. Trust is earned! Never forget that.

8. "Biopsies do not spread prostate cancer cells"! With the literature and some experts offering a conflicting opinion, you cannot afford to go into a biopsy without adequate knowledge, if not protection!

While every doctor is perceived as well-intentioned, physicians often struggle with the reality of patient treatment outcome. **Disease outcome prediction tables have been created to give a doctor and patient realistic odds of success based on validated patient data, but myopic physicians commonly ignore what the data predicts putting patients in harm's way.** Physicians find it difficult to send a seemingly qualified patient to a competitor for a second opinion based on many reasons including Ego, reputation, and/or a source of income. Finally, your PSA can only be normal if it is less than or equal to 0.5 ng/ml. Please get a copy of your PSA and keep it in your records.

NOTES:

APPENDIX—33

FOR IMMEDIATE RELEASE
AVENTURA, FLORIDA

Approval of Ground Breaking Clinical Trial for Chronic Prostatitis

Multidisciplinary team headed by the Krongrad Institute launches ground breaking trial of minimally invasive surgery for Chronic Prostatitis

Chronic prostatitis is associated with a cluster of potentially debilitating symptoms, including pain and bleeding upon urination and/or ejaculation, fever, malaise, and weakness. In severe cases, patients have pain from such mundane acts as sitting.

Chronic prostatitis is not only common and found always when the PSA value is 1.0 ng/ml or higher but potentially ruinous to quality of life at the personal level. It is also a huge public health problem costing millions in dollars spent as an estimated two million doctor visits a year in the United States alone is attributed to this inflammatory disorder.

The Krongrad Institute for Minimally Invasive Prostate Surgery has received IRB approval to conduct a prospective, longitudinal, non-randomized, single-arm Phase II study of patients with a diagnosis of chronic prostatitis before and after laparoscopic radical prostatectomy, **'a form of minimally invasive surgery'**.

"Individual clinical cases have shown that surgery using laparoscopic radical prostatectomy can eliminate the symptoms associated with chronic prostatitis. This represents a conceptual revolution for men who otherwise have no effective treatment option. The study—the first of its kind—aims to better characterize and quantify the effects of minimally invasive surgery on the symptoms of chronic prostatitis," said the study's principal investigator (Arnon Krongrad, MD).

The study is being led by Arnon Krongrad, MD, who in 1999 pioneered the use of laparoscopic prostatectomy in the United States; Dr. Krongrad will personally perform all the surgeries. The team also includes co-investigator and statistician Shenghan Lai, MD, PhD, Professor of Epidemiology, Medicine, Pathology, and Radiology at Johns Hopkins School of Medicine, and Rajiv Parti, MD, an anesthesiologist and Director of Advanced Pain Medicine at the Pain Institute of California; Dr. Parti himself had a 20-year history of chronic prostatitis, which was effectively treated by laparoscopic radical prostatectomy.

To learn more and to apply for participation please log on to:

http://ProstatitisSurgery.com/ or http://ClinicalTrials.gov/ct2/show/NCT00775515

Media Inquiries: Arnon Krongrad, MD email: ak@laprp.com
Phone: 305-936-0474

Dr. Wheeler's Commentary:

To suggest that patients undergo a prostatectomy using any methodology for the diagnosis of prostatitis is unconscionable in this physician's opinion. We have many tools that provide a much more favorable patient response or clinical outcome than removing a prostate. High Intensity Focused Ultrasound (HIFU) is one treatment option for these men that is extremely patient friendly, proven to be safe and effective while associated with minimal side effects if any. In my mind, HIFU should be the first choice as a definitive therapy for intractable prostatitis once all natural remedies (Peenuts®, as example) and conservative 'traditional therapies' have been exhausted. Selling this type of aggressive treatment to a patient for a relatively indolent disease that may one day become a cancer is far more caustic and potentially risky than offering HIFU to a patient with a progressively rising PSA that in all likelihood represents prostate cancer. **Stay tuned on this one as the final chapter for the treatment of intractable prostatitis has not been written yet as the 'jury is still out' on Dr. Krongrad's wisdom!**

APPENDIX—34

THE JOURNAL OF UROLOGY® Vol. 168, 2120, November 2002

RECTAL WALL RECURRENCE OF PROSTATIC ADENOCARCINOMA

THERESA M. KOPPIE, BRIAN P. GRADY* AND KATSUTO SHINOHARA†
From the Department of Urology, Mt. Zion Comprehensive Cancer Center, University of California, San Francisco, San Francisco, California

We report 2 cases of tumor recurrence in the rectal wall following prostate biopsy; while treating with radiation and cryoablation.

CASE REPORTS

Case 1. A 60-year-old man was treated with 72 Gy. external beam radiation therapy for a Gleason score 4 +3 = 7 adenocarcinoma of the prostate diagnosed by transrectal ultrasound guided biopsy. After treatment, prostate specific antigen (PSA) decreased to 1.3 ng./ml. One year later PSA had increased to 2.0 ng./ml. Transrectal ultrasound guided biopsy was performed revealing a recurrent prostatic adenocarcinoma. Salvage cryosurgical ablation of the prostate was then performed, after which PSA decreased to less than 0.5 ng./ml. Three years after primary therapy, a repeat transrectal ultrasound was performed for a superficial palpable nodule noted on digital rectal examination. At that time PSA was

1.8 ng./ml. Trans-rectal ultrasound demonstrated a fusiform mass in the rectal wall. Biopsy of the mass showed Gleason score 4 + 4 = 8 adenocarcinoma.

The patient subsequently received hormone ablation therapy. Six years after initial treatment he is still alive with hormone refractory prostate cancer.

Case 2. A 74-year-old man underwent cryosurgical ablation of the prostate for Gleason score 2 + 3 = 5 adenocarcinoma, which was detected by transrectal ultrasound guided biopsy. Sixteen months after cryotherapy PSA had increased to 6.0 ng./ml. and transrectal ultrasound guided biopsy revealed Gleason score 3 + 4 = 7adenocarcinoma. A secondary salvage cryosurgical ablation of the prostate was then performed, after which PSA decreased to less than 0.1 ng./ml. Forty-two months after the second cryoablation transrectal ultrasound was performed for increasing PSA and a palpable mass on digital rectal examination. The scan demonstrated a fusiform hypoechoic lesion within the muscularis propria of the rectum (see figure). Biopsies of the mass showed Gleason score 3 + 4 = 7 adenocarcinoma. The patient was subsequently treated with external beam radiation therapy, and PSA was undetectable 27 months after treatment.

DISCUSSION
Seeding from prostate needle biopsy is uncommon although cases have been reported in the literature.
Most cases have occurred following transperineal rather than transrectal prostate needle biopsy. (1, 2) It is speculated that perineal biopsy tract seeding can be attributed to the larger bore biopsy needles used in that approach. Generally such events have been associated with high grade, locally advanced tumors although seeding of a well differentiated tumor has also been

described.(1, 2) **Recurrence has been reported as late as 14 years after biopsy.**

Microscopic biopsy tract seeding has also been noted to occur after transrectal biopsy of the prostate. Bastacky et al. evaluated 350 consecutive clinical stage B prostatectomy specimens.(3) They identified 7 cases (2%) in which needle fusiform thickening of rectal muscularis propria as seen on trans-rectal ultrasound. **Biopsy associated tumor tracking was present on microscopic analysis, of which 6 occurred after transrectal biopsy.** To date, the clinical significance of such microscopic tracking remains unknown.

In both of our patients' biopsies were taken transrectally using an 18 gauge automated biopsy gun needle. Recurrences were noted at 13 and 42 months after secondary treatment (36 and 58 months after primary treatment), and were detected in response to increasing serum PSA. Pathology consisted of intermediate to high grade cancer. Interestingly in both cases either primary or salvage treatment consisted of cryosurgical ablation of the prostate. These procedures were performed transperineally without violation of or injury to the rectal wall. On ultrasound these masses were clearly isolated to the rectal wall, away from the prostate gland and transperineal cryoprobe tracts. **These findings suggest seeding of the transrectal needle tract rather than the cryosurgical ablation probe tract. To our knowledge we report the first 2 cases of rectal wall recurrence after transrectal ultrasound guided biopsy of the prostate.**

Dr. Wheeler's Commentary: Ignorance or not knowing does not constitute a valid medical opinion by any Medical doctor! With that said, does anyone still have any doubt

that needle biopsies can spread cancer cells? When you have your blood drawn, do you need to see a hematoma (bruise) to know blood cells have escaped? There must be a reason you have to keep pressure on the spot where the needle punctured the skin. Needle tracking with biopsies is intuitive and should not be doubted any longer! If you still have doubts, however, please reread the article and review the references or stick your finger 10 times with a needle and tell me what you see. How many times did you not see blood? The biopsy procedure has been implicated as a direct 'cause and effect' event and discussed, yet again, in Appendix 35. While the long term prognosis or clinical significance may not be well known (as opined by the authors), it is obvious that this misfortune and physician induced event cannot be healthy for any patient attempting to be cured of prostate cancer.

REFERENCES:

1. Moul, J. W., Bauer, J. J., Srivastava, S., Colon, E., Ho, C. K., Sesterhenn, I. A. et al: Perineal seeding of prostate cancer as the only evidence of clinical recurrence 14 years after needle biopsy and radical prostatectomy: molecular correlation. Urology, 51: 158, 1998

2. Haddad, F. S. and Somsin, A. A.: Seeding and perineal implantation of prostatic cancer in the track of the biopsy needle: three case reports and a review of the literature. J Surg Oncol, 35: 184, 1987

3. Bastacky, S. S., Walsh, P. C. and Epstein, J. I.: Needle biopsy associated tumor tracking of adenocarcinoma of the prostate. J Urol, 145: 1003, 1991 2120

0022-5347/02/1685-2120/0
THE JOURNAL OF UROLOGY *
Copyright © 2002 by AMERICAN UROLOGICAL ASSOCIATION , INC.*

Vol. 168, 2120, November 2002
Printed in U.S.A.
DOI: 10.1097/01.ju.0000032081.42658.ed

RECTAL WALL RECURRENCE OF PROSTATIC ADENOCARCINOMA

THERESA M. KOPPIE, BRIAN P. GRADY* AND KATSUTO SHINOHARA†

From the Department of Urology, Mt. Zion Comprehensive Cancer Center, University of California, San Francisco, San Francisco, California

We report 2 cases of tumor recurrence in the rectal wall following prostate biopsy and cryoablation.

CASE REPORTS

Case 1. A 60-year-old man was treated with 72 Gy. external beam radiation therapy for Gleason score 4 + 3 adenocarcinoma of the prostate diagnosed by transrectal ultrasound guided biopsy. After treatment prostate specific antigen (PSA) decreased to 1.3 ng./ml. One year later PSA had increased to 2.0 ng./ml. Transrectal ultrasound guided biopsy revealed recurrent prostatic adenocarcinoma. Salvage cryosurgical ablation of the prostate was then performed, after which PSA decreased to less than 0.5 ng./ml. Three years after primary therapy, repeat transrectal ultrasound was performed for a superficial palpable nodule noted on digital rectal examination. At that time PSA was 1.8 ng./ml. Transrectal ultrasound demonstrated a fusiform mass in the rectal wall. Biopsy of the mass showed Gleason score 4 + 4 adenocarcinoma. The patient subsequently received hormone ablation therapy. Six years after initial treatment he is living with hormone refractory prostate cancer.

Case 2. A 74-year-old man underwent cryosurgical ablation of the prostate for Gleason score 2 + 3 adenocarcinoma, which was detected by transrectal ultrasound guided biopsy. Sixteen months after cryotherapy PSA had increased to 6.0 ng./ml. and transrectal ultrasound guided biopsy revealed Gleason score 3 + 4 adenocarcinoma. Salvage cryosurgical ablation of the prostate was then performed, after which PSA decreased to less than 0.1 ng./ml. Forty-two months after the second cryoablation transrectal ultrasound was performed for increasing PSA and a palpable mass on digital rectal examination. The scan demonstrated a fusiform hypoechoic lesion within the muscularis propria of the rectum (see figure). Biopsies of the mass showed Gleason score 3 + 4 adenocarcinoma. The patient was subsequently treated with external beam radiation therapy, and PSA was undetectable 27 months after treatment.

DISCUSSION

Seeding of prostate needle biopsy tracts is exceedingly uncommon although cases have been reported in the literature. Most cases have occurred following transperineal rather than transrectal prostate needle biopsy.[1,2] It is speculated that perineal biopsy tract seeding can be attributed to the larger bore biopsy needles used in that approach. Generally such events have been associated with high grade, locally advanced tumors although seeding of a well differentiated tumor has also been described.[1,2] Recurrence has been reported as late as 14 years after biopsy.

Microscopic biopsy tract seeding has also been noted to occur after transrectal biopsy of the prostate. Bastacky et al evaluated 350 consecutive clinical stage B prostatectomy specimens.[3] They identified 7 cases (2%) in which needle

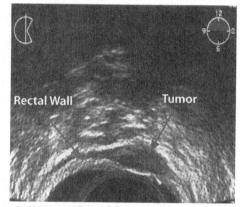

Fusiform thickening of rectal muscularis propria as seen on transrectal ultrasound.

biopsy associated tumor tracking was present on microscopic analysis, of which 6 occurred after transrectal biopsy. To date, the clinical significance of such microscopic tracking remains unknown.

In both of our patients biopsies were taken transrectally using an 18 gauge automated biopsy gun needle. Recurrences were noted at 13 and 42 months after secondary treatment (36 and 58 months after primary treatment), and were detected in response to increasing serum PSA. Pathology consisted of intermediate to high grade cancer. Interestingly in both cases either primary or salvage treatment consisted of cryosurgical ablation of the prostate. These procedures were performed transperineally without violation of or injury to the rectal wall. On ultrasound these masses were clearly isolated to the rectal wall, away from the prostate gland and transperineal cryoprobe tracts. These findings suggest seeding of the transrectal needle tract rather than the cryosurgical ablation probe tract. To our knowledge we report the first 2 cases of rectal wall recurrence after transrectal ultrasound guided biopsy of the prostate.

Accepted for publication June 7, 2002.
* Financial interest and/or other relationship with Pharmacia and Upjohn, Merck and Unimed.
† Financial interest and/or other relationship with ATI Medical, Endocare and NeoSeed.

REFERENCES

1. Moul, J. W., Bauer, J. J., Srivastava, S., Colon, E., Ho, C. K., Sesterhenn, I. A. et al: Perineal seeding of prostate cancer as the only evidence of clinical recurrence 14 years after needle biopsy and radical prostatectomy: molecular correlation. Urology, 51: 158, 1998
2. Haddad, F. S. and Somsin, A. A.: Seeding and perineal implantation of prostatic cancer in the track of the biopsy needle: three case reports and a review of the literature. J Surg Oncol, 35: 184, 1987
3. Bastacky, S. S., Walsh, P. C. and Epstein, J. I.: Needle biopsy associated tumor tracking of adenocarcinoma of the prostate. J Urol, 145: 1003, 1991

APPENDIX—35

Robotic Prostatectomy— A Race to Failure?

"There is currently no convincing evidence that early screening, detection, and treatment improve mortality. Limitations in prostate cancer screening include potential adverse health effects associated with false-positive and negative results, and treatment side effects." **ACPM Policy Statement, American Journal of Preventive Medicine, February 2008**

THERE WERE AN estimated 50,000 robotic prostatectomies performed in 2007[1]. It is projected that the number could double in 2008. While incredibly sad, even higher numbers are projected over the next 20 years and beyond! Robot assisted laparoscopic prostatectomy (RALP) is now accepted by Urology as the "gold standard" of curative treatment for Prostate Cancer. Robotic surgery is possible due to some amazing technology. One excellent example is the "da Vinci" system manufactured by Intuitive Medical, Inc. The device is remotely operated by the surgeon. Television cameras inserted into the abdomen provide multiple views and simulate three-dimensional vision. The robot consists of small, articulating arms which can perform multiple tasks, tools include suture, scalpel, cauterizing tool, etc. This is a laparoscopic surgical process and is considered to be minimally invasive. Promoters of robotic prostatectomy routinely use the term "promising" in their expectation that this device and procedure will eventually demonstrate improvement in the cure rate for prostate cancer. Their enthusiasm is generated by the awareness that other curative treatments have a poor track record to cure prostate cancer, accompanied by other negative side effects. **The reality is that robotic prostatectomy has yet to deliver any results or evidence that it will provide any improvement over other treatments to cure prostate cancer.** Granted, the technology and the procedure are still relatively new, but there is as yet nothing dramatically different in performing the procedure and in the results from the traditional laparoscopic surgery. Armed with hope for improved results, the urology community has increased the rate of these surgeries at an alarming rate. In 2000, there were 1500 robotic prostatectomies performed. In 2007, it was estimated that 50,000 robotic prostatectomies were performed.[1] The rate of procedures is still climbing, with upwards of 80,000 procedures performed in 2008. The number is staggering when you add robotic surgeries to all other curative procedures performed which include open prostatectomy, conventional laparoscopic prostatectomy, radiation in all forms, radiation seed implantation, cryosurgery, thermometry, high intensity focused ultrasound ablation (HIFU), etc. Additional economic pressure is applied due to the significant cost of the robotic system. A typical robotic surgery device costs $1.2M with annual maintenance of $120,000.00 per year.[2]

A great number of urologists and academic centers promote early detection and early curative treatment, citing a better cure rate. Nonetheless, the facts speak for themselves.

"These technical improvements would lead one to believe that improved results with continence, potency and oncologic outcomes should logically follow. Ultimately, long-term outcomes and possibly financial impact will determine the role of robotic-assisted laparoscopic prostatectomy."[1]

Published results of several studies simply do not support this . . .

"Cancer cure rate, measured by presence of cancerous cells at the surface of the removed prostate, and by PSA levels following surgery, was nearly identical for all three procedures (open, laparoscopic and robotic prostatectomy)."[2]

Concurrently, the leadership associated with Urology and academic institutions have for several years expressed concern regarding "over treatment" of prostate cancer. Retrospective studies have revealed that a very high percentage, (30-56%), of surgeries were performed for "insignificant" cancers.[3] In addition, physicians promote cure rates for robotic prostatectomy using statistics with only five years of data. **The failure rates become quite significant (40-60%) for all treatments by 7 to 10 years. Without any evidence for improvement in the rate of cure, surgeons are wagering on the hope that this new approach will deliver better results.** As the numbers of treatments escalates, so will increased numbers of treatment failures and the devastating side effects that accompany them. A seemingly incongruous announcement in a policy statement recently released by the American College of Preventive Medicine recommended against routine prostate screening. Does this announcement have any connection to the alarming escalation of treatment? Their policy statement details concern regarding the PSA blood test as cause for false positive and false negative diagnoses. However, it also recognizes concern over the inability to improve outcomes, to cure cancer predictably, or improve upon the negative side effects.

A conservative estimate is that 1,000,000 men are currently living as treatment failures as defined by a rising PSA result. A much greater number of men and their families suffer from debilitating side effects—incontinence, erectile dysfunction, diseases of the bowel, bleeding, infection, etc. At the current escalating rate of detection and treatment, notwithstanding, the associated needle biopsy issue, the number of failures could easily double within a few years. **Unfortunately, the sensationalism associated with robotic technology has been the driving force behind the escalation of treatment.**

Quality of Care

At what point does treatment go beyond quality of care and begin to cause greater harm than the disease itself? **Studies have already concluded that curative (radical) treatment of prostate cancer has provided no improvement in rate of cure and life expectancy when compared to doing nothing.** How can physicians ignore the facts, while noting the implications and continue to increase the rate of radical, so-called, curative treatments? Many surgeons now report that they "treat all cancers," even though a high percentage of cancers are determined to be insignificant or beyond treatment. Urologists generally diagnose, stage and grade the cancer according to location, extent and aggressiveness (Gleason Score) based on random 'blind biopsies'. Failure rates for Gleason 8 and above are very high within the first 5 years ($\geq 85\%$). Unfortunately, alternatives are presented to the patient in fewer and fewer cases leaving prostatectomy as the only option. **The goal, to cure cancer, is weighted with a higher degree of urgency and importance than a discussion of risk, loss of quality of life and outcomes.** In some cases, urologists present only one alternative, "watchful waiting," to the "curative" solution, i.e. radical treatment. Watchful waiting as it suggests, is watching PSA rise as we do nothing. Watchful waiting is a legitimate alternative, only due to the reality that all treatment approaches, including robotic prostatectomy; have yet to significantly improve upon doing nothing. Of course, a great majority of patients want to act with urgency, to have an enhanced chance to remove the cancer from their body before it has an opportunity to spread outside the prostate. Despite this thought, very few patients understand the need to insist on imaging with a 3 Tesla MRI scan to determine this. **Are urologists using this alternative as a "selling tool," to influence the patient to accept the physician's attempt at curative treatment?** Treatments, driven by robotic prostatectomy virtually doubled in 2008. The rate of needle biopsy has already doubled as well. [4]

> *"Our results suggest that tumor cell spillage and less frequently hematogenous dissemination may be associated with operative manipulation of the prostate during radical retropubic prostatectomy and may potentially represent mechanisms of failure after radical retropubic prostatectomy."* [5]

The patient and his urologist need to know that high PSA is driven primarily by non-bacterial prostatitis. Non-bacterial prostatitis is treatable and should be ruled out prior to any potentially harmful diagnostic testing, like random biopsies. A patient with an elevated PSA is typically referred by his general practitioner to a urologist. In almost every case, the urologist recommends exploratory needle biopsy. In 2007, the number of tissue "cores" taken from the prostate for an initial needle biopsy ranged between 6-8 cores. In 2008, the number of tissue samples taken in the initial biopsy has more than doubled, from 12-20 cores. **Exploratory needle biopsy is an extremely inefficient diagnostic procedure. Only 20-30% of needle cores return positive for prostate cancer, a failure rate of 70-80%.** Patients intuitively are suspicious of the invasive nature of needle biopsies. It is well documented, but rarely accepted by urologists, that needle biopsy spreads prostate cancer cells outside the prostate, a phenomenon termed "needle tracking." Additionally, needle biopsy inflicts trauma causing inflammation in prostate tumors. Inflammation has been documented to lead to prostate cancer and may cause prostate cancer tumors to metastasize. There is only one common denominator to all treatment methods that uniformly fail. It is prostate needle biopsy. To read more about needle tracking, review our article, *"Prostate Biopsy Spreads Prostate Cancer Cells.*[4]

Why are Surgeries Escalating?

Setting the Bar Too Low? Failure to cure cancer may be defined in different ways. The debate to define failure to cure is influenced by growing concern over increasing numbers of the failures, marked by a return of PSA following radical prostatectomy. **As the failures increase, the definition will become increasingly vague.** Urologists are encouraged that the five year rate of cure for robotic prostatectomy is "very good." **A PSA of 0.2ng/ml and above is defined as "biochemical failure."** Considering that all treatments perform well in the first five years, a 5 year cure rate of 84% for robotic prostatectomy does not sound very encouraging.[6] Other studies may report higher rates of cure.

Nevertheless, free from PSA elevation for five years is too short a time-frame to determine the effectiveness of any curative procedure.

Following radical prostatectomy (robotic surgery included), the body no longer has a prostate gland. **Any increase in PSA blood levels can only represent one reality; prostate cancer continues to exist and is growing in your body.** In medicine the debate is whether to treat regionally (pelvis) with radiation and globally with chemotherapy, or to do nothing but watch for a rise in PSA. Radiation and chemotherapy may, or may not be effective, can result in negative side effects and cannot be applied repeatedly. Some physicians, urologists and oncologists, recommend monitoring of the "PSA doubling time" as a logical representation for the growth of metastases. Others choose to go by the statistics, stating that it may take up to eight years for metastases to be detected on a bone scan. [7] While this may be true, a bone scan is notoriously poor in its detection of metastases while delivering a hefty dose of radiation. **With a PSA of 20 following curative treatment, a bone scan still can only detect metastases in 1 of 1000 cases.** [8]

Referencing a bone scan" In patients with a PSA <10.0 ng/ml, the chance of a positive scan is approximately 1:1000. While a bone scan may be used as a baseline study, 30-50% of bone mass being studied must be replaced for it to be positive." [8]

A statement difficult to accept by most patients, *"On average, it took eight years from the time a man's PSA first went up until he developed metastatic disease—which suggests that there is no need to panic at the first sign of a rise in PSA."* [7]

Brady Urological Institute, Johns Hopkins

"Even after developing metastatic cancer (detected by bone scans and other imaging techniques), men still lived an average of five years—." [7]

*"It could be argued that by 40 months after radical prostatectomy, obtaining an optimal outcome **in just over half of patients** is not as favorable a result as would be hoped from a widely practiced localized prostate cancer therapy."* [9]

If the patient did not accept "watchful waiting," why should he be asked to accept "waiting" as prostate cancer metastasizes in his body? The patient should know that if prostate cancer metastasizes to the point it can be discovered on a bone scan, it is already too late. In this scenario, patients typically have between 3 and 5 years to live. There is promising new technology in development to detect metastases at a much earlier stage. Additionally, there is research into improved ways to treat prostate cancer metastases.

Over-treatment of Prostate Cancer?

*"**I treat all cancers**" the same, states a Urologist to a Wall Street Journal Blog* [10]

*"Twenty nine out of 40 T1 stage histological cancers (67.5%), had tumor volume less than 1cc. The highest volume tumours were those of intermediate and high grade (Gleason scores of 5 through 8). Among tumours with volumes of less than 1 cc, 96.55% were confined within the prostatic capsule. According to our findings, there **is possibly a high over-treatment rate** in many patients with clinically insignificant PC."* [11]

"... the majority of impalpable prostate carcinomas are low volume, well differentiated tumours corresponding to **clinically insignificant** neoplasms, and that similar characteristics could be attributed to most of the impalpable carcinomas detected after prostatectomy for BPH in clinical practice. With such a high number of clinically insignificant PCs among T1 prostatectomy specimens, and with an extraordinarily slow tumour doubling time, there appear to be substantial consequences for therapeutic decisions." [3]

> "In the literature up to 31% of all non-palpable prostate cancers (stage T1c) diagnosed with needle biopsy and treated with radical prostatectomy are potentially insignificant tumors" [11]

> "Cancer-free status with full continence and potency was achieved in 30% of men at 12 months, 42% at 24 months, 47% at 36 months, and 53% at 48 months postoperatively." [9]

> Has Urology evolved to seek out smaller cancers, previously described as "insignificant?" One surgeon from a prestigious medical university advocates repeated biopsies to determine extent and grade of cancer. He also advocates aggressive treatment as best chance for cure. [12]

How can we predictably cure a man when we have spread prostate cancer cells with a biopsy? I guess this one surgeon (and many more) has not kept up with their reading! **This is the reason men must know their options and remain well informed if they want to avoid conveyor belt medicine!**

"Patients with significant, curable prostate cancer, e.g. those with at least 3 mm of Gleason 6 cancer, or any amount of Gleason 7 or greater tumors are probably best treated (radical prostatectomy or HIFU) rather than deferring treatment with active surveillance." [12]

"The Definition of a "clinically insignificant" tumor is Gleason 6 or less and less than 0.5 ccs volume."

"The arbitrariness of this is concerning. If the clinically significant prostate cancer rate was set at 4%, the clinically significant prostate cancer volume would be closer to 1 mL; conversely, if it were set at 12%, the clinically significant prostate cancer volume would be 0.2 mL. Nonetheless, this pathologic definition of clinically insignificant disease is widely used" [13], *thereby, confusing many, if not all of us!*

When is radical or curative treatment appropriate? A growing number of urologists believe when cancer is found, it should be treated. Their rationale, to discover and treat cancer in its earliest possible stage "is the best opportunity for cure." Of course, a great percentage of these cancers are called "insignificant" in retrospective studies. That is, the cancer was not expected to develop to a stage that it would be dangerous or life threatening. What of the dangerous or "aggressive" cancers? Prostate cancer is graded (Gleason Score) as a result of tissue analysis from needle biopsy. It has also been shown to be graded effectively with an MRI scanning sequence. Three categories emerge regarding the aggressiveness of prostate cancer. Cancers graded as "Gleason 6" and below are considered to be slow-growing and do not pose an immediate threat to most patients. An exception would be cancer location when it is near the capsular edge. Considering the poor outcomes of treatment, there is a strong argument that these cancers should not be treated radically. Gleason 6 cancers are believed to become weakened or less aggressive when inflammation associated with prostatitis is controlled. [14]

Cancers graded as "Gleason 8" and above are considered to be aggressive cancers. It would seem logical that these cancers be treated immediately in the hope that cancer has not yet escaped the prostate capsule and ventured into the body. Unfortunately, it has been demonstrated that these patients have an *85%* chance of cancer returning within 7-10 years of treatment (Biochemical Failure). Finally, you have the middle ground, the "Gleason 7" cancer. Are these cancers appropriate for curative treatment? The high percentage of failures within 7-10 years for these cancers may not appear to justify the excessive negative side effects. **A top physician representing a prestigious medical school in the U.S. presents in detail on his website that he treats all grades of prostate cancer with robotic prostatectomy. This is a disturbing trend.**

Robotic Prostatectomy is Still Surgery

Curative Intent

"The overly hasty and widespread adoption of this technique could set the field of early prostate cancer detection and treatment back 15 years as did the early application of ineffective open brachytherapy techniques in the 1970s."[15]

"... there is no evidence that the procedure (robotic prostatectomy) improves cure rates" [2] **Frankly, there is evidence, it does not!**

There is a steep Learning Curve for Robot Assisted Laparoscopic Prostatectomy. *"If you have to choose between someone who hasn't performed many robotic surgeries and a person who has performed many open procedures—take the open procedure," says Peter G. Schulam, M.D., Ph.D., a urology professor at the David Geffen School of Medicine at UCLA.*[2]

Robot Surgery is better due to potentially "fewer positive margins:" *"Several large studies have demonstrated that a positive surgical margin increases the chances that the prostate-specific antigen (PSA)—a protein produced by the cells of the prostate gland—will rise after surgery, and increase the chances that the disease will reoccur and progress." "Therefore, any intervention or technique to lower positive surgical margins,* **we think,** *will translate into a better long-term cure rate."*[16]

Fewer "Positive Margins" relates to the Experience of the Surgeon. *". . . positive margin rates in several laparoscopic prostatectomy series are concerningly high . . . Atug et al. reported a positive margin rate of 45.4% in the first 33 of 100 consecutive robotic prostatectomies . . . Baumert pointed out in an editorial comment, "the positive margin rate of the first group of patients is difficult to accept in this day and age. All surgical teams, new to robotic or laparoscopic surgery should initiate their programs with mentors to avoid 'sacrificing' the first (group) patients."*[15]

"Biochemical Failure"—Your Cancer has returned!!

When is surgery appropriate?

You need to know the potential outcomes of surgery. Gleason Score and PSA play an important role in determining the best opportunity to cure cancer. According to Johns Hopkins, James Buchanan Brady Urological Institute, **Biochemical Recurrence Probability after Radical Prostatectomy** was charted based upon Gleason Score and PSA. **According to the tables generated from the research, a Gleason 7 cancer with a PSA between 4.1 and 10 ng/ml, presents a 33% chance of biochemical recurrence (malignancy) in 10 years. For organ-confined Gleason 8-10 cancers with PSA between 4.1 and 10 ng/ml, there is a 43% probability of biochemical recurrence within 10 years. For non-organ confined disease, a Gleason 8 and above with PSA between 4.1 and 10 ng/ml, there is an 85% probability of failure within 10 years.** [17] For most radical prostatectomies, prior to surgery, it is unknown whether the disease is organ confined. **This is further reason that a 3 Tesla MRI scan must be performed prior to surgery.**

A study published in the Journal of Urology in 1996 revealed that in 92% of cases, prostate cancer cells were present in blood suctioned during surgical prostatectomy.[5] Authors of the study expressed concern and proceeded to speculate as to why this phenomenon existed. Robotic prostatectomy is promoted among physicians as having a lower rate of "positive margins." [16] Positive margins is an indication that not all of the cancerous tissue was removed during the surgery. The procedure may be promising, but it remains there is no evidence that robotic prostatectomy improves curative outcomes. It is still surgery and prostate cancer cells are still released into the blood stream.[5]

"In an attempt to understand the paradoxical observation of disease progression after radical

*retropubicprostatectomyinmenwithpathologically confined carcinoma several mechanisms have been hypothesized, including aggressive biological behavior with unrecognized metastases, **local and possibly distant dissemination associated with the surgical procedure**, faulty pathological assessment, and perhaps an antecedent event, such as multiple independent **puncture biopsies**"* [5]

Another advantage claimed by robotic surgery is the improved ability to perform the surgery while allowing the patient to retain sexual function. This is described as "nerve sparing" surgery. The robotic technology in theory has greater precision to separate the prostate gland from the delicate nerves and vessels of the neurovascular bundle from prostate glandular tissue. Unfortunately, the numbers have not yet demonstrated improved results over any other treatment method.[9,15,17] This surgery continues to be described as "extremely difficult" by the top surgeons in the country. They have good reason. In addition, it is now accepted that robotic surgery has a significant learning curve for surgeons. Some publications cite a requirement that as many as 200 surgeries must be performed before proficiency is achieved.

"Nerve Sparing," but what about Curative Intent?

"I try not to touch the nerves at all," said (urologist), a warm man with a gentle manner. He is, of course, limited by how far cancer has advanced. In 80 percent of cases he is able to perform maximum nerve-sparing, resulting in a return to continence for 97 percent of patients and sexual function for 87 percent, within 6 months." [18]

*Is **Open Radical Prostatectomy** a Better Method for Nerve-Sparing Surgery?* "For any surgeon, this procedure—technically, the anatomical radical retropubic prostatectomy—is a bumpy, treacherous road. There can be extreme blood loss. It takes years of training before a surgeon can handle the unexpected bleeding without panicking—and also without inadvertently damaging the fragile nerves. An experienced surgeon, too, **can tell much by tactile sensation**—literally, feeling the tissue for hardness, adherence, or other signs of cancer, and deciding how best to remove it."[19]

The benefit of a shorter hospital stay does not offset the high cost of the equipment or the procedure. [2] "It is costly. (Urologist) performs three robotic prostatectomies a day. His team nurse jokes that "we're heading for drive-thru surgery in this country" to cut down on hospital time. But the price can still reach $45,000.00 to more than $70,000.00 depending on who does the surgery"[18]

Has Robotic Prostatectomy Delivered on Its Promise? "Prostate cancer patients' biggest concerns—after cure—are the possible side effects of surgery, including urinary incontinence and sexual impotency. Data on these side effects from robotically assisted prostatectomy were sketchy at best, and no evidence was available to indicate that any surgical method emerged as better than another for these side effects." [2]

> "Although they may ultimately decide on treatment, there is no apparent gain to making this management decision quickly with the belief that a delay will compromise cure. Second, when selected carefully by use of criteria that suggest the presence of small-volume, lower-grade cancer

and then monitored with a rigorous protocol for disease progression, these patients appear to have the same risk of non-curable prostate cancer **for at least 2 years after diagnosis** *as those patients who received immediate prostate cancer surgery. Our data thus suggests that this expectant management approach (like CDM) should be used more frequently, given that approximately 50% of men today are diagnosed with low-risk prostate cancer."* [20]

Summary

The increasingly aggressive search for cancer by repeated needle biopsies will inevitably lead to more and more unnecessary surgeries, more failures to cure and a growing number of men and their families suffering from the devastating side effects of incontinence and sexual dysfunction. There exists no compelling evidence at this time that robotic prostatectomy will deliver any improvement whatsoever over the current poor rate of cure for all other radical, curative treatments. What is truly alarming is that the effort to find more cancers by more than doubling the rate of biopsy, will only serve to increase the devastation that exists today. **Ironically, increasing numbers of insignificant cancers included for treatment, will only serve to (falsely) indicate better cure rates for robotic prostatectomies.** Of course, this will only incentivize urologists to treat even more cancers. Additionally, urology is trending to treat more aggressive cancers, Gleason 8 and above, without confirming prior to actual surgery that the cancer is organ-confined with a 3 T MRI scans. The number of failures, exceeding 1,000,000 men, could easily double in the near future. What of these men and these families? The only reasonable conclusion is to discontinue curative treatments such as robotic prostatectomy, for the majority of positively diagnosed men until proof exists that these treatments can successfully cure prostate cancer. When will the cure become more dangerous than the disease? I think we have already reached that point!

References:

1. *Minimally Invasive Surgery in Urology*, Current Opinion in Urology. 18(2):173-179, March 2008, Box, Geoffrey N; Ahlering, Thomas E

2. *Robot-Assisted Prostate Surgery Has Possible Benefits, Higher Costs*, By Lisa Esposito, Editor, Health Behavior News Service, August 29, 2005

3. *Clinically Insignificant T1 Stage Tumors Of The Prostate*, Konstantinos Stamatiou, Vassilissa Karanassiou, Kavouras Nikolaos, Makris Vasilios, Lebren Fred, Emmanuel Agapitos: Clinically Insignificant T1 Stage Tumors Of The Prostate. *The Internet Journal of Urology*. 2007. Volume 4 Number 2.

4. *Prostate Biopsy Spreads Prostate Cancer Cells*, Diagnostic Center for Disease, February 28, 2008 & also in Chapter 6 in 'Men at Risk', the dirty little secret; prostate biopsies really do spread prostate cancer cells

5. *Molecular detection of prostate epithelial cells from the surgical field and peripheral circulation during radical prostatectomy*, Michael G. Oefelein, Karen Kaul,* Barbara Hew, Michael D. Blum, James M. Holland, Thomas C. Keeler, William A. Cook and Jeffrey m. Ignatoff, Departments of Urology and Pathology. McGaw Medical Center of Northwestern University, Evanston Hospital, Evanston, Illinois, Journal of Urology, 1996

6. *Largest Study Ever of Value of Robotic Prostate Surgery,* Research Team: Ketan Badani, M.D., Sanjeev Kaul, M.D., Mani Menon, M.D., Vattikuti Urology Institute, Henry Ford Health System

7. *What Happens if PSA Comes Back After Surgery?* Prostate Cancer Update, James Buchanan Brady Urological Institute Johns Hopkins Medical Institutions, Vol. V, Winter 2000

8. *Prostate Cancer—Diagnosis & Staging,* UroToday.com, 2007-05-02

9. *Achieving Optimal Outcomes after Radical Prostatectomy,* Jeffery W. Saranchuk, Michael W. Kattan, Elena Elkin, A. Karim Touijer, Peter T. Scardino, and James A. Eastham, Department of Urology, Sidney Kimmel Center for Prostate and Urologic Cancers; and Department of Epidemiology and Biostatistics, Memorial Sloan-Kettering Cancer Center, New York, NY, 2005 by the American Society of Clinical Oncology.

10. *Fastest-Growing Health Company: Intuitive Surgical,* Wall Street Journal, Posted by Jacob Goldstein September 5, 2007, 9:17 am

11. *Does Increased Needle Biopsy Sampling Of The Prostate Detect A Higher Number Of Potentially Insignificant Tumors?* Theresa Y. Chan, David Y. Chan, Kristen Lecksell, Ray E. Stutzman and Jonathan I.Epstein Departments of Pathology and Urology, The Johns Hopkins University School of Medicine and James Buchannan Brady Urological Institute, The Johns Hopkins Hospital, Baltimore, Maryland

12. *"Advanced Robotics Techniques"* Symposium, K.M. Slawin, MD, Urologist, Baylor Univeristy, Faculty 2006 symposium, hosted by Ash Tewari, M.D. at Weill Cornell School of Medicine in New York City

13. *Identification of Clinically Insignificant Disease,* 5(7):693-698. ©2007 Journal of the National Comprehensive Cancer Network

14. *Is It Necessary to Cure Prostate Cancer when It Is Possible?* Ronald E. Wheeler, MD, Clinical Interventions in Aging, Dove Press, Vol 2, Number 1, 2007

15. *"The value of robotic laparoscopic radical prostatectomy: Important vs. minimal use." Laparoscopic or Robotic Prostatectomy—Not There Yet,"* Stacy Loeb, M.D.[1] and William J.Catalona, M.D.[2,1] Department of Urology, Georgetown University School of Medicine, Washington, D.C. [2] Department of Urology and the Robert H. Lurie Comprehensive Cancer Center, Northwestern University Feinberg School of Medicine, Chicago, IL

16. **Robotic Procedure Improves Survival for Prostate Cancer Patients,** Thomas Jefferson University, news release, May 21, 2007

17. **Biochemical (prostate specific antigen) recurrence probability following radical prostatectomy for clinically localized prostate cancer,** Misop Han, alan w. Partin,* Marianna Zahurak, Steven Piantadosi, Jonathan I. Epstein and Patrick C. Walsh, The Journal of Urology® Vol. 169, 517–523, February 2003

18. **We're heading for drive-thru surgery,** Reuters News Services, Douglas Hamilton, January 31 2008 at 05:54PM

19. **The "Gold Standard" Treatment for Prostate Cancer,** Prostate Cancer Discovery, Brady Urological Institute, Johns Hopkins Medicine, Vol. I, Fall 2004

20. **Delayed Versus Immediate Surgical Intervention and Prostate Cancer Outcome,** Christopher Warlick, Bruce J. Trock, Patricia Landis, Jonathan I. Epstein, H. Ballentine Carter, Departments of Urology (CW, BJT, PL, HBC) and Pathology (JIE), Johns Hopkins University School of Medicine, James Buchanan Brady Urological Institute, Johns Hopkins Hospital, Baltimore, MD

APPENDIX 36

Benefits of Green Tea versus Prostate Cancer

Topic: *Green Tea Consumption May Reduce the Risk of Advanced Prostate Cancer*

Keywords: **PROSTATE CANCER**—*Green Tea, Camellia Sinensis, Catechin*

Reference: *"Green Tea Consumption and Prostate Cancer Risk in Japanese Men: A Prospective Study," Kurahashi N, Sasazuki S, et al, American Journal of Epidemiology, 2007; 167(1): 71-77. (Address: N. Kurahashi, Epidemiology and Prevention Division, Research Center for Cancer Prevention and Screening, National Cancer Center, 5-1-1 Tsukjii, Chuo-ku, Tokyo 104-0045, Japan. E-mail: nkurahas@gan2.res.ncc.go.jp).*

Summary: In a prospective study involving 49,920 men aged 40-69 years, consumption of green tea was found to be associated with a reduced risk of advanced prostate cancer. Subjects were followed from 1990 (cohort 1) and 1993 (cohort 2) through 2004. Four hundred and four (404) men were newly diagnosed with prostate cancer during that time, out of which 114 had advanced stage prostate cancer, 271 had localized, and 19 had undetermined stage prostate cancer. Green tea consumption was assessed via questionnaires at baseline and through the follow up period. Results found that while green tea consumption was not associated with localized prostate cancer, it was associated, in a dose-dependent manner, with advanced prostate cancer. Men who consumed more than 5 cups/day of green tea were found to have a multivariate relative risk of 0.53, compared with men consuming less than 1 cup per day. The authors conclude, "Green tea may be associated with a decreased risk of advanced prostate cancer."

Effects of Dietary Changes on Prostate Cancer Growth

Dietary Changes May Slow Prostate Cancer Growth
Study in mice shows increasing the ratio of omega-3 to omega-6 fatty acids slows the progression of prostate cancer
By Anthony J. Brown, MD

TUESDAY, August 1 (Reuters Health)—Increasing the ratio of omega-3 to omega-6 fatty acids in the diet appears to slow the progression of prostate cancer, according to the results of an animal study.

The so-called Western diet commonly consumed in the US contains mostly omega-6 fatty acids, derived from corn oil and other sources. Omega-3 fatty acids, by contrast, are abundant in cold-water fish, a food source missing in the diets of many Americans.

"Our study showed that altering the fatty acid ratio found in the typical Western diet to include more omega-3 fatty acids and decreasing the amount of omega-6 fatty acids reduced prostate cancer tumor growth rates and PSA levels in mice," senior author Dr. William J. Aronson, from the University of California, Los Angeles School of Medicine, told Reuters Health.

Aronson noted that the Western diet usually contains an omega-6 to—3 ratio of about 15 to 1. In the current study, comparison animals received a diet containing a similar ratio, while intervention animals were given a diet with a ratio of about 1 to 1.

Aronson believes that with dietary changes and the use of fish oil supplements, an omega-6 to—3 ratio of 2 to 1 or possibly lower is attainable in prostate cancer patients.

The new study, reported in Clinical Cancer Research, involved mice implanted with human prostate cancer cells. Aside from the difference in the omega-6 to 3 ratio, all of the animals received identical 20 percent fat diets.

Tumor growth rates, the final tumor size, and PSA levels were all lower in the intervention group compared with mice given Western diets. Laboratory testing showed that cancer cells grew 22 percent slower in culture dishes containing body fluid from the intervention group. Consumption of the increased omega-3 diet was also associated with an 83% reduction in tumor prostaglandin E (PGE)-2 levels, a chemical known to promote inflammation.

"This is an initial animal-model study that is one of the first to show the impact of diet on lowering an inflammatory response known to promote prostate tumor progression in tumors. More research needs to be done before clinical recommendations can be made, but the finding is significant," Aronson noted.

"At this point we would not recommend changing fatty acid intake for prostate cancer patients. However, we are conducting a randomized study in men to test if dietary changes affect prostate tissue levels of COX-2 and PGE-2," he added.

SOURCE: Clinical Cancer Research, August 1 2006.

APPENDIX 38

SYNOPSIS OF PROFESSIONAL ACHIEVEMENTS (Curriculum Vitae)

Ronald E. Wheeler, M.D.
Medical Director of the Diagnostic Center for Disease™,
Sarasota, Florida

Author of a book entitled, 'Men at Risk; the Dirty Little Secret', 'Prostate biopsies really do spread prostate cancer cells'; in Press for release in early 2012

Named **Medical Director (May 2011) of CZ Biomed**, a Tampa, Florida based research group specializing in vaccine therapy for Prostate Cancer, Breast Cancer, Colon Cancer and Lung Cancer using an Oncolytic virus (RSV). www.czbiomed.com

Recognized world leader in the Subspecialties of Prostate Ultrasound, Magnetic Resonance Spectroscopy Imaging (MRSI) and High Intensity Focused Ultrasound (HIFU) Internationally. Featured Urology Consultant for HIFU in London, England and Cancun, Mexico.

Featured Speaker for the Society of Naturopaths in Vancouver, Canada in 2010

Keynote Speaker at Confirma Corporation in Seattle, Washington (www.Confirma.com) associated with their launch of a Prostate related technology, Dynamic Contrast Enhancement (DCE) and its role in MRI-Spectroscopy Imaging—November 2007

Member of the American Urologic Association (AUA) since 1985

Recipient of Post-Graduate Continuing Medical Education Achievement Awards

Member of the National Institutes of Health (NIH) 'Prostatitis Collaborative'

Internationally recognized Urologist invited to speak at the 1st National Men's Health Conference sponsored by Penn State (May 21, 2004); Topic: "Can Education and Awareness on Prostate Disease Alter the Death Rate from Prostate Cancer in the State of Florida?"

Practicing Urologist for more than 25 years with practice focus on male health related issues including Impotency and Prostate Diseases associated with BPH, Prostatitis, and Prostate Cancer

Post Graduate Urology Residency Training at **LSU Medical Center** in New Orleans, Louisiana

Member of the Esteemed Royal College of Alternative Medicine (RCAM), Dublin, Ireland

Featured Speaker (Master's Series at A4M **(The Society of Anti-Aging)**—Las Vegas, December, 2007—Topic: Perils Associated with Testosterone Replacement

Medical Director of the Diagnostic Center for Disease™ located in Sarasota, Florida, featuring 3.0 T MRI-Spectroscopy, "the next greatest diagnostic test for prostate cancer", according to Peter Scardino, M.D. from Memorial Sloan-Kettering; this technology helps men to avoid unnecessary prostate biopsies

Certified treating expert in High Intensity Focused Ultrasound (HIFU), a novel prostate cancer treatment, that is currently involved in Phase 3 trials at the FDA; this therapy is currently available in Canada, Dominican Republic, Mexico, Bermuda and the Bahamas having treated more than 250 patients in 5 years

Medical Director of Preferred Health Foundation...speaking to better choices in health care through awareness and education

Runner-up in the "**Physician Educator of the Year**" award sponsored by **AFUD (American Foundation of Urologic Disease)**

Post Graduate 3T MRI Educational Symposia: Why and What You Need to Know About 3T MRI—Sponsored by General Electric (March, 2007)

Post Graduate MRI-S Physician Review Course Sponsored by UCSF—December, 2006

Principal Investigator (PI) in a "Neo-Adjuvant Study for Organ Confined Prostate Cancer", sponsored in part by Schering

Pharmaceuticals and accepted for presentation at the Western Section of the American Urology Association (AUA); comparing clinical utilization of an LHRH-analalog + Antiandrogen versus an Antiandrogen + a 5-alpha Reductase Inhibitor with PSA nadir as an end point

Owner of two Patents on Prostatitis Detection and Resolution; Prostatitis is a Precursor disease process known to evolve into Prostate Cancer (reference: American Association of Cancer Research; AACR)

Inventor of Peenuts®, a branded prostatitis formula that has been patented in the USA, Canada and Europe and expects to be the featured formula in the ProCap Trial as we endeavor to prove that prostatitis resolution can prevent prostate cancer

Invited Speaker at the National Institutes of Health (Bethesda, Maryland) in 1999 and 2000 discussing the topics of: "Voiding Symptoms Predict Prostatitis, Not BPH" and "For the Prostate to be Healthy, Your PSA Must Be Less than One"

Featured Speaker at the Florida Osteopathic Sectional Meeting; Topic: "Anti-Aging Solutions to Prostate Health" 2002 as well as a featured speaker on the topic, "The Truth about Prostate Disease"—2007

Featured Speaker at the American College of Advanced Medicine (ACAM), November 2002 & October 2008

Featured Speaker at Age Management Medicine Group (AMMG), November 2008

Featured Speaker at the Navigators National Conference in Colorado Springs, Colorado– September 2008

Featured Speaker at the Cancer Control Society, September 2003 on "Prostatitis as a Cause of Prostate Cancer and why the PSA (blood test) Must be Less than One"

Patient advocate for "Prostate Health" and sponsor of "The Drive for Prostate Health", a Motor Coach that offers Early Detection for Prostate Disease to businesses and individuals throughout the State of Florida and Nationally

Frequent Speaker at Prostate Cancer Support Meetings including Man to Man events throughout Florida, PAACT, and the State of New Mexico's Prostate Cancer Survival Group

Author of numerous Prostate related Articles including: "Everything You Ever Wanted to Know about Prostatitis", "PSA—A Barometer of Prostate Health or a License to Biopsy", "Anti-Androgen Monotherapy is Our Signature Treatment for Prostate Cancer" at the Prostatitis and Prostate Cancer Center, and "Straight Talk on Impotency"

Participant Physician in a Vaccine Study (sponsor: Dendrion) for Hormone Refractive Prostate Cancer utilizing "Provenge"; now FDA approved effective 2011

Current member or previous member of the Advisory Board For Several Health-Related Corporations and Foundations including: Sanofi-Aventis Oncology, Urology Times, PAACT, Prostate Awareness Foundation, Glaxo Smith Kline, Abbott, and Radiation Centers of America

Developer of 5 Websites: accessed at: www.TheProstateCenter. com, www.ProstateCancerPreventionFoundation.org, www. MrisUSA.com, www.PanAmHIFU.com and www.Peenuts.com

Frequent Guest of Health Radio Broadcasts including: The David Darbro Show, The Deborah Ray Show, Western Health Radio, Dr. Burton live in Philadelphia, Frank Tabino Show, Eva Herr's Show from Atlanta and Public Health Radio

Featured Expert on a nationally acclaimed Radio Talk Show, "PJ and the Doc, Let's Talk Prostate"; www.1490wwpr.com; Launched December 2007 until September 2008

Author of Research article, entitled, "Is it Necessary to Cure Prostate Cancer When it is Possible? Published in the Peer Reviewed Journal, "Clinical Interventions in Aging", Volume 2, Number 1—April 2007

(Edited: 03/15/2012)

APPENDIX—39

Data Regarding Benefit of the Peenuts® formula on the White blood cell count of the Expressed Prostatic Secretion (EPS); a consecutive series of patients

(A lower white blood cell count indicates decreased inflammation with continued use)

INITIALS	EPS (Mean)	F/U EPS	% CHANGE	TIME TO SURVEILLANCE	COMMENTS
D.L.	310	210	32%	12 mo.	HGPIN
A.C.	125	6	95%	12 mo.	PC
R.D.	160	36	78%	12 mo.	PC
J.F.	400	185	54%	18 mo.	PC
K.H.	275	27	90%	12 mo.	PC
G.H.	100	75	25%	14 mo.	PC
R.P.	300	200	33%	6 mo.	PC
R.D.	500	50	90%	12 mo.	PC
C.H.	113	70	38%	6 mo.	
B.P.	200	38	81%	12 mo.	
D.S.	268	25	91%	18 mo.	
R.A.	90	35	61%	9 mo.	
M.H.	150	95	37%	6 mo.	
I.R.	256	70	73%	14 mo.	

INITIALS	EPS (Mean)	F/U EPS	% CHANGE	TIME TO SURVEILLANCE	COMMENTS
L.M.	300	263	12%	6 mo.	
S.W.	295	70	76%	12 mo.	
W.P.	83	60	28%	6 mo.	
B.M.	400	125	69%	12 mo.	
C.M.	300	100	67%	13 m	
B.R.	165	160	3%	6 mo.	
S.S.	150	95	37%	12 mo.	
A.M.	256	70	73%	15 mo.	
S.A.	42	11	74%	12 mo.	
N.F.	65	100	54%(+)	6 mo.	
S.G.	160	26	84%	11 mo.	
R.G.	400	38	91%	14 mo.	
F.H.	20	7	65%	48 mo.	
S.H.	50	8	84%	8 mo.	
B.H.	450	110	76%	10 mo.	
M.H.	300	65	78%	9 mo.	
B.I.	450	70	84%	11 mo.	
J.K.	210	135	36%	8 mo.	
M.K.	190	48	75%	8 mo.	
E.L.	105	15	86%	18 mo.	
T.L.	325	155	52%	48 mo.	
B.M.	20	12	40%	9 mo.	
K.M.	48	35	27%	15 mo.	
D.G.	325	12	96%	36 mo.	
J.M.	105	85	19%	36 mo.	
E.M.	290	30	90%	10 mo.	
W.M.	300	35	88%	25 mo.	
S.K.	210	10	95%	12 mo.	
W.M.	350	140	60%	24 mo.	
W.M.	140	45	68%	18 mo.	
J.N.	275	100	64%	5 mo.	
A.D.	80	25	69%	4 mo.	
D.A.	70	16	77%	4 mo.	
C.B.	80	13	84%	4 mo.	

INITIALS	EPS (Mean)	F/U EPS	% CHANGE	TIME TO SURVEILLANCE	COMMENTS
B.C.	235	154	35%	4 mo.	
C.F.	170	35	79%	4 mo.	
F.C.	340	65	81%	4 mo.	
F.W.	256	113	56%	12 mo.	
J.B.	85	15	82%	12 mo.	
S.A.	325	190	42%	12 mo.	
S.A.	190	60	68%	12 mo.	
J.C	350	158	55%	12 mo.	
W.G.	TNTC	5	99%	24 mo.	
R.J.	268	17	94%	12 mo.	
D.S.	375	150	60%	12 mo.	
G.P.	205	9	96%	24 mo.	
C.B.	350	30	91%	12 mo.	
L.R.	275	70	75%	12 mo.	
E.E.	185	35	81%	12 mo.	
R.N.	175	60	66%	18 mo.	
P.R.	400	130	68%	9 mo.	
D.S.	131	15	89%	14 mo.	
J.R.	50	31	38%	6 mo.	
W.S.	80	40	50%	13 mo.	
D.S.	225	140	38%	14 mo.	
T.S.	400	40	90%	13 mo.	
W.S.	TNTC	28	94%	22 mo.	
D.S.	110	70	36%	6 mo.	
J.W.	105	16	85%	36 mo.	PC
M.W.	88	35	60%	8 mo.	
W.W.	TNTC	50	90%	9 mo.	PC
K.W.	200	25	88%	24 mo.	
J.M.	TNTC	105	79%	10 mo.	PC
T.M.	175	90	49%	36 mo.	
J.K.	268	156	42%	24 mo.	
R.S.	80	40	50%	12 mo.	
D.S.	225	140	38%	26 mo.	
A.W.	278	40	86%	5 mo.	

INITIALS	EPS (Mean)	F/U EPS	% CHANGE	TIME TO SURVEILLANCE	COMMENTS
S.P.	110	30	73%	1 mo.	
J.M.	125	70	44%	3 mo.	
J.W.	90	40	56%	2 mo.	
F.R.	238	175	27%	1 mo.	
R.S.	60	21	65%	2.5 mo.	
R.A.	30	10	67%	2 mo.	
J.M.	45	4	91%	9.5 mo.	
R.G.	110	93	16%	2 mo.	
D.I.	25	13	48%	1.5 mo.	
R.D.	22	5	77%	1.5 mo.	
M.P.	500	50	90%	8 mo.	
R.M.	175	30	83%	1.5 mo.	
R.K.	500	130	74%	6 mo.	
F.B.	48	13	73%	4 mo.	
N.E.	140	55	61%	2 mo.	
J.S.	45	7	84%	6 mo.	
J.F.	110	25	77%	12 mo.	
P.H.	90	50	44%	6 mo.	
J.Q.	38	13	66%	15 mo.	
R.V.	130	35	73%	9 mo.	
N=102	Mean:208	Mean:65	69% Mean EPS Reduction on Peenuts®		

Data regarding PSA variation following the use of the Peenuts® Formula at varying intervals

INITIALS	PSA	F/U PSA	% CHANGE	TIME TO SURVEILLANCE	COMMENTS
S.S.	16.6	11.3	32%	37 mo.	Biopsy Negative x 2
M.S	14.9	6.7	55%	6 mo.	Biopsy Negative
D.J.	33.9	5.7	83%	6 mo.	Biopsy Negative
D.L.	5.6	1.8	68%	14 mo.	HGPIN
D.S.	7	2.6	63%	14 mo.	HGPIN (Biopsy x 3)
B.L.	5.8	4.9	16%	1 mo.	PC
R.L.	5.3	4.9	8%	4 mo.	PC
S.K.	4.2	1.6	62%	12 mo.	PC
R.P.	8.4	2.9	65%	13 mo.	PC
F.W.	8.5	3.1	64%	72 mo.	PC; + Avodart®
J.B.	7	2.4	66%	60 mo.	PC
S.A.	4.7	2.1	55%	41 mo.	PC; + Avodart®
J.W.	11.7	5.8	50%	60 mo.	PC
R.C.	2.9	1.7	41%	72 mo.	PC
J.C.	2.1	2.8	33%(+)	42 mo.	PC; + Avodart®
W.G.	7.3	4.5	38%	40 mo.	PC; + Avodart®
R.V.	6.9	6	13%	38 mo.	PC
D.S.	9.1	5.5	40%	58 mo.	PC
J.G.	3.2	2	38%	21 mo.	PC; + Avodart®
G.D.	6.2	4.4	29%	21 mo.	PC
C.B.	4.4	1.7	61%	39 mo.	PC; + Avodart®
J.S.	11.4	12.3	8%(+)	34 mo.	PC

INITIALS	PSA	F/U PSA	% CHANGE	TIME TO SURVEILLANCE	COMMENTS
L.R.	6.8	1.9	72%	49 mo.	PC; + Avodart®
E.E.	6.6	1.8	73%	24 mo.	PC
J.M.	14.4	1.5	90%	29 mo.	PC; + Avodart®
J.C.	8.4	1.8	79%	18 mo.	PC; + Avodart®
R.W.	4.4	4.7	7%(+)	14 mo.	PC; + Avodart®
R.C.	6.1	1.3	79%	13 mo.	PC
R.W.	0.5	0.3	40%	84 mo.	
A.C.	3.6	1.4	61%	4.5 mo.	
B.R.	1.2	0.58	52%	6 mo.	
R.A.	0.9	0.7	22%	6 mo.	
C.B.	6.9	5.8	16%	6 mo.	
L.A.	3.4	2.7	21%	6 mo.	
P.R.	3.9	3	23%	6 mo.	
B.D.	9.26	8.44	9%	3 mo.	
R.C.	7	4.6	34%	19 mo.	
N.F.	6.8	2.5	63%	16 mo.	
S.G.	3.5	2.6	26%	12 mo.	
R.G.	4.4	4.9	11%(+)	9 mo.	
R.H.	9.1	3.36	63%	27 mo.	
G.H.	13	9.6	26%	2 mo.	
F.H.	6.5	3.9	40%	12 mo.	
S.H.	1.16	0.92	21%	12 mo.	
R.H.	13	11.4	12%	7 mo.	
D.H.	5.8	4.7	19%	2 mo.	
D.J.	13.8	5.23	62%	4 mo.	
D.G.	3.3	0.97	71%	26 mo.	
E.L.	7.6	4.3	43%	47 mo.	
B.M.	0.6	0.4	33%	41 mo.	
K.M.	4.8	1.9	60%	15 mo.	
J.M.	11.79	6.7	43%	24 mo.	
E.M.	10.6	8.8	17%	8 mo.	
W.M.	0.7	0.7	0%	25 mo.	
W.M.	3.8	2	47%	48 mo.	
R.M.	6.3	4.4	30%	22 mo.	
C.M.	3.7	1.6	57%	24 mo.	
R.M.	6.6	3.2	46%	39 mo.	
R.S.	1.64	0.9	45%	4 mo.	

INITIALS	PSA	F/U PSA	% CHANGE	TIME TO SURVEILLANCE	COMMENTS
R.N.	2.89	1.77	39%	7 mo.	
R.N.	5.8	2.43	58%	32 mo.	
F.R.	10.8	5.2	52%	6 mo.	
J.R.	9.84	4.3	56%	12 mo.	
F.R.	5.2	3.1	40%	6 mo.	
J.R.	7.1	2.8	61%	44 mo.	
W.S.	2.4	1.6	33%	56 mo.	
D.S.	11.7	3.7	68%	19 mo.	
M.W.	7.1	5.6	21%	8 mo.	
T.M.	7.7	3.8	51%	48 mo.	Biopsy Negative
S.G.	0.6	0.6	0%	42 mo.	
J.K.	5.4	2.6	48%	48 mo.	
D.S.	9.8	3.7	62%	15 mo.	Plus Avodart®
R.E.	24.1	9.2	62%	9 mo.	Bx.X(2)(Neg); Plus Avodart®
L.W.	6.4	0.7	89%	> 6 mo.	
T.G.	43	7.4	83%	4 mo.	
R.D.	16	3.8	76%	11 mo.	
R.V.	2.9	2.1	28%	> 6 mo.	
B.C.	2.1	0.9	57%	> 6 mo.	
B.M.	7.9	7	11%	> 6 mo.	
H.M.	11.4	4.1	64%	10 mo.	
C.A.	14	2.7	81%	> 6 mo.	
J.S.	8.4	4.2	50%	8 mo.	
M.S.	3.8	0.8	79%	> 6 mo.	
R.V.	25	16	36%	9 mo.	Biopsy Negative X 2
G.S.	6.8	4.7	31%	> 6 mo.	
G.M.	8.8	5.4	39%	> 6 mo.	
D.E.	25.3	3	88%	8 mo.	Biopsy Negative
C.R.	4.7	3.7	21%	> 6 mo.	
B.G.	2.5	2.1	16%	> 6 mo.	
C.P.	4.1	2.8	32%	> 6 mo.	
V.J.	4.5	3.6	20%	> 6 mo.	
L.V.	15.6	5.4	65%	> 6 mo.	
D.V.	3.8	1.2	68%	> 6 mo.	
J.C.	10	3.1	69%	> 6 mo.	
C.C.	22	19	14%	> 6 mo.	

INITIALS	PSA	F/U PSA	% CHANGE	TIME TO SURVEILLANCE	COMMENTS
H.F.	5.3	4.6	13%	> 6 mo.	
F.J.	7.5	5.2	31%	> 6 mo.	
R.H.	8.5	5.4	37%	> 6 mo.	
R.A.	2.5	2.2	12%	> 6 mo.	
R.G.	5.9	5.5	7%	> 6 mo.	
G.T.	1.4	0.8	43%	6 mo.	
G.H.	36	1.6	96%	> 6 mo.	
V.S.	3.8	2.9	24%	> 6 mo.	
C.C.	5.6	4.3	23%	> 6 mo.	
R.L.	7.4	4.1	45%	> 6 mo.	
C.D.	3.6	2.4	33%	> 6 mo.	
J.L.	4.0	3.5	13%	4 mo.	
L.G.	1.3	0.9	31%	12 mo.	
R.S.	11.0	5.8	47%	4 mo.	
E.L.	6.7	4.2	37%	3.5 mo.	
M.L.	11.4	7.4	35%	3 mo.	
C.T.	2.6	2.0	23%	5 mo.	
L.S.	4.1	3.4	17%	10 mo.	
E.S.	4.3	3.2	26%	6 mo.	
J.B.	4.6	3.9	15%	9 mo.	
B.D.	9.3	4.8	48%	5 mo.	
M.S.	7.5	5.4	28%	9 mo.	
R.N.	7.0	2.1	69%	8 mo.	
E.G.	4.7	4.1	13%	3 mo.	
L.L.	2.6	1.3	50%	13 mo.	
D.L.	18.0	10.5	42%	4 mo.	**Negative Biopsy X 2**
H.K.	5.6	2.6	54%	6 mo.	
P.H.	1.0	0.9	10%	6 mo.	
A.A.	4.5	0.8	82%	9 mo.	
C.C.	5.9	3.7	37%	14 mo.	
J.A.	7.5	4.9	35%	2 mo.	
R.A.	0.8	0.5	38%	10 mo.	
E.H.	0.9	0.6	33%	20 mo.	
R.D.	13.6	7.2	47%	2 mo.	
E.H.	1.5	1.2	20%	12 mo.	
T.M.	8.1	1.7	79%	2 mo.	
R.K.	25	16	36%	> 6 mo.	

INITIALS	PSA	F/U PSA	% CHANGE	TIME TO SURVEILLANCE	COMMENTS
L.T.	6.8	4.7	31%	> 6 mo.	
A.B.	8.8	5.4	39%	> 6 mo.	
D.M.	3.8	0.8	79%	> 6 mo.	
A.S.	2.9	2.1	28%	> 6 mo.	
L.M.	8.4	4.2	50%	> 6 mo.	
C.B.	14	2.7	81%	> 6 mo.	
K.T.	11.4	4.1	64%	> 6 mo.	
S.R.	7.9	7.0	11%	> 6 mo.	
I.B.	25.3	3.0	88%	> 6 mo.	
S.W.	4.7	3.7	21%	> 6 mo.	
C.F.	2.5	2.1	16%	> 6 mo.	
E.C.	4.5	3.6	20%	> 6 mo.	
B.R.	4.1	2.8	32%	> 6 mo.	
S.H.	15.6	5.4	65%	> 6 mo.	
R.R.	3.8	1.2	68%	> 6 mo.	
T.S.	10	3.1	69%	> 6 mo.	
J.D.	22	19	14%	> 6 mo.	
C.L.	5.3	4.6	13%	> 6 mo.	
A.L.	7.5	5.2	31%	> 6 mo.	
A.R.	8.5	5.4	37%	> 6 mo.	
M.M.	2.5	2.2	12%	> 6 mo.	
N.S.	5.9	5.5	7%	> 6 mo.	
N=154	Mean 7.8	Mean 3.9	50%		

APPENDIX—41

Data regarding the varying improvement of Voiding Symptoms with the continuous use of the Peenuts® Formula of 6-12 months or longer

MILD SYMPTOMS (1-7)			MODERATE SYMPTOMS (8-19)			SEVERE SYMPTOMS (20-35)		
Pre-Peenuts	Post-Peenuts	% Change	Pre-Peenuts	Post-Peenuts	% Change	Pre-Peenuts	Post-Peenuts	% Change
1.5	0.5	67%	16.5	4	76%	20.5	9	56%
4	0.5	88%	13.5	4.5	67%	20	11.5	43%
2.5	0.5	80%	15.5	5.5	65%	30.5	13.5	56%
7.5	3.5	53%	8.5	0.5	94%	20.5	10	51%
7.5	3.5	53%	13	2	85%	20.5	8.5	59%
6	1	83%	12.5	2	84%	21	0.5	98%
5.5	0	100%	10	2.5	75%	21.5	8	63%
4.5	2	56%	10.5	1.5	86%	23.5	16.5	30%
5.5	2.5	55%	11	1.5	86%	25	16	36%
6.5	2	69%	13	2	85%	23	10.5	55%
4	0	100%	15	1.5	90%	22.5	10	56%
5.5	2.5	55%	11.5	1.5	87%	25.5	15.5	40%
7.5	1.5	80%	18.5	5.5	70%	20	4.5	78%
7	0	100%	5.5	0	100%	22	15.5	30%
5	2	60%	16.5	8.5	48%	21.5	2	91%
3.5	0.5	86%	11	2.5	77%	21	4.5	79%
2.5	2	20%	17	1.5	91%	23.5	12	49%
6	3	50%	11.5	4.5	61%	28.5	12.5	57%
7.5	2	73%	14	2.5	82%	20.5	7	66%
7	0.5	93%	11.5	6.5	43%	23.5	10	57%
5.5	0	100%	9.5	1.5	84%	20	7	65%

MILD SYMPTOMS (1-7)			MODERATE SYMPTOMS (8-19)			SEVERE SYMPTOMS (20-35)		
Pre-Peenuts	Post-Peenuts	% Change	Pre-Peenuts	Post-Peenuts	% Change	Pre-Peenuts	Post-Peenuts	% Change
N=21			8	1.5	81%	24.5	16	34%
		72%	14	6.5	53%	25	4.5	86%
	Improved		14	5	64%	22	5	77%
			12	3.5	71%	25.5	3.5	86%
			15	5	67%			
			19.5	4	80%	N=25		60%
			9.5	3.5	63%			Improved
			18.5	10	46%			
			16	5	69%			
			9.5	2.5	74%			
			16.5	8	52%			
			20	7	65%			
			10.5	3.5	67%			
			11.5	1.5	87%			
			14.5	4.5	69%			
			19.5	8.5	56%			
			10.5	6	43%			
			11.5	7.5	35%			
			11	7	36%			
			9.5	2	79%			
			15.5	10	35%			

MILD SYMPTOMS (1-7)			MODERATE SYMPTOMS (8-19)			SEVERE SYMPTOMS (20-35)		
Pre-Peenuts	Post-Peenuts	% Change	Pre-Peenuts	Post-Peenuts	% Change	Pre-Peenuts	Post-Peenuts	% Change
			8.5	1.5	82%			
			15.5	5.5	65%			
			14.5	10.5	28%			
			12.5	1	92%			
			11.5	3	74%			
			13.5	7.5	44%			
			15.5	8.5	45%			
			14	2.5	82%			
			16.5	11.5	70%			
			10	3.5	65%			
			15.5	5	68%			
			15	3	80%			
			15.5	5.5	65%			
			13.5	4	71%			
			15.5	7	55%			
			15	1	94%			
			14.5	4.5	69%			
			16	2.5	85%			
			9	5	45%			
			17	4.5	74%			
			9.5	2.5	74%			

MILD SYMPTOMS (1-7)			MODERATE SYMPTOMS (8-19)			SEVERE SYMPTOMS (20-35)		
Pre-Peenuts	Post-Peenuts	% Change	Pre-Peenuts	Post-Peenuts	% Change	Pre-Peenuts	Post-Peenuts	% Change
			17	3.5	79%			
			12	7.5	38%			
			16	5.5	67%			
			13.5	3.5	74%			
			16.5	7.5	55%			
			14.5	0.5	97%			
			11	2.5	78%			
			8.5	0.5	95%			
			11.5	3.5	70%			
			19	6	68%			
			10.5	2.5	76%			
			18.5	11.5	38%			
			17.5	5.5	69%			
			16.5	8.5	48%			
			16.5	6.5	61%			
			15.5	5	61%			
			9	2	78%			
			10.5	0	100%			
			17	1.5	91%			
			11.5	4.5	61%			
			12.5	2	84%			

MILD SYMPTOMS (1-7)			MODERATE SYMPTOMS (8-19)			SEVERE SYMPTOMS (20-35)		
Pre-Peenuts	Post-Peenuts	% Change	Pre-Peenuts	Post-Peenuts	% Change	Pre-Peenuts	Post-Peenuts	% Change
			14	2.5	82%			
			18.5	4	79%			
			17	10.5	39%			
			15.5	7	55%			
			17	7	59%			
			17	9	47%			
			16.5	8.5	49%			
			14	2	86%			
			13.5	4	71%			
			8.5	3.5	59%			
			11.5	3.5	70%			
			15	2	87%			
			17.5	5	72%			
			10	3	70%			
			14	3	79%			
			10	5	50%			
			17	5.5	68%			
			13	7.5	43%			
			9	1	89%			
			17.5	7	60%			
			17	3	83%			

MILD SYMPTOMS (1-7)			MODERATE SYMPTOMS (8-19)			SEVERE SYMPTOMS (20-35)		
Pre-Peenuts	Post-Peenuts	% Change	Pre-Peenuts	Post-Peenuts	% Change	Pre-Peenuts	Post-Peenuts	% Change
			17	6.5	62%			
			16	6	63%			
			18.5	7.5	60%			
			12	6	50%			
			11.5	3.5	70%			
			13.5	2.5	82%			
			12	2.5	80%			
			11	5	55%			
			16	3.5	79%			
			11	3	73%			
			18.5	12.5	33%			
			15	3	80%			
			15.5	5.5	65%			
			13.5	4	71%			
			15.5	7	55%			
			15	1	94%			
			14.5	4.5	69%			
			16	2.5	85%			
			9	5	45%			
			17	4.5	74%			
			9.5	2.5	74%			

MILD SYMPTOMS (1-7)			MODERATE SYMPTOMS (8-19)			SEVERE SYMPTOMS (20-35)		
Pre-Peenuts	Post-Peenuts	% Change	Pre-Peenuts	Post-Peenuts	% Change	Pre-Peenuts	Post-Peenuts	% Change
			17	3.5	74%			
			12	7.5	38%			
			16.5	5.5	67%			
			13.5	3.5	74%			
			16.5	7.5	55%			
			14.5	0.5	97%			
			11	2.5	78%			
			8.5	0.5	95%			
			11.5	3.5	70%			
			19	6	68%			
			10.5	2.5	76%			
			18.5	11.5	38%			
			17.5	5.5	69%			
			16.5	8.5	48%			
			16.5	6.5	61%			
			9	2	78%			
			10.5	0	100%			
			17	1.5	91%			
			11.5	4.5	61%			
			12.5	2	84%			
			14	2.5	82%			

MILD SYMPTOMS (1-7)			MODERATE SYMPTOMS (8-19)			SEVERE SYMPTOMS (20-35)		
Pre-Peenuts	Post-Peenuts	% Change	Pre-Peenuts	Post-Peenuts	% Change	Pre-Peenuts	Post-Peenuts	% Change
			16.5	4	76%			
			13.5	4.5	67%			
			15.5	5.5	65%			
			8.5	0.5	94%			
			13	2	85%			
			12.5	2	84%			
			10	2.5	75%			
			10.5	1.5	86%			
			11	1.5	86%			
			13	2	85%			
			15	1.5	90%			
			11.5	1.5	87%			
			18.5	5.5	70%			
			16.5	8.5	48%			
			11	2.5	77%			

N=162

70% Improvement

CPSIA information can be obtained
at www.ICGtesting.com
Printed in the USA
BVOW03s2133020118

504283BV00001B/17/P